Idiopathic Pulmonary Fibrosis

Idiopathic Pulmonary Fibrosis

JEFFREY J. SWIGRIS, DO, MS
Director, Interstitial Lung Disease Program
Division of Pulmonary, Critical Care and Sleep Medicine
National Jewish Health
Denver, CO, USA

KEVIN K. BROWN, MD
Professor and Vice Chair
Department of Medicine
National Jewish Health
Denver, CO, USA

ELSEVIER

ELSEVIER

3251 Riverport Lane
St. Louis, Missouri 63043

IDIOPATHIC PULMONARY FIBROSIS

Content Strategist: Robin Carter
Content Development Manager: Christine McElvenny
Content Development Specialist: Jennifer Horigan
Publishing Services Manager: Deepthi Unni
Project Manager: Janish Ashwin Paul
Designer: Gopalakrishnan Venkatraman

Printed in United States of America

Last digit is the print number: 9   8   7   6   5   4   3   2   1

Working together
to grow libraries in
developing countries

www.elsevier.com • www.bookaid.org

List of Contributors

Jeffrey J. Swigris, DO, MS
Director, Interstitial Lung Disease Program
Division of Pulmonary, Critical Care and Sleep
  Medicine
National Jewish Health
Denver, CO, USA

Kevin K. Brown, MD
Professor and Vice Chair
Department of Medicine
National Jewish Health
Denver, CO, USA

Amy L. Olson, MD, MSPH
Associate Professor of Medicine
Medical Director, Pulmonary Physiology Unit
Division of Pulmonary, Critical Care and
  Sleep Medicine
Department of Medicine
National Jewish Health
Denver, CO, USA

Associate Professor of Medicine
Department of Medicine
University of Colorado Denver
Aurora, CO, USA

David Sprunger, MD
Research Fellow
Interstitial Lung Disease Program
National Jewish Health
Denver, CO, USA

Michael Mohning, MD
Assistant Professor
Department of Medicine
National Jewish Health
Denver, CO, USA

Gregory P. Downey, MD
Executive Vice President, Academic Affairs
Department of Medicine
National Jewish Health
Denver, CO, USA

Professor
Department of Medicine and Integrated Department of
  Immunology
University of Colorado Denver
Denver, CO, USA

Gregory P. Cosgrove, MD
Professor of Medicine
Division of Pulmonary, Critical Care and
  Sleep Medicine
National Jewish Health
Denver, CO, USA

Elizabeth F. Redente, PhD
Instructor, Department of Pediatrics
Division of Cell Biology
National Jewish Health
Denver, CO, USA

Rebecca Keith, MD
Assistant Professor
Division of Pulmonary and Critical Care Medicine
University of Colorado
Denver School of Medicine
Aurora, CO, USA

National Jewish Health
Denver, CO USA

Rocky Mountain Regional Veterans Affairs
Aurora, CO, USA

Tasha Fingerlin, PhD
Associate Professor
Department of Biomedical Research
Director, Center for Genes, Environment & Health
Director, Program in Quantitative Genetics

J. Caleb Richards, MD
Assistant Professor of Radiology
Department of Radiology
National Jewish Health
Denver, CO, USA

Tilman Koelsch, MD
Assistant Professor of Radiology
Department of Radiology
National Jewish Health
Denver, CO, USA

Rosane Duarte Achcar, MD, FCAP, FASCP
Associate Professor
Department of Medicine, Division of Pathology
National Jewish Health
Denver, CO, USA

Tristan Huie, MD
Assistant Professor of Medicine
Division of Pulmonary, Critical Care and Sleep
   Medicine
National Jewish Health
Denver, CO, USA

Stephen K. Frankel, MD, FCCM, FCCP
Chief Medical Officer
National Jewish Health

Professor of Medicine
National Jewish Health and University of Colorado
   School of Medicine
Aurora, CO, USA

Joshua J. Solomon, MD
Associate Professor of Medicine
Division of Pulmonary Sciences and Critical Care
   Medicine
National Jewish Health
Denver, CO, USA

Evans R. Fernández Pérez, MD, MS, FCCP
Associate Professor of Medicine
Division of Pulmonary, Critical Care and Sleep
   Medicine
Interstitial Lung Disease Program and Autoimmune
   Lung Center
National Jewish Health
Denver, CO, USA

Associate Professor of Medicine
University of Colorado School of Medicine
Aurora, CO, USA

Amen Sergew, MD
Assistant Professor of Medicine
Department of Medicine, Division of Pulmonary,
   Critical Care and Sleep Medicine
National Jewish Health
Denver, CO, USA

Zulma Yunt, MD
Assistant Professor of Medicine
Division of Pulmonary, Critical Care and Sleep
   Medicine
National Jewish Health
Denver, CO, USA

Bridget A. Graney, MD
Fellow
Division of Pulmonary, Critical Care and Sleep
   Medicine
National Jewish Health
Denver, CO, USA

Fellow
Division of Pulmonary Sciences and Critical Care
   Medicine
University of Colorado
Aurora, CO, USA

Patricia George, MD
Associate Professor
Division of Pulmonary
Critical Care and Sleep Medicine
Department of Medicine
National Jewish Health
Denver, CO, USA

Isabelle Amigues, MD, MS
Assistant Professor
Division of Rheumatology
National Jewish Health
Denver, CO, USA

Yael Aschner, MD
Assistant Professor of Medicine
Division of Pulmonary Sciences & Critical Care
   Medicine
University of Colorado

Preface

With the increased awareness of idiopathic pulmonary fibrosis (IPF) and the hope and enthusiasm generated by recent discoveries, we believe the time is right to summarize the state of knowledge of IPF. In this book, you will find chapters that review IPF from pathogenesis to patient care. Each chapter provides an informative summary that will be of interest to anyone involved in the evaluation or care of patients with IPF.

Kevin K. Brown, MD and
Jeffrey J. Swigris, DO, MS
Interstitial Lung Disease Program
National Jewish Health
Denver, Colorado

Contents

1 **Introduction**, *1*
Jeffrey Swigris, DO, MS and Kevin K. Brown, MD

2 **Idiopathic Pulmonary Fibrosis Epidemiology**, *3*
Amy L. Olson, MD, MSPH and David Sprunger, MD

3 **Mechanisms of Fibrosis**, *9*
Michael P. Mohning, MD, Gregory P. Downey, MD, Gregory P. Cosgrove, MD, and Elizabeth F. Redente, PhD

4 **Genetics of Pulmonary Fibrosis**, *33*
Rebecca Keith, MD, Kevin K. Brown, MD, and Tasha Fingerlin, PhD

5 **Imaging of Idiopathic Pulmonary Fibrosis**, *39*
J. Caleb Richards, MD and Tilman Koelsch, MD

6 **The Pathology of Usual Interstitial Pneumonia**, *55*
Rosane Duarte Achcar, MD

7 **Making the Diagnosis**, *65*
Tristan Huie, MD and Stephen K. Frankel, MD, FCCM, FCCP

8 **IPF Look-Alikes: Chronic Hypersensitivity Pneumonitis, Connective Tissue Disorder—Related Pulmonary Fibrosis, and Other Fibrosing Interstitial Pneumonias**, *73*
Evans R. Fernández Pérez, MD, MS, FCCP, Isabelle Amigues, MD, and Joshua J. Solomon, MD

9 **Natural History of Idiopathic Pulmonary Fibrosis and Disease Monitoring**, *89*
Amen Sergew, MD and Kevin K. Brown, MD

10 **Biomarkers in IPF**, *99*
Zulma Yunt, MD, Yael Aschner, MD, and Kevin K. Brown, MD

11 **Therapeutic Options for Patients With Idiopathic Pulmonary Fibrosis**, *113*
Deepa Ramadurai, MD, Yosafe Wakwaya, MD, Bridget A. Graney, MD, Marjorie Patricia George, MD, Amy L. Olson, MD, MSPH, and Jeffrey J. Swigris, DO, MS

INDEX, *127*

CHAPTER 1

Introduction

JEFFREY SWIGRIS, DO, MS • KEVIN K. BROWN, MD

The medical community is now firmly seated in a new era of intensified awareness of fibrosing interstitial lung disease (fILD). The ubiquitous use of computed tomography (CT) of the chest to screen for lung cancer, to measure coronary artery calcification, or to rule out acute pulmonary thromboembolic disease has identified a growing number of people with lung abnormalities ranging from so-called interstitial lung abnormalities to clinically significant fILDs, like the one that affects more people than any other, idiopathic pulmonary fibrosis (IPF). The era has ushered in an improved understanding of the pathophysiologic underpinnings of IPF; the discovery of genetic factors that predispose to the development of IPF; the completion of several, large-scale, multinational, meticulously performed treatment trials; and the approval, by regulatory agencies around the world, of drugs to treat IPF.

Given the increased awareness of the condition and the enthusiasm generated by these accomplishments, we believe now is a good time to create a book that summarizes the field's knowledge of IPF. This volume includes a collection of chapters that span a broad range of topics on IPF, from pathogenesis to patient care. In each chapter, authors review and critique scientific data to yield informative yet practical synopses that we believe will be of interest to clinicians and researchers alike.

In Chapter 2, Drs. Sprunger and Olson describe the breadth of the problem of IPF from an epidemiologic perspective, reminding the reader that IPF's footprint will continue to expand as the world's aging human population increases. In Chapter 3, Drs. Mohning, Cosgrove, Downey, and Redente review what is known about the molecular and cellular mechanisms involved in generating lung fibrosis, an area of the field that has witnessed exponential growth in knowledge over the last decade. In Chapter 4, Drs. Keith and Fingerlin

discuss the genetic polymorphisms or mutations that predispose people to the development of fILD. In Chapter 5, Drs. Richards, Koelsch, and Lynch describe the central role that high-resolution CT scans play in the evaluation of patients with IPF and detail the radiologic appearance of the disease. In Chapter 6, a chapter rich with exemplary figures, Drs. Achcar and Groshong highlight the characteristic pathologic appearance of usual interstitial pneumonia (UIP), the histologic pattern in IPF, and detail how to differentiate UIP from other lung injury patterns. In Chapter 7, Drs. Huie and Frankel guide the reader through a systematic approach to integrating clinical data used in making the diagnosis of IPF in a patient presenting with fILD. In Chapter 8, Drs. Solomon and Fernandez-Perez highlight how making a confident diagnosis of IPF can be a challenging endeavor that requires the exclusion of IPF look-alikes, including connective tissue disease–related ILD and chronic, fibrotic hypersensitivity pneumonitis. Next, the reader will discover a chapter by Drs. Sergew and Brown in which the authors describe the natural history of IPF and offer recommendations for carefully monitoring patients with IPF over time. In Chapter 10, Drs. Yunt, Aschner and Brown review what is known about biomarkers in IPF, an area of intense research in which investigators are striving to identify circulating molecules that can be used to more accurately and efficiently diagnose IPF and determine prognosis or response to therapeutic intervention. In Chapter 11, Drs. Ramadurai, Wakwaya, Graney, Olson, George, and Swigris cover pharmacologic and nonpharmacologic therapeutic interventions for patients with IPF.

Thank you for accessing a copy of this book. We appreciate your interest and hope you find it an enjoyable and informative reference guide to IPF.

CHAPTER 2

Idiopathic Pulmonary Fibrosis Epidemiology

AMY L. OLSON, MD, MSPH • DAVID SPRUNGER, MD

THE EPIDEMIOLOGY OF IDIOPATHIC PULMONARY FIBROSIS

Background

Idiopathic pulmonary fibrosis (IPF) is the most common of the idiopathic interstitial pneumonias[1] and was once considered a rare, orphan disease. Epidemiologic studies suggest that the disease burden attributable to IPF is growing, underlining the importance of ongoing research into this devastating disease.

Historically, several factors have hampered investigators in their conduct of large-scale, epidemiologic studies in IPF as follows: (1) the condition was thought to be too rare to study easily; (2) diagnostic criteria and disease assessment modalities were evolving, making the case definition a bit of a moving target; and (3) there was no specific code in the International Classification of Diseases (ICD) for IPF. The identification or, in some cases, development of large, population-level databases have helped to overcome some of these factors. For example, health insurance care claims databases have been used to determine incidence and prevalence estimates, and investigators have used death certificate databases to determine mortality rates. In addition, the generation of ICD codes that allow researchers to specifically identify IPF or other fibrotic lung diseases have been instrumental in promoting epidemiologic research using large databases. However, there are limitations associated with the use of these large datasets, including the inability to assess the fidelity of diagnostic codes.

Trends in Idiopathic Pulmonary Fibrosis Incidence and Prevalence

The incidence of disease is the number of new cases that occur during a specified period of time in a population at risk for developing the disease, whereas the prevalence of disease is a ratio of the number of affected cases present in the population at a specific time divided by the number of persons in the population at that time.[2]

The United States

In the early 1990s, a summary of the National Heart, Lung, and Blood Institute workshop stated that few data were available on the occurrence of IPF in the general population.[3] In the wake of this summary, in 1994, Coultas and colleagues published a regional epidemiologic investigation into the incidence and prevalence of interstitial lung diseases (ILDs), including IPF, occurring in persons over the age of 18 years in the United States.[4] Using data from 1988 through 1993, the authors established a population-based registry in Bernalillo County, New Mexico. In it, they examined primary care and pulmonary physician records, pathology reports, hospital discharge diagnoses, death certificates, and autopsy reports. The authors reported the incidence of IPF as 10.7 per 100,000 person-years in men and 7.4 per 100,000 person-years in women. The prevalence of IPF was 20.2 cases per 100,000 persons in men and 13.2 cases per 100,000 persons overall. When stratified by age and gender, both the incidence and prevalence of IPF was higher in men than in women, and each increased with increasing age.

Raghu and colleagues examined the incidence and prevalence of IPF using data from a healthcare claims processing center from 1996 through 2000.[5] The center services a plan that covers nearly 3 million people across 20 states—mostly in the South Atlantic, South Central, and North Central regions of the United States. The authors estimated IPF incidence and prevalence for the entire United States. Using broad case-finding criteria (age > 18, at least one medical encounter for IPF [ICD-9 code 516.3], and no encounters with diagnostic codes for any other ILD after an encounter coded as IPF), they estimated an incidence of 16.3 per 100,000 persons/year and a prevalence of 42.7 per 100,000 persons, respectively. Employing narrow case-finding criteria (the broad criteria plus at least one claim with a procedure code for a surgical lung biopsy, transbronchial biopsy, or thoracic computed tomography [CT]), they estimated the incidence and prevalence at 6.8 per 100,000 persons/year and 14.0 per 100,000 persons, respectively. Like Coultas and his coinvestigators, Raghu and colleagues found that both the incidence and prevalence of IPF increased with age, and both were higher in men than in women. Based on these two landmark studies, the incidence and prevalence of IPF appeared to increase over time, but as with any study using claims data, questions remained: were cases with non-IPF ILDs counted as IPF, and were cases of IPF missed?

Using data from patients evaluated at the Mayo Clinic in Rochester from 1997 to 2005, Fernández-Pérez and colleagues completed a population-based, historical cohort study in Olmsted County, Minnesota.[6] These authors also used both narrow and broad case-finding criteria. The narrow criteria included a usual interstitial pneumonia (UIP) pattern on surgical lung biopsy or a definite UIP pattern on thoracic high-resolution CT (HRCT), whereas broad criteria included the less-strict pattern on HRCT scan of possible UIP. Using the narrow definition, the age- and sex-adjusted incidence (for people over the age of 50) was 8.8 cases per 100,000 person-years (95% CI = 5.3−12.4), and using the broad definition, it was 17.4 cases per 100,000 person-years (95% CI = 12.4−22.4). The age- and sex-adjusted prevalence (for those over the age of 50) was 27.9 cases per 100,000 persons (95% CI = 10.4−45.4) and 63 cases per 100,000 persons (95% CI = 36.4−89.6). Over the last 3 years of the study, incidence was on the decline. Given the low number of incidence cases (47 according to broad case-finding criteria), confidence is low that these statistics accurately reflected national trends during the study period (1997−2005).

In a random sample of 5% of Medicare beneficiaries (65 years of age or older), Raghu and colleagues performed another study to generate estimates for the annual incidence and cumulative prevalence of IPF.[7] Using ICD-9 codes 516.3 (IPF) and 515 (postinflammatory pulmonary fibrosis [PIPF]), they determined that from 2001 to 2011 the incidence of IPF remained stable (overall 93.7 cases per 100,000 person-years [95% CI = 91.9−95.4]). But, the annual cumulative prevalence rose from 202.2 cases per 100,000 persons in 2001 to 494.2 cases per 100,000 persons in 2011. The authors also found that cases diagnosed in 2007 had

longer survival times (4.0 years [95% CI = 3.8−4.5]) than those diagnosed before 2007 (3.3 years [95% CI = 3.0−3.8]) and suggested that longer survival after diagnosis might explain the discrepancy between incidence and prevalence.

In another epidemiologic study of IPF, investigators used an administrative, patient claims, insurance dataset that included data from more than 45 managed healthcare plans covering more than 89 million people for the years 2005−10.[8] Using a narrow case definition, they determined that the annual incidence of IPF among people 18−64 years old decreased from 2.9 to 2.4 new cases per 100,000 person-years, while the annual prevalence ranged from 4.6 to 6.7 per 100,000 person-years from 2005 to 2010. Using a broad case definition, they reported that the annual incidence decreased from 5.1 to 3.6 new cases per 100,000 person-years from 2005 to 2010, and the annual prevalence ranged from 8.4 to 11.3 per 100,000 person-years over that time. In contrast to the stable incidence and increasing prevalence noted in the older Medicare population, the incidence declined in this younger cohort over time, while the prevalence plateaued. The results appeared to be driven by changes in statistics for younger patients (18−44 years): the likelihood of them being diagnosed (inappropriately, as patients younger than 50 years old rarely develop the disease) with IPF declined over time. Presumably, they were being appropriately diagnosed with known cause of pulmonary fibrosis (PF) (e.g., connective tissue disease−related)—a condition far more likely than IPF to cause PF in patients younger than 50 years.

In a large research database, a case definition of IPF (defined as a diagnosis by a physician and no alternative diagnosis within the 6 months before or after) had a positive predictive value (PPV) of only 44.4% (95% CI = 29.6−60.0%).[9] This suggests incidence and prevalence estimates determined by using healthcare claims databases are likely to be overestimated. Correcting for the PPV and standardizing the claims cohort to the US population, for 2006−12, the incidence of IPF was calculated to be 14.6 per 100,000 person-years, and the prevalence was estimated at 125.2 per 100,000 persons.

The United Kingdom
Epidemiologic studies from investigators in the United Kingdom also suggest an increase in the incidence of IPF over time. Gribbin and colleagues used a general practice database and applied diagnostic codes for "cryptogenic fibrosing alveolitis" and "idiopathic pulmonary fibrosis"—terms used interchangeably until

recently—to find that the overall incidence of IPF had doubled from 1991 to 2003.[10] They estimated an over-all crude incidence of IPF at 4.6 cases per 100,000 person-years, which equaled a yearly increase in inci-dence of 11% (rate ratio 1.11; 95% CI = 1.09−1.13).

Navaratnam and colleagues used the same database and a similar approach (included cases coded as "cryp-togenic fibrosing alveolitis" or "idiopathic pulmonary fibrosis," but also included cases coded as "diffuse pul-monary fibrosis," "idiopathic fibrosing alveolitis NOS," or "Hamman-Rich syndrome") to determine statistics for the entity they termed IPF-clinical syndrome (IPF-CS).[11] Between 2000 and 2008, the overall crude incidence of IPF-CS was 7.44 per 100,000 person-years—nearly double the incidence rate of the prior decade. They estimated that the incidence of IPF-CS increased by 5% annually over this time period (rate ratio 1.05; 95% CI = 1.03−1.06), although at a some-what slower rate than the prior decade. Experts have posited that reasons for the increased incidence could be an uptick in the use of CT of the chest and/or the conduct of multinational drug trials for IPF, which could serve to raise awareness of the disease.[12]

Canada

Hopkins and colleagues used two national administra-tive databases from the Canadian Institute for Health Information to estimate the incidence and prevalence of IPF in Canada from 2007 through 2011.[13] For their broad case definition, incidence and prevalence in men was 21.3 per 100,000 person-years) and 45.3 per 100,000 persons, respectively. Their narrow case defini-tion yielded incidence and prevalence estimates in men of 10.5 per 100,000 person-years and 22.3 per 100,000 persons, respectively. For women, the broad case defini-tion yielded incidence and prevalence estimates of 16.2 per 100,000 persons-years and 38.2 per 100,000 persons, respectively, whereas the narrow case defini-tion produced incidence and prevalence estimates of 7.4 per 100,000 person-years and 17.7 per 100,000 persons, respectively. These estimates are similar to those generated for the United States and the United Kingdom.

Other countries

Hyldgaard and coauthors conducted a single-center, observational cohort study of 431 patients with various ILDs (121 with IPF) living in Denmark between 2001 and 2011.[14] The authors estimated an overall crude incidence rate for IPF of 4.1 cases per 100,000 person-years. And they found the incidence rose from 3.8 to 6.8 per 100,000 persons over the study period. The

authors attribute this increase to centralized, specialized referral centers within the Danish healthcare system and increased access to HRCT over the study period. Other data, including those from a systematic review on the global incidence of IPF, suggest the worldwide inci-dence of IPF is increasing, and rates across countries appear to be converging. As more countries begin to collect large-scale data on IPF, a better understanding of the global incidence and disease burden of IPF will be possible.

Mortality Rates and Trends Over Time

Mortality rate is the total number of deaths from a particular cause in 1 year divided by the number of people alive within the population at midyear. In the era of ICD-10 coding, using death certificate coding from 1999 onward, Hutchinson and colleagues recently examined the death certificates from 124 decedents whose deaths the authors had confirmed as due to IPF. Of these, 82% had a diagnostic code somewhere on the death certificate for IPF (J84.1) or ILD unspeci-fied (ILD-U) (J84.9). This suggests that death certificate data may underestimate mortality rates by ~ 20%.[15] It is unclear if these findings apply to death certificate data outside of the United Kingdom, and more research on the validity of death certificate data is needed.

The United States

Mannino and colleagues used US death certificate data from 1979 to 1991 to calculate age-adjusted mortality from PF (ICD-9 codes 516.3 [IPF] and 515 [PIPF]).[16] They determined that mortality from PF had increased from 48.6 deaths per million to 50.9 deaths per million from the late 1970s to the early 1990s. They found a 4.7% increase in mortality among men and a 27.1% increase among women. This study was the first in which PF mortality was reported to vary between regions of the United States: mortality rates were highest in the West and Southeast and lowest in the Midwest and Northeast.

Using the same database, our group examined US death certificate data from 1992 to 2003. We observed an increase from 49.7 deaths per million to 64.3 deaths per million (for a relative 29.4% increase) among men, and from 42.3 deaths per million to 58.4 deaths per million (for a relative 38.1% increase) among women. We also found that mortality rates increased with increasing age and were higher in men than in women but were increasing more steeply in women than in men.[17]

Hutchinson and coinvestigators examined the same dataset for the years 2000−10.[18] Including only decedents in whom J84 (includes IPF and ILD-U) was coded as the "underlying cause of death" (UCD), they observed that mortality rates had increased by 1% per year (annual increase 1.01; 95% CI = 1.011−1.014). The age-adjusted mortality rate in 2010 for decedents whose UCD was coded as J84 was 7.8 per 100,000 persons (which equates to 78 deaths per million). Like other UCD analyses, these estimates are subject to potential extreme underreporting bias.

Other countries
In a study of death certificates from England and Wales, Australia, Canada, Japan, Northern Ireland, New Zealand, Scotland, Spain, and Sweden collected between 2000 and 2010, deaths in which J84 was the UCD increased between 1% and 4% per year in all countries except Northern Ireland where data were limited (only available from 2009 to 2011) and the increases were much larger (25%).[18] In a metaanalysis of data from the United States and these eight countries, there was a 2% annual increase in mortality over time (rate ratio, 1.02; 95% CI = 1.01−1.03). Age-standardized mortality rates varied by country: those with the lowest mortality rates included Sweden (4.68 per 100,000) and New Zealand (5.55 per 100,000); those with mortality rates similar to the United States included Australia (6.49 per 100,000) and Canada (7.52 per 100,000); and those with the highest mortality rates included England and Wales (9.84 per 100,000) and Japan (10.26 per 100,000). The reasons for this apparent global heterogeneity remain unclear, but if real, are presumably due at least in part to genetic variation.

Risk Factors
Like many other epidemiologic studies, those conducted to examine risk factors for IPF have been subject to a number of limitations, including recall and misclassification biases.

Cigarette smoking
Cigarette smoking is a risk factor for IPF and familial pulmonary fibrosis (FPF). In a study of 248 cases of IPF identified between 1989 and 1993 and 491 controls matched for age, sex, and geography, ever-smoking was associated with a 60% increased odds of IPF (OR = 1.6; 95% CI = 1.1−2.2).[19] Among former smokers, those who had recently quit (within 2.5 years) had the highest risk for the development of IPF (OR = 3.5%; 95% CI = 1.1−11.9), whereas those who quit more remotely (at least 25 years prior) had the lowest risk (OR = 1.3; 95% CI = 0.7−2.3).

In a Japanese cohort, smokers with a 20.0−39.9 pack-year history had an increased risk for IPF (OR = 2.26; 95% CI = 1.3−3.8). Those with a less than 20.0 pack-year history or a 40.0 pack-year history or greater were not at increased risk.[20]

Authors of a metaanalysis that included US and Japanese studies and another three studies from the United Kingdom or Japan found ever-smoking conferred a 58% increase in the odds of IPF (summary OR = 1.58; 95% CI = 1.27−1.97).[21] They estimated that 49% of cases of IPF could be prevented by eliminating cigarette smoking.

Data are similar for FPF. In a study of 309 cases of FPF and 360 unaffected family members, ever-smoking was associated with a greater than threefold odds of developing FPF (OR = 3.6; 95% CI = 1.3−9.8) while adjusting for age and gender.[22]

Occupational and environmental exposures
Results from several studies suggest an association between dust and/or dusty environments and IPF.

In a metaanalysis of five case-controlled studies published between 1990 and 2005, results suggested a significant association between metal dust exposure and the development of IPF (summary OR = 2.44, 95% CI = 1.74−3.40).[21,23] In one study, the association held only for those with ≥5 years of exposure, suggesting a dose-response relationship.[24] In an analysis of the pension fund archives from a metal engineering company, investigators found no relationship between metal dust exposure and IPF, except in people exposed for greater than 10 years (OR = 1.71; 95% CI = 1.09−2.68).[25] In two other studies, there was no relationship between exposure to metal dusts and IPF, but the investigators did not consider the extent or duration of exposure.[26,27]

According to a metaanalysis of five case-control studies, there is an association between exposure to wood dusts and IPF (summary OR = 1.94; 95% CI = 1.34−2.81).[23] However, in two of the five individual studies, no association was identified, suggesting the risk may be relevant for only certain woods. In support of this, in another study, there was an association between birch or hardwood dust and IPF; there was no association between fir dust exposure and IPF.[26]

Exposure to livestock has been found to be associated with IPF (summary OR = 2.17; 95% CI = 1.20−2.26).[23] Results from one study suggest a dose-response relationship: for the subgroup of subjects with <5 years of exposure, there was no association; however, for the subgroup with more than 5 years of exposure, there was a strong association with the development of IPF (OR = 3.3; 95% CI = 1.3−8.3).[24] Other studies of farming (or residing in a region in which farming is common) corroborate these findings.[23,24,28] In one study, there was an association between exposure to agricultural chemicals specifically and IPF (OR = 3.32; 95% CI = 1.22−9.05).[28]

Exposure to sand, stone, or silica dusts have been found to be associated with the development of IPF (summary OR = 1.97; 95% CI = 1.09−3.55).[23,29] Other exposures with associations with IPF include hair dressing, raising birds, or residing in an urban/polluted area.[23,29]

In sum, inhalational exposures of various kinds are associated with IPF; however, whether these exposures have roles in the pathogenesis of IPF is uncertain and warrants additional evaluation.

SUMMARY

Although IPF was once considered an orphan disease, studies suggest that mortality rates are similar to certain common malignancies. Epidemiologic research has helped elevate knowledge of IPF at the population level, but many questions remain to be explored. Doing so will likely lead to an even greater understanding of accurate epidemiologic trends and by extension, risk factors will increase understanding of IPF pathobiology.

REFERENCES

1. Raghu G. Idiopathic pulmonary fibrosis: guidelines for diagnosis and clinical management have advanced from consensus-based in 2000 to evidence-based in 2011. *Eur Respir J.* 2011;37(4):743−746.
2. Gordis L. Measuring the occurrence of disease. In: Leon G, ed. *Epidemiology.* Philadelphia, PA: Elsevier Saunders; 2004: 32−47.
3. Cherniack RM, Crystal RG, Kalica AR. NHLBI workshop summary. Current concepts in idiopathic pulmonary fibrosis: a road map for the future. *Am Rev Respir Dis.* 1991;143(3):680−683.
4. Coultas D, et al. The epidemiology of interstitial lung disease. *Am J Respir Crit Care Med.* 1994;150:967−972.
5. Raghu G, et al. Incidence and prevalence of idiopathic pulmonary fibrosis. *Am J Respir Crit Care Med.* 2006; 174(7):810−816.
6. Fernandez Perez ER, et al. Incidence, prevalence, and clinical course of idiopathic pulmonary fibrosis: a population-based study. *Chest.* 2010;137(1):129−137.
7. Raghu G, et al. Idiopathic pulmonary fibrosis in US Medicare beneficiaries aged 65 years and older: incidence, prevalence, and survival, 2001-11. *Lancet Respir Med.* 2014; 2(7):566−572.
8. Raghu G, et al. Incidence and prevalence of idiopathic pulmonary fibrosis in US adults 18-64 years old. *Eur Respir J.* 2016;48(1):179−186.
9. Esposito DB, et al. Idiopathic pulmonary fibrosis in United States automated claims. Incidence, prevalence, and algorithm validation. *Am J Respir Crit Care Med.* 2015; 192(10):1200−1207.
10. Gribbin J, et al. Incidence and mortality of idiopathic pulmonary fibrosis and sarcoidosis in the UK. *Thorax.* 2006;61(11):980−985.
11. Navaratnam V, et al. The rising incidence of idiopathic pulmonary fibrosis in the U.K. *Thorax.* 2011;66(6):462−467.
12. American Thoracic Society. Idiopathic pulmonary fibrosis: diagnosis and treatment. International consensus statement. American Thoracic Society (ATS), and the European Respiratory Society (ERS). *Am J Respir Crit Care Med.* 2000; 161(2 Pt 1):646−664.
13. Hopkins RB, et al. Epidemiology and survival of idiopathic pulmonary fibrosis from national data in Canada. *Eur Respir J.* 2016;48(1):187−195.
14. Hyldgaard C. A cohort study of Danish patients with interstitial lung diseases: burden, severity, treatment and survival. *Dan Med J.* 2015;62(4):B5069.
15. Hutchinson J, et al. Global incidence and mortality of idiopathic pulmonary fibrosis: a systematic review. *Eur Respir J.* 2015;46(3):795−806.
16. Mannino DM, Etzel RA, Parrish RG. Pulmonary fibrosis deaths in the United States, 1979-1991. An analysis of multiple-cause mortality data. *Am J Respir Crit Care Med.* 1996;153(5):1548−1552.
17. Olson AL, et al. Mortality from pulmonary fibrosis increased in the United States from 1992 to 2003. *Am J Respir Crit Care Med.* 2007;176(3):277−284.
18. Hutchinson JP, et al. Increasing global mortality from idiopathic pulmonary fibrosis in the twenty-first century. *Ann Am Thorac Soc.* 2014;11(8):1176−1185.
19. Baumgartner K, et al. Cigarette smoking: a risk factor for idiopathic pulmonary fibrosis. *Am J Respir Crit Care Med.* 1997;155:242−248.
20. Miyake Y, et al. Occupational and environmental factors and idiopathic pulmonary fibrosis in Japan. *Ann Occup Hyg.* 2005;49(3):259−265.
21. Taskar V, Coultas D. Exposures and idiopathic lung disease. *Semin Respir Crit Care Med.* 2008;29(6):670−679.
22. Steele MP, et al. Clinical and pathologic features of familial interstitial pneumonia. *Am J Respir Crit Care Med.* 2005; 172(9):1146−1152.
23. Taskar VS, Coultas DB. Is idiopathic pulmonary fibrosis an environmental disease? *Proc Am Thorac Soc.* 2006;3(4): 293−298.
24. Baumgartner KB, et al. Occupational and environmental risk factors for idiopathic pulmonary fibrosis: a multicenter case-control study. Collaborating Centers. *Am J Epidemiol.* 2000;152(4):307−315.
25. Hubbard R, et al. Risk of cryptogenic fibrosing alveolitis in metal workers. *Lancet.* 2000;355(9202):466−467.

26. Gustafson T, et al. Occupational exposure and severe pulmonary fibrosis. *Respir Med.* 2007;101(10):2207–2212.
27. Harris JM, Cullinan P, McDonald JC. Occupational distribution and geographic clustering of deaths certified to be cryptogenic fibrosing alveolitis in england and wales. *Chest.* 2001;119(2):428–433.
28. Iwai K, et al. Idiopathic pulmonary fibrosis: epidemiologic approaches to occupational exposure. *Am J Respir Crit Care Med.* 1994;150:670–675.
29. Scott J, Johnston I, Britton J. What causes cryptogenic fibrosing alveolitis? A case control study of environmental exposure to dust. *BMJ.* 1990;301:1015–1017.

CHAPTER 3

Mechanisms of Fibrosis

MICHAEL P. MOHNING, MD • GREGORY P. DOWNEY, MD •
GREGORY P. COSGROVE, MD • ELIZABETH F. REDENTE, PHD

INTRODUCTION

Idiopathic pulmonary fibrosis (IPF) is a devastating and relentlessly progressive fibrosing disease of the lung. The characteristic histopathologic pattern associated with IPF is "usual interstitial pneumonia" (UIP). The hallmark findings of a UIP pattern are temporal heterogeneity, fibroblastic foci (clusters of fibroblasts and myofibroblasts), and honeycombing (subpleural cystic airspaces).[1] Collagen and extracellular matrix are overproduced and deposited in a disorganized fashion. These pathologic findings are important as we consider the pathophysiology of IPF and the correlative findings in animal models of pulmonary fibrosis.

While the etiology of IPF remains elusive, there are many risk factors that are known to contribute to the pathologic fibrogenic response. Smoking is one of the most commonly recognized risk factors for the development of IPF.[2] Repetitive microinjuries, such as through aspiration and tobacco smoking, are also thought to play an important pathogenic role.[2] There are genetic predispositions which may contribute to the disease process, including the MUC5B promoter variant rs35705950.[3] Other genetic abnormalities associated with familial forms of pulmonary fibrosis include mutations in genes coding for telomerase[4] and surfactant proteins.[5,6]

The current paradigm in IPF pathophysiology is that repetitive injuries initiate repair processes, which then become dysregulated, resulting in a pathologic fibrogenic response that goes unchecked (Fig. 3.1). There are many contributing factors and cells that mediate both the initiation of the injury as well as the fibrotic response. Those that will be discussed in the following section include fibroblasts, myofibroblasts, and fibrocytes, which are cells crucial to the fibrotic response and involved in the deposition of collagen and extracellular matrix. The respiratory epithelium response is critical in the initiation phase of injury, and immune cells such as macrophages and lymphocytes are implicated in both the injury and the fibrotic response.

ANIMAL MODELS OF PULMONARY FIBROSIS

The use of animal models of pulmonary fibrosis has contributed significantly to our understanding of the pathogenesis of pulmonary fibrosis.[7,8] There are noteworthy limitations, however, in regard to how well they replicate IPF. Specifically, the most commonly used model of pulmonary fibrosis, the early phase after the intratracheal instillation of bleomycin, more accurately reflects the pathophysiology of acute respiratory distress syndrome than IPF. In this model, there is a massive influx of inflammatory cells in the lungs, but inflammation is not seen in IPF patients when then initially come to clinical attention.[9] Furthermore, during the fibrotic response in the bleomycin model, there is a lack of fibroblastic foci, subpleural fibrosis, and honeycombing, each of which are typical features of the UIP pattern of IPF.[8] Notably, unlike human disease in which the fibrotic response is progressive, in the bleomycin model, fibrosis is self-resolving.

For decades, rodents, mostly mice, have been the predominate animal used in the study of pulmonary fibrosis.[7] They have many important characteristics that make them useful. From a practical standpoint, their small size makes them an ideal species for medical research because they can be housed easily and inexpensively and breed rapidly. Inbreeding of mice allows for minimization of genetic heterogeneity, which could otherwise complicate the interpretation of studies. Genetic modifications, which are increasingly easy to perform in mice, have been an extremely important tool in studying both the initiation and propagation of fibrosis.[10]

In animal models, there are several endpoints that are useful to assess the degree of fibrosis. Collagen levels

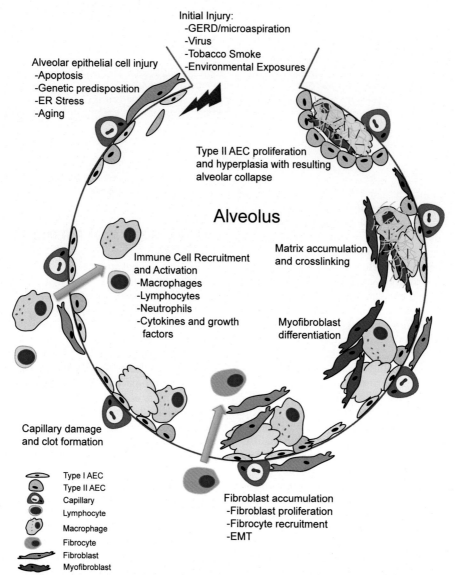

FIG. 3.1 Pathophysiology of pulmonary fibrosis. Initial recurrent injury from various causes triggers epithelial cell damage and apoptosis. Immune cell activation occurs, leading to cytokine and growth factor release. Activation of clotting factors occurs simultaneously further promoting fibrosis. Fibroblast accumulation and differentiation into myofibroblasts leads to increased extracellular matrix deposition and stiffening of the alveolus, with eventual alveolar collapse. *AEC*, alveolar epithelial cell; *GERD*, gastroesophageal reflux disease; *ER*, endoplasmic reticulum; *EMT*, epithelial to mesenchymal transition. (Adapted from Ahluwalia N, Shea BS, Tager AM. New therapeutic targets in idiopathic pulmonary fibrosis. Aiming to rein in runaway wound-healing responses. *Am J Respir Crit Care Med.* 2014;190(8):867–878.)

(as measured through hydroxyproline), lung compliance, and histologic examination are all important endpoints to consider when studying experimental pulmonary fibrosis.[10] Fig. 3.2 demonstrates typical findings on histology and collagen staining in the bleomycin model of fibrosis at various timepoints.[11]

Besides the bleomycin murine model, there are a number of other useful models that have been

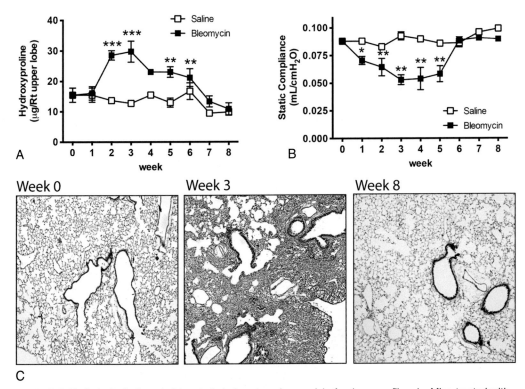

FIG. 3.2 Pathologic findings in bleomycin-induced murine model of pulmonary fibrosis. Mice treated with intratracheal bleomycin demonstrate a fibrotic response with increased hydroxyproline (A) and decreased static compliance (B) peaking around week 3 (C). Collagen deposition (*blue*) can be seen on histology, peaking at week 3 and resolving by week 8. (Adapted from Redente EF, et al. Tumor necrosis factor-α accelerates the resolution of established pulmonary fibrosis in mice by targeting profibrotic lung macrophages. *Am J Respir Cell Mol Biol.* 2014;50(4):825–837.)

developed to study the pulmonary fibrotic response. Table 3.1 highlights some of the findings in the different animal models that will be discussed. Each model has important uses and limitations that need to be considered when interpreting the data they yield.

Bleomycin Model

As noted earlier, the bleomycin model of pulmonary fibrosis remains the most commonly used preclinical model and is the recommended model for therapeutics testing.[10] Bleomycin is a chemotherapeutic antibiotic that has been used to treat lymphomas and other malignancies for decades. An important side effect that has been seen in humans undergoing chemotherapy is pulmonary fibrosis,[12] which led to its use in the experimental model. Intratracheal administration is

the most typical method of delivery, but other routes have included intraperitoneal, intravenous, and subcutaneous administrations.[7] The C57BL/6J mouse has been the strain of choice in this model, as they are uniquely sensitive to the fibrotic response. Interestingly, aged males appear to be more prone to fibrosis than females.[13] While young mice (8–12 weeks old) have been studied most frequently, aged mice may more closely match human IPF.[8,13]

The typical findings after administration of intratracheal bleomycin are early (day 1–3) death of epithelial cells followed by a robust inflammatory response with neutrophils and lymphocytes. Fibrosis develops between days 10–21 following fibroblast activation, with peak fibrosis typically occurring around days 14–21 (See Fig. 3.2). The fibrosis then resolves over the ensuing 6–8 weeks.

TABLE 3.1
Animal Models of Pulmonary Fibrosis

Model	Mechnism of Injury	Strengths	Limitations
Bleomycin	Intratracheal, intravenous, subcutaneous, or intraperitoneal instillation of bleomycin	Well characterized and most frequently used	Patchy fibrosis, self-resolving, marked early inflammatory response
Recurrent bleomycin	Repetitive intratracheal instillations of bleomycin	More accurately reflects human disease, with persistent fibrosis	Multiple treatments, prolonged time course
TGF-β overexpression	TGF-β overexpression via transgene or viral vector	Able to use inducible systems, study direct affect of TGF-β	Viral vectors can promote inflammatory response, not clinically relevant
Silica	Intratracheal or aerosolized instillation of silica	Clinically relevant cause of fibrosis, persistent fibrosis	Slow-developing fibrosis, nodular fibrosis does not mimic IPF
Asbestos	Intratracheal administration or inhalation of asbestos	Clinically relevant, histology with fibroblastic foci, able to visualize particle deposition	Patchy fibrosis, inhalation model can have prolonged time course of fibrosis development
FITC	Intratracheal administration of FITC	Affected area fluoresces allowing accurate study of areas of injury, persistent fibrosis	Not a clinically relevant model, variable fibrotic response, initial inflammatory response
Irradiation	Lung irradiation	Relevant to human disease	Prolonged time course of fibrosis development requiring several months to develop
Hermansky-Pudlak	Gene deletion	Clinically relevant to certain familial cases of pulmonary fibrosis	Requires "second hit" which is typically bleomycin
Humanized murine model	Intravenous instillation of IPF fibroblasts into immunodeficient mice	Allows labeling of fibroblasts for trafficking purposes, persistent and fairly rapid fibrosis	Mice lack immune cells which is not seen in humans, limiting clinical relevance

FITC, fluorescein isothiocyanate; *IPF*, idiopathic pulmonary fibrosis; *TGF-β*, transforming growth factor beta.

Repetitive Bleomycin Model

Given the self-resolving nature of the bleomycin model, several groups have developed a model that utilizes repetitive dosing of bleomycin over several weeks to more closely recapitulate the human disease in which it is thought that repetitive injury is a major contributor to the fibrotic response.[14,15] This model uses 3–8 installations of bleomycin given intratracheally over a period of a few months. Initial studies have shown that the resultant fibrosis is long-lasting.[16] A major limitation of this model is the prolonged duration (up to several months) of treatment, as compared with the single bleomycin instillation model.

Acid Instillation

Instillation of hydrochloric acid, a common model of acute lung injury,[9] generates a small amount of fibrosis, and recently, repetitive dosing of hydrochloric acid has been shown to produce sustained fibrosis.[17] A repetitive acid instillation model is promising in that it may more closely replicate what is thought to be a risk factor in IPF, recurrent stomach acid aspiration;[18] however, experience with this model is limited.

Transforming Growth Factor-β Overexpression

As a major profibrotic cytokine and a driver of pulmonary fibrosis, the role of transforming growth factor-β

(TGF-β) in the pathogenesis of pulmonary fibrosis has been studied extensively in rodent models. Given its importance in the pathophysiology of pulmonary fibrosis,[19,20] groups have developed transgenic mice that overexpress TGF-β in lung epithelial cells.[21] Similarly, overexpression of TGF-β can be induced via the administration of recombinant adenovirus that produces active TGF-β.[22] These models demonstrate a fibrotic response developing at day 7, peaking at day 14–21, and lasting up to 2 months.[8] While this model does result in persistent fibrosis (as compared with the single-dose bleomycin model which resolves), the response is variable, thus limiting its reproducibility. Given the absence of an injurious agent, this method of fibrosis initiation does not adequately replicate human disease.

Silica

Occupational inhalation of silica particles can lead to fibrosis in humans.[23] While this disease process differs from the pathogenesis of IPF, much can be learned from studying this disease model in rodents. Silica particulates can be given experimentally via the intratracheal, inhalational, or oropharyngeal aspiration routes.[24] C3H/HeN and C57Bl/6 mice are more susceptible to silica-induced fibrosis than other strains.[8] This model leads to fibrotic nodules,[25] occurring as early as 4 weeks after administration. There is a coexistent inflammatory response with macrophages and neutrophils. While this model can be used to study fibrotic mediators, the fibrosis of this model does not closely replicate what is seen in human IPF.

Asbestosis

Inhaled asbestos fibers can cause pulmonary fibrosis in humans.[26] While asbestosis has some similarities to IPF (such as having a UIP pattern), unlike IPF, asbestosis has a clear precipitant. In the murine model of asbestosis, asbestos fibers (chrysotile or amphibole) are given either intratracheally or via inhalation. While the inhalational model takes longer (up to a month) to develop fibrosis than the intratracheal model, the inhalational model more closely replicates human disease.[7] Specifically, inhalation of asbestos fibers promotes a more peripheral and uniform fibrotic response. In vitro, asbestos leads to endoplasmic reticulum (ER) stress and apoptosis of epithelial cells, processes important in the development of lung fibrosis in humans.[27] These processes have been demonstrated in vivo as well and are followed by the initiation of fibrosis.[28]

Fluorescein Isothiocyanate

Fluorescein isothiocyanate (FITC) can be given through intratracheal administration to promote a fibrotic response.[29] While this chemical is not associated with human disease, it produces a prolonged fibrotic response, up to 6 months, which makes it potentially useful in studying the mechanisms of the fibrotic response.[7] Following administration, this agent leads to an early inflammatory response, followed by the development of fibrosis that is patchy. Because FITC is fluorescent, areas of deposition and injury can be viewed via microscopy.[7,30] A limitation of the model is that the variability in dosing limits its reproducibility.

Radiation-Induced Fibrosis

Another animal model that is relevant to human disease is radiation-induced fibrosis.[31] Ionizing radiation is a known cause of pneumonitis and pulmonary fibrosis in humans.[32] In rodent models, a single exposure of irradiation can promote fibrosis approximately 24 weeks later. There are significant differences in mouse strain susceptibility, and C57BL/6 is the most fibrosis-prone inbred strain of mice.[31] These animals also develop a subacute pneumonitis after radiation, similar to human disease. For the initial injury, this model is dependent on damage to DNA induced by free radicals, and later there is induction of TGF-β.[33] A factor for the widespread applicability of this model is the long duration between injury and fibrosis.

Hermansky-Pudlak Models

Hermansky-Pudlak syndrome (HPS) is a rare autosomal recessive disorder that is manifest in albinism, bleeding disorders, and pulmonary fibrosis. A newly described model of pulmonary fibrosis uses known mutations in HPS genes and recreates the human disease.[34] The mutations increase the susceptibility of alveolar epithelial cells (AECs) to undergo apoptosis following bleomycin-induced injury,[35] resulting in a more robust fibrotic response and increased mortality of exposed mice. The response seen in this model is dependent on TGF-β signaling.[36]

EPITHELIAL CELLS IN FIBROSIS

As the initial barrier of defense, AECs play a crucial role in protecting the lung from invading microbial pathogens and inhaled particulate matter on a daily basis.[37] The thin layer of Type I cells, which cover the greatest surface area of the alveoli, enables the exchange of oxygen and carbon dioxide between the alveolar space and the bloodstream.[38] Type II AECs produce surfactant, which prevents collapse of the alveoli. It is now thought that injuries, particularly frequent microinjuries to the alveolar epithelium, serve as the trigger for IPF.[39] These injuries may be related to exposures to smoke, pollution particulates, viruses, or acid microaspirations, resulting in damage to and loss of type I AECs. Type II cells, which are responsible for replacing injured type I cells,[40] become increasingly taxed and unable to cover the denuded basement membrane of the injured alveoli.

Epithelial cells also contribute to the recruitment of fibroblasts and immune cells through the release of a variety of cytokines, chemokines, and growth factors,[37,39] which will be discussed further in this chapter. Aside from their signaling properties, a number of epithelial cell processes are now recognized to contribute to the initiation of fibrosis.

Endoplasmic Reticulum Stress

Apoptosis of AECs is a typical finding in pulmonary fibrosis.[2] One mechanism by which apoptosis occurs is through the ER stress response. The ER is the organelle responsible for the folding and packaging of proteins in the cell. When a cell's demand for protein synthesis is greater than the capacity of the cell to produce, misfolding of proteins occurs due to ER stress. Misfolded proteins then activate the unfolded protein response, which tries to restore normal folding and degrade the misfolded proteins.[41] If the cell is unable to compensate, this pathway can lead to apoptosis of the cell. Notably, markers of ER stress and the unfolded protein response are seen in type II AECs obtained from patients with IPF; thus, this response has been implicated in its pathogenesis.[42]

Interestingly, proteins from herpesviruses have been noted in type II AECs from patients with IPF, leading to the hypothesis that viral infection contributes to the apoptosis of AECs in IPF.[43] Inhaled asbestos are taken up by epithelial cells and promote ER stress.[27] In the setting of surfactant protein C mutations, which leads to pulmonary fibrosis,[5,6] the misfolding of the mutated surfactant protein leads to ER stress and likely contributes to the pathogenesis of fibrosis seen in these individuals.[44] Other triggers for ER stress and the unfolded protein response may exist, and additional study is needed to identify them.

Developmental Program Reactivation

The aberrant reactivation of developmental signaling programs in epithelial cells is increasingly being recognized as a contributor to the pathogenesis of pulmonary fibrosis. The Wnt,[45,46] Sonic hedgehog,[47] and notch pathways[17] are all thought to be activated following alveolar injury. These pathways, important in proliferation, survival, and differentiation, are activated to aid in the repair process but become dysregulated, leading to a fibrogenic response.[48] As an example, the Wnt signaling pathway is important in the transdifferentiation of type II AECs to type I cells. Persistent activation, however, leads to release of cytokines, including TGF-β, a key mediator in pathologic fibrosis.[49] Concordant with this, aberrant Wnt activation has been noted at sites of fibroblastic foci and honeycomb cysts in IPF lungs.[50,51] Another pathway, Sonic hedgehog signaling, has also been shown to be upregulated in IPF lung tissue.[52] These pathways are now being explored as possible therapeutic targets.

Epithelial-Mesenchymal Transition

An intriguing but controversial cell process is epithelial to mesenchymal transition (EMT), whereby epithelial cells acquire features of mesenchymal cells such as fibroblasts and myofibroblasts. This reprogramming of epithelial cells occurs in the setting of TGF-β-mediated activation,[53,54] hypoxia,[55] and in response to ER stress.[56,57] While this process can be reproduced in vitro, it has been more difficult to examine in vivo,[58] and the degree to which it contributes to the pathogenesis of IPF remains unresolved. In humans, alveolar type II epithelial cells from IPF lungs have demonstrated costaining of the epithelial markers thyroid transcription factor 1 (TTF-1) and prosurfactant protein C, as well as the mesenchymal proteins αSMA (α-smooth muscle actin) and N-cadherin.[59] While epithelial cells have demonstrated the expression of mesenchymal proteins, there are few data in humans showing fibroblasts expressing epithelial cell markers, which raise the question of whether the epithelial cells can fully differentiate into fibroblasts. However, type II AECs isolated from IPF lungs have also shown high expression of mRNA for type I collagen,[59] so it does appear that these cells are able to produce important mediators of fibrosis. The study of EMT remains an important and active area of research.

FIBROBLASTS AND COLLAGEN DEPOSITION

Fibroblasts

A hallmark finding on pathology in IPF patients' lungs is the fibroblastic focus, which represents an area of accumulated fibroblasts and myofibroblasts. Fibroblasts are a mesenchymal cell population that resides in the lung during homeostasis, and they are responsible for the production of extracellular matrix materials such as collagen and elastin.[60] These materials provide the structural framework for the lung and allow for its unique physiologic properties of compliance and resistance. Fibroblasts are a crucial cell involved in wound healing, and they differentiate into myofibroblasts during tissue repair.[60]

Fibroblasts accumulate in lung tissue of IPF patients through a number of mechanisms (see Fig. 3.3). Given their ability to produce collagen and other extracellular matrix components, fibroblasts and myofibroblasts are one of the major areas of research in pulmonary fibrosis. IPF fibroblasts have abnormally increased proliferative capacity and an invasive phenotype.[61,62] This is thought to be due to chronic activation signals produced by the alveolar epithelium in the setting of recurrent injury.

Myofibroblasts

Fibroblasts that have undergone differentiation into myofibroblasts have the capacity to produce αSMA, a protein that gives the myofibroblast the ability to contract, an important process in wound repair.[60] Myofibroblasts can be differentiated from fibroblasts

in the setting of excess TGF-β, and as discussed earlier, EMT may be another source of myofibroblast-like cells.[60] Myofibroblasts produce most of the collagen and other extracellular matrix proteins in the IPF lung, further contributing to the fibrosis and remodeling of the lung.

Interestingly, myofibroblasts in IPF lungs develop resistance to apoptosis, a normal process of cell death in resolving tissue injury.[63] Apoptosis of fibroblasts and myofibroblasts in normal wound healing limits the deposition of excessive extracellular matrix material. The reason for apoptotic resistance in IPF is thought to be multifactorial, including pathologic activation of the PI3K/Akt pathway,[64] which promotes cell survival; alterations in apoptosis pathways;[65–67] and a deficiency in prostaglandin E2, or resistance to PGE2,[68] which is an important mediator in the apoptosis pathway,[69] and prevents fibroblast to myofibroblast transition.[70] In IPF, myofibroblasts also become more invasive, further promoting the spread of fibrosis in the lung.[71]

Fibrocytes

Fibrocytes are a newly described cell that arise from the bone marrow and are thought to traffic to sites of injury in the lung.[72,73] They comprise a very small percentage of circulating leukocytes (0.1%–0.5%) in healthy

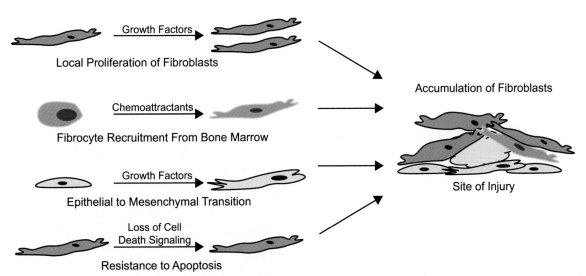

FIG. 3.3 Mechanisms for fibroblast accumulation in pulmonary fibrosis. Fibroblast numbers increase in idiopathic pulmonary fibrosis (IPF) lung tissue, occurring through a variety of mechanisms. IPF fibroblasts show an increased proliferative capacity, thereby increasing their numbers locally, whereas fibrocytes from the bone marrow can traffic to the lung and differentiate into fibroblasts. Epithelial-to-mesenchymal transition may be a source of fibroblasts; however, this remains controversial. Finally, IPF fibroblasts demonstrate resistance to apoptosis (programmed cell death), thereby helping maintain their numbers.

controls. These cells express markers of leukocytes (CD45) and stem cells (CD34).[72] Notably, they also express collagen-1. On arrival to a site of injury, these cells can differentiate into fibroblasts and myofibroblasts, while also activating resident fibroblasts, thereby promoting lung fibrosis.[74,75] Fibrocytes have been found in increased numbers in the circulation of IPF patients, and their levels independently predicted mortality.[76] These cells can produce a number of profibrotic mediators, including growth factors, cytokines, and extracellular matrix components.[72,77] In animals, the antifibrotic drug pirfenidone inhibits the accumulation of fibrocytes in the bleomycin model.[78]

Pericytes

Pericytes are a unique mesenchymal cell type that exists in perivascular spaces throughout the lung.[79] Fate mapping performed in mice using the bleomycin fibrosis model demonstrated a large number of pericytes differentiating into myofibroblasts and producing collagen.[80] While intriguing, there is currently no identified role for pericytes in human pulmonary fibrosis pathogenesis.

Collagen and Extracellular Matrix

A hallmark finding of IPF is the excessive production and deposition of collagen. Collagen is produced and then deposited by myofibroblasts and fibroblasts in the extracellular matrix in a disorganized manner. This deposition leads to alterations in the structure of distal airways and alveoli. While there are several types of collagen, in the normal lung, types I and III are the major isoforms.[81] Types II, IV, and VI are also present but in lesser amounts. In normal lungs, the fibroblast is the major source of both collagen production as well as collagen degradation. Collagen turnover is a continuous process, with collagen being taken up by fibroblasts and degraded intracellularly.[81]

Matrix metalloproteinases (MMPs) (discussed later) are also involved in the extracellular degradation of

---

TABLE 3.2
Growth Factors, Cytokines, and Chemokines in Pulmonary Fibrosis Pathogenesis

Molecule	Cell of Origin	Function
TGF-β	Macrophages, epithelial cells, fibroblasts	Promotes activation and proliferation of fibroblasts, release of fibrogenic growth factors and cytokines
CTGF	Macrophages, epithelial cells, fibroblasts, smooth muscle cells	Production of connective tissue, ECM remodeling, angiogenesis, EMT
PDGF	Platelets, macrophages, endothelial cells, epithelial cells	Fibroblast proliferation, fibrocyte migration, collagen deposition, and angiogenesis
FGF	Macrophages, fibroblasts, endothelial cells, epithelial cells	Fibrogenesis, epithelial mesenchymal transition, some family members may be antifibrotic
VEGF	Macrophages, monocytes, epithelial cells	Angiogenesis, endothelial repair
IL-13	T lymphocytes, mast cells, basophils, eosinophils, NK cells	Stimulate collagen production, enhance TGF-β production, alter MMP and TIMP production
TNF-α	Macrophages	Proinflammatory which may promote fibrotic environment, promotes apoptosis of macrophages which may limit fibrosis
IFN-γ	T lymphocytes, NK cells, macrophages, epithelial cells	Inhibit fibroblast proliferation, suppress Th2 signaling
MCP-1 (CCL2)	Monocytes, alveolar macrophages, dendritic cells	Recruitment of monocytes and fibrocytes to site of injury, mediate angiogenesis, regulate production of MMPs
CCL18	Monocytes, alveolar macrophages, dendritic cells	Immune cell trafficking, stimulate collagen production

CCL18, chemokine (C-C motif) ligand 18; *CCL2*, chemokine (C-C motif) ligand 2; *CTGF*, connective tissue growth factor; *EMT*, epithelial to mesenchymal transition; *FGF*, fibroblast growth factor; *IFN-γ*, interferon-gamma; *IL-13*, interleukin 13; *MCP-1*, monocyte chemoattractant protein 1; *MMP*, matrix metalloproteinase; *PDGF*, platelet derived growth factor; *TGF-β*, transforming growth factor-β; *TIMP*, tissue inhibitors of metalloproteinases; *TNF-α*, tumor necrosis factor-α; *VEGF*, vascular endothelial growth factor.

collagen.[82] In the setting of pulmonary fibrosis, collagen III deposition occurs early, with collagen I being deposited at later stages of fibrosis.[83] Fibroblastic foci, a characteristic feature in the UIP pattern of lung injury, is the predominate site of collagen production.[84] Collagen cross-linking is an important step in the pathogenesis of pulmonary fibrosis. This process is carried out via lysyl oxidase–like enzymes.[85] While inhibiting lysyl oxidase–like 2 experimentally reversed fibrosis in a bleomycin fibrosis model,[86] a recent clinical trial in IPF using a monoclonal antibody against lysyl oxidase–like 2 failed to show a benefit.[87]

While there is an increased production of collagen occurring in the fibrotic lung due to increased fibroblast and myofibroblast numbers, there may also be a decrease in the degradation of collagen, further increasing the overall collagen content in the extracellular matrix. Although fibroblasts are important in collagen uptake and degradation,[81] macrophages are also involved in scavenging collagen fragments. Milk fat globule-epidermal growth factor 8 (Mfge8) is a glycoprotein that binds collagen and facilitates uptake into macrophages.[88] Mice deficient in Mfge8 demonstrated more severe fibrosis following bleomycin treatment. Whether this pathway is impaired in humans is unknown.

Collagen is a major component of the extracellular matrix, but other molecules such as fibronectin and elastin are present as well.[83] Along with collagen, fibronectin is responsible for the tensile strength of the matrix, whereas elastin is important in determining the elastic recoil of the lung. The matrix is extensively modified in pulmonary fibrosis, resulting in an extremely stiff matrix, which contributes to the restrictive physiology seen in IPF. Interestingly, the stiff matrix can act as a positive feedback mechanism:[89] fibroblasts cultured on stiff matrices develop a myofibroblast phenotype and promote fibroblast invasion.[90] Furthermore, TGF-β is bound in matrix, and a stiffer matrix promotes the activation of this important growth factor.

Matrix Metalloproteinases

MMPs are enzymes involved in the degradation of extracellular matrix molecules, including collagen.[91] Currently there are 23 known MMPs, and these molecules are typically classified based on the substrate they degrade in vitro (collagen, gelatin, etc.). Along with their inhibitors, tissue inhibitors of metalloproteinases (TIMPs)[92] are thought to be involved in the pathogenesis of pulmonary fibrosis.[82,91] Based on their degradative properties, it was initially believed they would be antifibrotic in nature; however, multiple lines of evidence have shown the opposite. In patients with IPF, serum and bronchoalveolar lavage (BAL) fluid have shown elevated levels of multiple MMPs.[93] In fact, MMP-7 has been evaluated as a potential biomarker for IPF.[94,95] MMPs are expressed by a variety of cells, including neutrophils, macrophages, epithelial cells, and fibroblasts, making their study in animal models more challenging. In pulmonary fibrosis models, results from multiple studies have shown decreased fibrosis in mice deficient in particular MMPs, including MMP-3,[96] MMP-7,[97] and MMP-8;[98] however, data on a number of other MMPs (MMP-9, MMP-12, and MMP-13) are conflicting.[99] Some of the conflicting data may be due to redundancies in the MMPs, differences in MMP expression between rodents and humans, cell specific expression, or a temporal issue. Further study is needed to clarify these questions before targeting of these molecules could be systematically assessed in IPF patients.

GROWTH FACTORS, CYTOKINES, AND CHEMOKINES

There is a complex network of growth factors, cytokines, and chemokines that interact in the pathogenesis of IPF. Many of these molecules are becoming targets for possible therapies. Both parenchymal cells (fibroblasts and epithelial cells) as well as immune cells (alveolar macrophages) release many of these potential target molecules during the fibrotic response. We will discuss a few of the main mediators thought to have major roles in fibrogenesis.

Transforming Growth Factor-β

One of the major drivers, and most studied growth factors, implicated in pulmonary fibrosis is TGF-β. It is produced and released by a variety of cells, including macrophages, epithelial cells,[100] and fibroblasts. Normally important in repair after injury, it promotes the activation, proliferation, and differentiation of fibroblasts, leads to release of extracellular matrix from fibroblasts,[101] and can promote the release of other fibrogenic growth factors and cytokines. Elevated levels of TGF-β are found in the BAL of IPF patients, and it is upregulated in animal models of fibrosis. Notably, overexpression of TGF-β, as discussed earlier, can lead to the spontaneous development of pulmonary fibrosis in animals, whereas blockade of TGF-β signaling is enough to inhibit fibrosis in animal models.

TGF-β signaling is highly regulated. TGF-β is released in a latent form and must be activated by enzymatic cleavage of a latency-associated peptide attached to TGF-β; this may occur through MMPs. Both canonical signaling (through Smad proteins) and noncanonical signaling (involving Src and MAP kinases) transduce TGF-β-dependent signals, further complicating its study.[20] Protein tyrosine phosphatase-α (PTP-α) can augment TGF-β signaling in fibroblasts and is highly expressed in IPF lungs. Intriguingly, blockade of PTP-α in animal models prevents pulmonary fibrosis.[102]

Connective Tissue Growth Factor

Connective tissue growth factor (CTGF) is another important mediator of fibrogenesis, residing downstream of TGF-β. CTGF, a matricellular protein, is a member of the CCN family of extracellular matrix–associated proteins. It functions to promote fibroblast-mediated production of connective tissue, extracellular matrix (ECM) remodeling, angiogenesis, and is also involved in EMT.[103] While CTGF signaling is quite complex, one of the mechanisms by which it functions is via its interaction with other growth factors and cytokines, whose signaling CTGF may alter. Like TGF-β, CTGF expression is increased in IPF patients.[104] Overexpression of CTGF can promote pulmonary fibrosis in animal models,[105] and blockade of CTGF signaling can prevent and may even reverse fibrosis in animal models.[103] Blockade of CTGF is currently being evaluated as a potential therapy in IPF.[106]

Platelet-Derived Growth Factor

While its name is platelet-derived growth factor (PDGF), PDGF can also be released from cells such as macrophages, epithelial cells, lymphocytes, and endothelial cells.[107] PDGF exists as four separate proteins (A, B, C, and D) that dimerize to signal through PDGF receptors, which are receptor tyrosine kinases.[108] PDGF signaling is crucial for lung development; PDGF-deficient mice die during embryogenesis due to arrested lung development.[107]

Expression of PDGF is increased in IPF lungs,[109] particularly in macrophages,[110] and fibroblasts from patients with IPF express increased levels of PDGF receptor.[111] PDGF signaling increases the mobility of fibrocytes in bleomycin-induced pulmonary fibrosis in mice[112] and promotes fibroblast proliferation and collagen deposition in the silica murine model.[113] Blockade of PDGF signaling decreases experimental pulmonary fibrosis.[114] Notably, nintedanib, an antifibrotic drug approved for the treatment of IPF, is a tyrosine kinase inhibitor and is known to inhibit PDGF receptor signaling.[108,111]

Fibroblast Growth Factor

Fibroblast growth factor (FGF), another growth factor in IPF, also signals through a nintedanib-sensitive receptor tyrosine kinase.[108] FGFs represent a family of 22 molecules, and there are a number of reports suggesting that some FGF members are profibrotic, whereas others may be antifibrotic. Specifically, levels of FGF2 are elevated in the BAL of IPF patients[115] and at least partially mediate the effect of TGF-β; however, loss of FGF2 signaling had no effect on fibrogenesis in the bleomycin model.[116] FGF9 may be important in fibrocyte recruitment;[117] however, its role in human disease has not been determined. Alternatively, FGF1,[118] FGF7,[119] and FGF10[120] appear to be protective in experimental lung injury models. Given these complex interactions, further study will be important to better determine whether blockade of broad FGF signaling, as in the case of nintedanib, is beneficial.

Vascular Endothelial Growth Factor

Vascular endothelial growth factor (VEGF) has a complex role in pulmonary fibrosis pathogenesis. VEGF, which represents a family of five isoforms, is crucial in angiogenesis and is important in the repair processes after injury. VEGFs also signal through receptor tyrosine kinases, which can be inhibited by nintedanib.[108] In mouse models of pulmonary fibrosis, VEGF has been shown to have both antifibrotic[121,122] and profibrotic effects.[123] There have also been conflicting data in humans, whereby there are reports of both increased and decreased levels of circulating VEGF in IPF patients[124] and decreased levels in the BAL[93] and lung tissue.[121] Furthermore, it has recently been shown that splicing variants of VEGF-A behave differently in pulmonary fibrosis,[125] further complicating our understanding of VEGF signaling in IPF.

Interleukin 13

Interleukin 13 (IL-13) is a profibrotic cytokine responsible for Th2 responses in humans. Released by T cells, mast cells, and eosinophils, IL-13 is typically associated with allergic inflammation, including asthma. However, Th2-type inflammatory responses are also important in fibrosis pathogenesis, and multiple animal models have demonstrated that blockade of IL-13 signaling decreases fibrogenesis.[126–128] IL-13 can induce collagen expression by fibroblasts, stimulate production of TGF-β,[129] and alter production of MMPs and their inhibitors (TIMPs). While animal models have demonstrated this antifibrotic effect, recent clinical trials of agents that block IL-13 signaling have unfortunately not demonstrated a benefit in patients with IPF.[130]

Tumor Necrosis Factor-α

Tumor necrosis factor-α (TNF-α) is a cytokine released predominately from macrophages, but it is also released from a variety of other immune cells. As a pyrogen, TNF-α is important in the acute phase of inflammation and infection, with signaling through NF-κB. It also serves as a proapototic signal through the TNF receptor death domain.[131] In humans, TNF-α expression is elevated in IPF patients,[132] and there is an increased risk of developing IPF in people with TNF-α gene polymorphisms[133] that are known to promote exaggerated inflammatory responses. Despite these findings, the role of TNF-α in IPF remains uncertain. TNF-α can promote production of TGF-β,[134] and overexpression of TNF-α in mouse epithelial cells promoted spontaneous fibrosis.[135] Furthermore, blocking TNF receptor signaling prevents fibrosis in the bleomycin murine model of fibrosis.[136,137] However, paradoxically, addition of TNF-α in established fibrosis accelerates the resolution of fibrosis through apoptosis of alveolar macrophages,[11] and TNF-α can sensitize fibroblasts to apoptosis.[66] These conflicting reports are likely due to the known role that inflammation plays in the generation of fibrosis in the bleomycin model.[138] These processes may not be relevant to human IPF. Notably, a randomized controlled trial assessing the effectiveness of etanercept, which blocks TNF-α signaling, did not demonstrate benefits in patients with progressive IPF.[139]

Interferon-γ

Interferon-γ (IFN-γ) is an important cytokine that is found in decreased amounts in patients with IPF. IFN-γ is produced by NK and T cells and is an important antiviral cytokine and activator of macrophages. It has been shown to inhibit fibroblast proliferation[140] and to suppress proinflammatory Th2 signaling. While a clinical trial of subcutaneous IFN-γ failed to show clinical benefit,[141] a trial assessing the use of nebulized IFN-γ is ongoing.

Monocyte Chemoattractant Protein 1

Monocyte chemoattractant protein 1 (MCP-1), also known as chemokine (C-C motif) ligand 2 (CCL2), is a chemokine involved in recruiting monocytes[142] to sites of injury and inflammation and has been shown to play a role in fibrosis pathogenesis.[143] Similar to other cytokines, it is found in elevated levels in the BAL of patients with IPF.[143] MCP-1 signals through

the receptor C-C chemokine receptor type 2 (CCR2), and blockade of CCR2 (through genetic deletion) in both the bleomycin murine model and the FITC model of pulmonary fibrosis mitigates the fibrotic response.[144] It has been shown to promote the recruitment of fibrocytes to the lung,[74] mediate angiogenesis, and may regulate the production of certain MMPs. Unfortunately, a phase two trial of carlumab, a neutralizing antibody directed against CCL2, did not show clinical benefit.[145]

Chemokine (C-C motif) Ligand 18

Chemokine (C-C motif) ligand 18 (CCL18) is another chemokine that has been implicated in the pathogenesis of IPF. It too is found in elevated levels in the BAL fluid and serum of patients with IPF.[146] The association between disease activity and CCL18 levels in the serum has led to its consideration as a possible biomarker in IPF,[147] and CCL18 levels appear to correlate with progression of fibrosis.[146] In the lung, CCL18 is released from alveolar macrophages, either on stimulation with Th2 cytokines or with collagen, and protein expression is upregulated in IPF macrophages.[148] CCL18 is predominately involved in immune cell trafficking and also appears to increase collagen expression on cultured fibroblasts.[149] The rodent orthologue of CCL18 is not known, so this has limited the ability to study CCL18 in animal models.

Other Cytokines

IL-8 levels are elevated in alveolar macrophages and in BAL[93,150] of IPF patients, and this cytokine appears to be detrimental, as high serum IL-8 levels are predictive of poor outcomes.[151] CCL7, which is highly expressed in IPF fibroblasts,[152] and CCL12, which recruits fibrocytes,[153] both signal through CCR2, which was discussed earlier.

INFLAMMATION AND IMMUNE CELLS

Treatment of IPF with antiinflammatory or immunosuppressant therapies have shown no benefit,[154,155] which has led many experts to dismiss the idea of inflammation or immune response involvement in the pathogenesis of IPF. However, there is some evidence as discussed later, both in humans and animal models, that inflammatory cells may play important roles in the development and progression of fibrosis.

Macrophages

Macrophages are a crucial immune cell in the lung. Alveolar macrophages are responsible for the daily clearance of millions of particles, viruses, and apoptotic cells, while preventing a robust inflammatory response from developing.[156] Macrophages in the lung are thought to be present in a number of locations. Resident alveolar macrophages reside in the alveolus and do a large amount of the clearance. Interstitial macrophages are below the basement membrane, in areas around the vasculature.[157] In the setting of inflammation, it is thought that monocytes from the systemic circulation influx into the lung mature into a form of recruited macrophages.[158] Animal models suggest that these recruited macrophages are both reparative and profibrotic.[159,160] Much of this information has been elucidated in murine models, and additional research needs to be done to correlate findings with human macrophage subtypes, especially in a disease setting.

Macrophages are noteworthy in their ability to be both inflammatory and antiinflammatory.[161] In the past, this has often been described as macrophage polarization, where M1 macrophages were described as proinflammatory and M2 macrophages were described as antiinflammatory or reparative macrophages. It is the M2 macrophages that are thought to be involved in the fibrotic response.[162] Unfortunately, this paradigm does not hold up well in vivo, and now it is thought that macrophages actually exist in a continuum along the inflammatory-repair scale.[163]

Macrophages have the ability to produce a number of pro- and antifibrotic cytokines and growth factors.[161] An important role for alveolar macrophages is the ingestion of apoptotic cells (efferocytosis).[142] Interestingly, in IPF patients, the efferocytic ability of macrophages appears to be diminished,[164] which could lead to many downstream effects. Specifically, failed clearance of apoptotic cells can lead to increased inflammation, as these cells then undergo secondary necrosis. Furthermore, efferocytosis typically promotes the release of reparative molecules.[165] Other important roles of macrophages include the production of MMPs,[91] which play a role in collagen degradation and ingestion of collagen fragments in the extracellular matrix.[88]

Lymphocytes

There is an abundance of data in animal models of pulmonary fibrosis that T cells play an important role in the pathogenesis of fibrosis.[166] There are several T cell populations that have now been studied in fibrosis, including Th1, Th2, Th17, and regulatory T cells (Tregs).[117,167] In mouse models, there is a significant Th2 response that appears to drive fibrosis through release of the profibrogenic cytokines IL-4, IL-5, and IL-13.[168] This Th2 response counters the

antifibrotic Th1 response in which IFN-γ and IL-12 have been shown to limit fibrosis. The roles of these cytokines were discussed earlier. In addition to Th1 and Th2 cells, Th17 cells have also been identified as potential mediators of fibrosis as well: blocking IL-17,[169] which is released by Th17 cells, dampens the fibrotic response. There have been conflicting data regarding the role of Tregs in pulmonary fibrosis, with some indicating an antifibrotic role[117] and others demonstrating a profibrotic role.[167] This is likely due to the complex interactions of Tregs with other T cell populations. While there are strong data in animal models of fibrosis, there are currently limited data demonstrating T lymphocyte involvement in IPF.

While B cells likely play a role in connective tissue disease–related interstitial lung disease (CTD-ILD), their role in IPF is less clear.[170] Germinal centers containing B cells are frequently seen in CTD-ILD,[171] but their presence in suspected IPF is less common. A significant number of patients with IPF will have circulating autoantibodies, however,[172] raising the possibility that B cells could play a role in the pathogenesis of pulmonary fibrosis. Recent proteomic analysis of ILD lung tissue, including from IPF patients, demonstrated the presence of plasma B cells in increased numbers compared with controls.[173] Furthermore, CXCL13, a chemokine important in B cell trafficking, is elevated in the serum of IPF patients and correlates inversely with outcomes.[174] Animal models have demonstrated a potential role, as mice lacking B cells were protected from bleomycin-induced pulmonary fibrosis.[175]

Neutrophils

Neutrophils are the most abundant white blood cell in the body. With a short life span, they are typically present in the early stages of inflammation or in chronic inflammatory conditions. Neutrophils are found in the BAL fluid of patients with IPF, and their numbers are associated with mortality.[176] In the milieu of the IPF lung, neutrophils release neutrophil elastase,[177] which has the ability to break down many extracellular matrix components, including elastin, collagen, and fibronectin. Interestingly, blocking or genetic deletion of neutrophil elastase in animal models of fibrosis resulted in decreased fibrosis and fibroblast accumulation.[178,179] Neutrophil elastase promotes myofibroblast differentiation and fibroblast proliferation[180] and may also lead to TGF-β activation[178] and secretion.[181] Neutrophils are also able to produce a number of MMPs[182] as well as IL-17,[183,184] which can promote upregulation of CTGF, an important fibrogenic growth factor.

Infections

While there is no evidence that acute viral infection leads to IPF, a number of studies of animal models using γ-herpesvirus[185–188] demonstrated a possible role for chronic or latent viral infections in the promotion of pulmonary fibrosis. In some animal studies, viral infection preceding fibrosis-inducing lung injury resulted in an augmented fibrotic response.[189,190] Data from human studies have demonstrated some evidence of a potential link between viral infection and IPF. Human herpesvirus 7 (HHV-7) and HHV-8, Epstein-Barr virus, and human cytomegalovirus latent infections have been demonstrated in human IPF.[191] Torque teno virus DNA has been found in serum from IPF patients and was associated with worse outcomes.[192] In another study, herpesvirus saimiri proteins were found in the lung tissue of 21/21 patients with IPF.[193] Notably, herpesvirus saimiri is a γ-herpesvirus similar to that used in the animal models of fibrosis discussed earlier. These viruses may infect lung epithelial cells, causing dysfunction years later. Interestingly, at-risk but asymptomatic family members of pulmonary fibrosis patients, who had early interstitial abnormalities on CT of lung, were also found to have herpesvirus DNA in BAL fluid and makers of ER stress in AECs.[43] As discussed earlier, viral proteins produced in alveolar type II cells may contribute to ER stress[44] and promote apoptosis of these cells. Age may play an important role: aged mice infected with herpesvirus developed fibrosis, whereas young mice did not,[194] and herpesvirus infection was associated with an increased responsiveness to TGF-β in fibroblasts.

Viral infection may also promote acute worsening in IPF patients. A number of studies have shown that patients with acute worsening have evidence of viral infection.[195–198] However, the majority of cases in these studies did not demonstrate an infectious etiology.

New data implicate changes in the lung microbiome as a possible contributor to pulmonary fibrosis.[199–201] It is noteworthy that a number of genes that predispose to pulmonary fibrosis, toll-like receptor 3,[202] toll interacting protein,[203] and MUC5B,[3] are involved in lung defense. While it is certainly possible that ongoing bacterial infection may perpetuate epithelial injury, clarifying data are needed. Interestingly, in an animal model of fibrosis, *Pseudomonas aeruginosa* did not worsen fibrosis. Currently there are ongoing studies addressing the possible role of infectious drivers in IPF patients through the use of antimicrobial therapies.[204]

COAGULATION

An important component of wound healing is activation of the coagulation cascade (Fig. 3.4). While this essential process limits bleeding and aids in repair of injured tissue, an imbalance in coagulation can promote an aberrant fibrotic response. This is believed to play an important role in the pathophysiology of pulmonary fibrosis. Specific mediators that have been studied in IPF patients include tissue factor,[205] factor X,[206] thrombin,[207] activated protein C, and the antifibrinolytic molecules plasminogen activator inhibitors 1 and 2 (PAI-1, PAI-2).[93,208] Studies in patients with IPF demonstrate an increase in procoagulant and fibrinolytic activity.[208,209] Specifically, BAL fluid from patients with IPF demonstrated elevated levels of tissue factor as compared with normal controls.[205,208] Increased expression levels of tissue factor were seen in both fibroblasts[210] and epithelial cells of IPF lungs.[205] Likewise, increased expression of factors X[206] and VII[210] have been measured in IPF lungs, and PAI-1 and PAL-2 levels are elevated in BAL fluid of IPF patients.[93,208] Thrombin lies downstream in the coagulation cascade and signals through the protease activated receptors PAR-1 and PAR-2. PAR-1 is highly expressed in IPF epithelium, fibroblasts, and macrophages,[211] and PAR-2 expression has also been shown to be elevated in IPF lung specimens.[210] These findings are consistent with a procoagulant environment in the IPF lung and likely, systemically, as evidence by the increased risk of thromboembolic events in IPF patients.[212,213]

In vitro and animal studies corroborate the human findings. In the bleomycin model, treatment with the anticoagulants heparin,[214] activated protein C,[215] and factor Xa inhibitors[206] all decreased the degree of fibrosis, whereas overexpression of PAI-1 led to increased fibrosis.[216] In vitro, thrombin inhibits fibroblast apoptosis and leads to increased collagen and CTGF production (via its effect on PAR-1[217]) while also transforming them to myofibroblasts.[218] In the bleomycin model, PAR-2 signaling was shown to induce myofibroblast differentiation, and PAR-2-deficient animals were protected from fibrosis.[219] Factor Xa has been found to promote proliferation of fibroblasts and to stimulate collagen production in vitro.[220] While these findings are intriguing, treatment of IPF patients with the indirect anticoagulant warfarin did not demonstrate a mortality benefit.[221] Novel anticoagulants that inhibit thrombin and factor Xa are now available, however, and results from in vitro and animal studies suggest they may warrant additional investigation in IPF patients.[222–225]

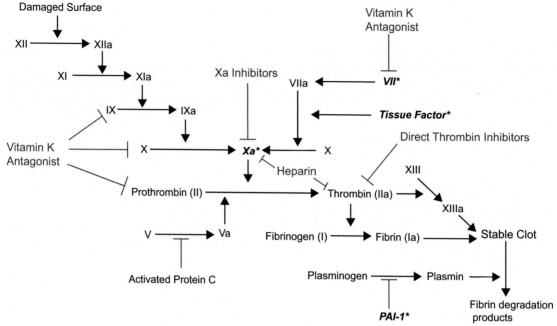

FIG. 3.4 Clotting cascade. The idiopathic pulmonary fibrosis (IPF) lung contains a procoagulant environment that contributes to fibrogenesis. Asterisks (*) indicates molecules that are seen in elevated concentrations in IPF tissue or BAL fluid. Molecules labeled in red inhibit clot formation and may be potential therapies in IPF.

MUCOCILIARY DYSFUNCTION

With the finding that a gain of function promoter variant of MUC5B (rs35705950) was associated with IPF, there has been new research assessing how this mucin may be involved in the pathogenesis of pulmonary fibrosis. The MUC5B promoter variant is the strongest known risk factor for the development of IPF, with homozygotes for the polymorphism having a 20-fold increased risk of IPF and heterozygotes having a sevenfold increase in risk. Interestingly, these common variants are also associated with improved outcomes in IPF patients.[226] How increased MUC5B expression promotes pulmonary fibrosis is not fully understood at this time.[227] MUC5B is produced by airway epithelial cells in the distal airways and, along with MUC5AC, is one of the main mucins in the lung.[228] Mucins are critically important in airway defense by trapping and helping to clear inhaled particles and pathogens.[229]

In the setting of IPF, MUC5B can be found in the microscopic honeycomb cysts and in the distal airways.[230] Interestingly, upregulation of cilium genes[231] has been associated with histologic honeycombing, further implicating mucociliary dysfunction in the peripheral airways in the pathogenesis of pulmonary fibrosis. Currently there are a few hypotheses as to the role of MUC5B in the pathogenesis of pulmonary fibrosis.[227] One possibility is that overproduction of MUC5B may lead to the entrapment of inflammatory particles that have reduced clearance as the mucus layer has become thicker and more viscous. In turn, this leads to increased inflammation and injury in the distal airway and bronchoalveolar junction. Another possibility is that, as a large and heavily glycosylated molecule, the overproduction of MUC5B may promote ER stress and the unfolded protein response or, has been previously shown, ER stress may be required for the production of mucins.[232] As discussed earlier, ER stress has been shown to be involved in the pathogenesis of IPF.[233] A third possibility is that stem cells in the distal airway, which are required to regenerate injured epithelium, are disrupted due to excessive production of MUC5B, potentially by modifying growth factor signaling pathways or altering the stem cell differentiation through metabolic stress from the production of MUC5B. These are hypotheses that are currently being evaluated and promoting the possible development of new therapeutic approaches to the treatment of IPF.

AGING LUNG

It is noteworthy that IPF typically presents in the 6—7th decades, with incidence increasing as patients age. This is also seen in animal models, where aged mice have more severe fibrosis in response to bleomycin.[13] Fibroblasts from IPF lungs also have a senescence phenotype that may contribute to fibrosis.[234,235] Recent genetic studies in familial cases of IPF have implicated telomere maintenance in the pathogenesis of pulmonary fibrosis. Specifically, rare variants in the TERT, TERC,[4] PARN,[236,237] and RTEL[238] genes are associated with the development of familial pulmonary fibrosis, which can occur in patients younger than those with sporadic IPF.[239]

Telomerases are enzymes that function to add nucleotide caps to the ends of chromosomes, protecting them from degradation during repetitive cell divisions. These loss-of-function variants in the associated proteins are associated with telomere shortening and cell senescence. Interestingly, shortened telomeres have also been seen in patients with sporadic IPF[240,241] and are associated with worse survival,[242] suggesting some potential role for telomerase dysfunction in the pathogenesis of pulmonary fibrosis. Whether this directly contributes to the pathogenesis is unclear, and notably in animal models, mice with these mutations do not have spontaneous, more severe, or prolonged fibrosis.[243] However, there are a number of potential explanations for this finding, including longer telomeres in mice.[244] Therefore, mouse models may not be useful in studying the importance of this pathway in pulmonary fibrosis.

THERAPEUTIC PERSPECTIVES

While many therapies have been tried, only two have shown any benefit in slowing progression of IPF. Pirfenidone and nintedanib are the only two Food and Drug Administration—approved therapies at this time.[245—247] While the mechanism by which pirfenidone works remains unclear,[204] nintedanib is a tyrosine kinase inhibitor that blocks VEGF receptor, PDGF receptor, and FGF receptor[108,248] while also having nontyrosine kinase—related antifibrotic effects.[249,250]

Some therapies that are currently undergoing testing include direct inhibition of CTGF through the use of monoclonal antibody.[106] This has shown promise in early testing as a potential therapy. Serum amyloid P is also being developed as a potential antifibrotic[251] through its role in altering macrophage and fibrocyte function.[252,253] Despite efficacy in preclinical models,[86,126] recent studies aimed at blocking IL-13[130] and LOXL2[87] in IPF have been less successful. Other agents currently under study include those that target $\alpha v \beta 6$ integrin,[254] Sonic hedgehog pathway,[255] and ROCK2.[256] Unfortunately, there has been little success to date in finding therapies for IPF, likely due to the overall complexity of the disease process as highlighted earlier. Therefore, continuing to improve our knowledge on the pathogenesis of IPF will hopefully foster new and promising treatments in the future.

CONCLUSIONS

While IPF is, by definition, due to unknown causes, our understanding of the mechanisms leading to fibrosis has expanded significantly over the past several years. The pathogenesis of IPF is complex, with the currently accepted dogma promoting the idea that IPF is the result of repetitive injury that leads to an aberrant fibrotic response with multiple cell types and mechanisms involved. Continued study of the mechanisms of pulmonary fibrosis is imperative to the development of effective therapies aimed at treating this deadly disease.

REFERENCES

1. American Thoracic Society/European Respiratory Society International Multidisciplinary Consensus classification of the idiopathic interstitial pneumonias. *Am J Respir Crit Care Med.* 2002;165(2):277—304.
2. King TE, Pardo A, Selman M. Idiopathic pulmonary fibrosis. *Lancet.* 2011;378(9807):1949—1961.
3. Seibold MA, et al. A common MUC5B promoter polymorphism and pulmonary fibrosis. *New Engl J Med.* 2011;364(16):1503—1512.
4. Tsakiri KD, et al. Adult-onset pulmonary fibrosis caused by mutations in telomerase. *Proc Natl Acad Sci USA.* 2007;104(18):7552—7557.
5. Hamvas A, et al. Progressive lung disease and surfactant dysfunction with a deletion in surfactant protein C gene. *Am J Respir Cell Mol Biol.* 2004;30(6):771—776.
6. Lawson W, et al. Genetic mutations in surfactant protein C are a rare cause of sporadic cases of IPF. *Thorax.* 2004;59(11):977—980.
7. Moore BB, Hogaboam CM. Murine models of pulmonary fibrosis. *Am J Physiol Lung Cell Mol Physiol.* 2008;294(2):L152—L160.
8. Moore BB, et al. Animal models of fibrotic lung disease. *Am J Respir Cell Mol Biol.* 2013;49(2):167—179.
9. Matute-Bello G, Frevert CW, Martin TR. Animal models of acute lung injury. *Am J Physiol Lung Cell Mol Physiol.* 2008; 295(3):L379—L399.

10. Jenkins RG, et al. An Official American Thoracic Society Workshop Report: use of animal models for the preclinical assessment of potential therapies for pulmonary fibrosis. *Am J Respir Cell Mol Biol.* 2017;56(5):667−679.

11. Redente EF, et al. Tumor necrosis factor-α accelerates the resolution of established pulmonary fibrosis in mice by targeting profibrotic lung macrophages. *Am J Respir Cell Mol Biol.* 2014;50(4):825−837.

12. Sleijfer S. Bleomycin-induced pneumonitis. *Chest.* 2001;120(2):617−624.

13. Redente EF, et al. Age and sex dimorphisms contribute to the severity of bleomycin-induced lung injury and fibrosis. *Am J Physiol Lung Cell Mol Physiol.* 2011;301(4):L510−L518.

14. Degryse AL, et al. Repetitive intratracheal bleomycin models several features of idiopathic pulmonary fibrosis. *Am J Physiol Lung Cell Mol Physiol.* 2010;299(4):L442−L452.

15. Chung MP, et al. Role of repeated lung injury and genetic background in bleomycin-induced fibrosis. *Am J Respir Cell Mol Biol.* 2003;29(3):375−380.

16. Degryse AL, Lawson WE. Progress toward improving animal models for Ipf. *Am J Med Sci.* 2011;341(6):444−449.

17. Cao Z, et al. Targeting of the pulmonary capillary vascular niche promotes lung alveolar repair and ameliorates fibrosis. *Nat Med.* 2016;22(2):154−162.

18. Lee JS, et al. Anti-acid therapy and disease progression in idiopathic pulmonary fibrosis: an analysis of data from three randomized controlled trials. *Lancet Respir Med.* 2013;1(5):369−376.

19. Fernandez IE, Eickelberg O. The impact of TGF-β on lung fibrosis. *Proc Am Thorac Soc.* 2012;9(3):111−116.

20. Aschner Y, Downey GP. Transforming growth factor-β: master regulator of the respiratory system in health and disease. *Am J Respir Cell Mol Biol.* 2016;54(5):647−655.

21. Lee CG, et al. Early growth response gene 1−mediated apoptosis is essential for transforming growth factor β(1)−induced pulmonary fibrosis. *J Exp Med.* 2004;200(3):377−389.

22. Sime PJ, et al. Adenovector-mediated gene transfer of active transforming growth factor-beta1 induces prolonged severe fibrosis in rat lung. *J Clin Investig.* 1997;100(4):768−776.

23. Leung CC, Yu IT, Chen W. Silicosis. *Lancet.* 2012;379(9830):2008−2018.

24. Lacher SE, et al. Murine pulmonary inflammation model: a comparative study of anesthesia and instillation methods. *Inhal Toxicol.* 2010;22(1):77−83.

25. Dauber JH, et al. Experimental silicosis: morphologic and biochemical abnormalities produced by intratracheal instillation of quartz into guinea pig lungs. *Am J Pathol.* 1980;101(3):595−612.

26. Kamp DW. Asbestos-induced lung diseases: an update. *Transl Res.* 2009;153(4):143−152.

27. Kamp DW, et al. Asbestos-induced alveolar epithelial cell apoptosis. The role of endoplasmic reticulum stress response. *Am J Respir Cell Mol Biol.* 2013;49(6):892−901.

28. Kim S-J, et al. The role of mitochondrial DNA in mediating alveolar epithelial cell apoptosis and pulmonary fibrosis. *Int J Mol Sci.* 2015;16(9):21486−21519.

29. Roberts SN, et al. A novel model for human interstitial lung disease: hapten-driven lung fibrosis in rodents. *J Pathol.* 1995;176(3):309−318.

30. Christensen PJ, et al. Induction of lung fibrosis in the mouse by intratracheal instillation of fluorescein isothiocyanate is not T-cell-dependent. *Am J Pathol.* 1999;155(5):1773−1779.

31. Karvonen RL, et al. An animal model of pulmonary radiation fibrosis with biochemical, physiologic, immunologic, and morphologic observations. *Radiat Res.* 1987;111(1):68−80.

32. Movsas B, et al. Pulmonary radiation injury. *Chest.* 1997;111(4):1061−1076.

33. Mancini ML, Sonis ST. Mechanisms of cellular fibrosis associated with cancer regimen-related toxicities. *Front Pharmacol.* 2014;5:51.

34. Atochina-Vasserman EN, et al. Early alveolar epithelial dysfunction promotes lung inflammation in a mouse model of Hermansky-Pudlak syndrome. *Am J Respir Crit Care Med.* 2011;184(4):449−458.

35. Young LR, et al. The alveolar epithelium determines susceptibility to lung fibrosis in Hermansky-Pudlak syndrome. *Am J Respir Crit Care Med.* 2012;186(10):1014−1024.

36. Young LR, et al. Epithelial-macrophage interactions determine pulmonary fibrosis susceptibility in Hermansky-Pudlak syndrome. *JCI Insight.* 2016;1(17):e88947.

37. Camelo A, et al. The epithelium in idiopathic pulmonary fibrosis: breaking the barrier. *Front Pharmacol.* 2014;4(173).

38. Rackley CR, Stripp BR. Building and maintaining the epithelium of the lung. *J Clin Investig.* 2012;122(8):2724−2730.

39. Selman M, Pardo A. Role of epithelial cells in idiopathic pulmonary fibrosis. *Proc Am Thorac Soc.* 2006;3(4):364−372.

40. Barkauskas CE, et al. Type 2 alveolar cells are stem cells in adult lung. *J Clin Investig.* 2013;123(7):3025−3036.

41. Hetz C. The unfolded protein response: controlling cell fate decisions under ER stress and beyond. *Nat Rev Mol Cell Biol.* 2012;13:89.

42. Lawson WE, et al. Endoplasmic reticulum stress enhances fibrotic remodeling in the lungs. *Proc Natl Acad Sci USA.* 2011;108(26):10562−10567.

43. Kropski JA, et al. Extensive phenotyping of individuals at risk for familial interstitial pneumonia reveals clues to the pathogenesis of interstitial lung disease. *Am J Respir Crit Care Med.* 2015;191(4):417−426.

44. Lawson WE, et al. Endoplasmic reticulum stress in alveolar epithelial cells is prominent in IPF: association with altered surfactant protein processing and herpesvirus infection. *Am J Physiol Lung Cell Mol Physiol.* 2008;294(6):L1119−L1126.

45. Königshoff M, et al. Functional Wnt signaling is increased in idiopathic pulmonary fibrosis. *PLoS One.* 2008;3(5): e2142.
46. Pfaff E-M, et al. Dickkopf proteins influence lung epithelial cell proliferation in idiopathic pulmonary fibrosis. *Eur Respir J.* 2011;37(1):79−87.
47. Kugler MC, et al. Sonic hedgehog signaling in the lung. From development to disease. *Am J Respir Cell Mol Biol.* 2015;52(1):1−13.
48. Chanda D, et al. Developmental reprogramming in mesenchymal stromal cells of human subjects with idiopathic pulmonary fibrosis. *Sci Rep.* 2016;6:37445.
49. Spanjer AIR, et al. TGF-β-induced profibrotic signaling is regulated in part by the WNT receptor Frizzled-8. *FASEB J.* 2016;30(5):1823−1835.
50. Chilosi M, et al. Aberrant Wnt/β-catenin pathway activation in idiopathic pulmonary fibrosis. *Am J Pathol.* 2003; 162(5):1495−1502.
51. Meuten T, et al. WNT7B in fibroblastic foci of idiopathic pulmonary fibrosis. *Respir Res.* 2012;13(1):62.
52. Bolaños AL, et al. Role of Sonic Hedgehog in idiopathic pulmonary fibrosis. *Am J Physiol Lung Cell Mol Physiol.* 2012;303(11):L978−L990.
53. Willis BC, et al. Induction of epithelial-mesenchymal transition in alveolar epithelial cells by transforming growth factor-β1: potential role in idiopathic pulmonary fibrosis. *Am J Pathol.* 2005;166(5):1321−1332.
54. Jayachandran A, et al. SNAI transcription factors mediate epithelial−mesenchymal transition in lung fibrosis. *Thorax.* 2009;64(12):1053−1061.
55. Guo L, et al. Hypoxia-induced epithelial-mesenchymal transition is involved in bleomycin-induced lung fibrosis. *BioMed Res Int.* 2015;2015:232791.
56. Tanjore H, et al. Alveolar epithelial cells undergo epithelial-to-mesenchymal transition in response to endoplasmic reticulum stress. *J Biol Chem.* 2011; 286(35):30972−30980.
57. Zhong Q, et al. Role of endoplasmic reticulum stress in epithelial−mesenchymal transition of alveolar epithelial cells: effects of misfolded surfactant protein. *Am J Respir Cell Mol Biol.* 2011;45(3):498−509.
58. Kim KK, et al. Alveolar epithelial cell mesenchymal transition develops in vivo during pulmonary fibrosis and is regulated by the extracellular matrix. *Proc Natl Acad Sci USA.* 2006;103(35):13180−13185.
59. Marmai C, et al. Alveolar epithelial cells express mesenchymal proteins in patients with idiopathic pulmonary fibrosis. *Am J Physiol Lung Cell Mol Physiol.* 2011;301(1): L71−L78.
60. Kendall RT, Feghali-Bostwick CA. Fibroblasts in fibrosis: novel roles and mediators. *Front Pharmacol.* 2014;5(123).
61. Ahluwalia N, et al. Fibrogenic lung injury induces non−cell-autonomous fibroblast invasion. *Am J Respir Cell Mol Biol.* 2016;54(6):831−842.
62. Ramos C, et al. Fibroblasts from idiopathic pulmonary fibrosis and normal lungs differ in growth rate, apoptosis, and tissue inhibitor of metalloproteinases expression. *Am J Respir Cell Mol Biol.* 2001;24(5):591−598.
63. Thannickal VJ, Horowitz JC. Evolving concepts of apoptosis in idiopathic pulmonary fibrosis. *Proc Am Thorac Soc.* 2006;3(4):350−356.
64. Kulasekaran P, et al. Endothelin-1 and transforming growth factor-β1 independently induce fibroblast resistance to apoptosis via AKT activation. *Am J Respir Cell Mol Biol.* 2009;41(4):484−493.
65. Ajayi IO, et al. X-linked inhibitor of apoptosis regulates lung fibroblast resistance to Fas-mediated apoptosis. *Am J Respir Cell Mol Biol.* 2013;49(1):86−95.
66. Frankel SK, et al. TNF-α sensitizes normal and fibrotic human lung fibroblasts to Fas-induced apoptosis. *Am J Respir Cell Mol Biol.* 2006;34(3):293−304.
67. Huang SK, et al. Histone modifications are responsible for decreased Fas expression and apoptosis resistance in fibrotic lung fibroblasts. *Cell Death Dis.* 2013;4(5): e621.
68. Huang SK, et al. Hypermethylation of PTGER2 confers prostaglandin E(2) resistance in fibrotic fibroblasts from humans and mice. *Am J Pathol.* 2010;177(5):2245−2255.
69. Huang SK, et al. Prostaglandin E(2) induces fibroblast apoptosis by modulating multiple survival pathways. *FASEB J.* 2009;23(12):4317−4326.
70. Kolodsick JE, et al. Prostaglandin E2 inhibits fibroblast to myofibroblast transition via E. Prostanoid receptor 2 signaling and cyclic adenosine monophosphate elevation. *Am J Respir Cell Mol Biol.* 2003;29(5):537−544.
71. Li Y, et al. Severe lung fibrosis requires an invasive fibroblast phenotype regulated by hyaluronan and CD44. *J Exp Med.* 2011;208(7):1459−1471.
72. Reilkoff RA, Bucala R, Herzog EL. Fibrocytes: emerging effector cells in chronic inflammation. *Nat Rev Immunol.* 2011;11:427.
73. Loomis-King H, Moore BB. Fibrocytes in the pathogenesis of chronic fibrotic lung disease. *Curr Respir Med Rev.* 2013; 9(1):34−41.
74. Moore BB, et al. CCR2-Mediated recruitment of fibrocytes to the alveolar space after fibrotic injury. *Am J Pathol.* 2005;166(3):675−684.
75. Ashley SL, et al. Periostin regulates fibrocyte function to promote myofibroblast differentiation and lung fibrosis. *Mucosal Immunol.* 2016;10:341.
76. Moeller A, et al. Circulating fibrocytes are an indicator of poor prognosis in idiopathic pulmonary fibrosis. *Am J Respir Crit Care Med.* 2009;179(7):588−594.
77. Kleaveland KR, Moore BB, Kim KK. Paracrine functions of fibrocytes to promote lung fibrosis. *Expert Rev Respir Med.* 2014;8(2):163−172.
78. Inomata M, et al. Pirfenidone inhibits fibrocyte accumulation in the lungs in bleomycin-induced murine pulmonary fibrosis. *Respir Res.* 2014;15(1):16.
79. Barron L, Gharib SA, Duffield JS. Lung pericytes and resident fibroblasts: busy multitaskers. *Am J Pathol.* 2016; 186(10):2519−2531.
80. Rock JR, et al. Multiple stromal populations contribute to pulmonary fibrosis without evidence for epithelial to mesenchymal transition. *Proc Natl Acad Sci USA.* 2011; 108(52):E1475−E1483.

81. Glasser SW, et al. Mechanisms of lung fibrosis resolution. *Am J Pathol*. 2016;186(5):1066—1077.

82. Pardo A, Selman M. Matrix metalloproteases in aberrant fibrotic tissue remodeling. *Proc Am Thorac Soc*. 2006; 3(4):383—388.

83. Burgess JK, et al. The extracellular matrix — the under-recognized element in lung disease? *J Pathol*. 2016; 240(4):397—409.

84. Bensadoun ES, et al. Proteoglycan deposition in pulmonary fibrosis. *Am J Respir Crit Care Med*. 1996;154(6): 1819—1828.

85. Tjin G, et al. Lysyl oxidases regulate fibrillar collagen remodelling in idiopathic pulmonary fibrosis. *Dis Model Mech*. 2017;10(11):1301—1312.

86. Barry-Hamilton V, et al. Allosteric inhibition of lysyl oxidase—like-2 impedes the development of a pathologic microenvironment. *Nat Med*. 2010;16:1009.

87. Raghu G, et al. Efficacy of simtuzumab versus placebo in patients with idiopathic pulmonary fibrosis: a randomised, double-blind, controlled, phase 2 trial. *Lancet Respir Med*. 2017;5(1):22—32.

88. Atabai K, et al. Mfge8 diminishes the severity of tissue fibrosis in mice by binding and targeting collagen for uptake by macrophages. *J Clin Investig*. 2009;119(12): 3713—3722.

89. Liu F, et al. Feedback amplification of fibrosis through matrix stiffening and COX-2 suppression. *J Cell Biol*. 2010;190(4):693—706.

90. Chen H, et al. Mechanosensing by the $\alpha(6)$-integrin confers an invasive fibroblast phenotype and mediates lung fibrosis. *Nat Commun*. 2016;7:12564.

91. Pardo A, et al. Role of matrix metalloproteinases in the pathogenesis of idiopathic pulmonary fibrosis. *Respir Res*. 2016;17:23.

92. García-Alvarez J, et al. Tissue inhibitor of metalloproteinase-3 is up-regulated by transforming growth factor-β1 in vitro and expressed in fibroblastic foci in vivo in idiopathic pulmonary fibrosis. *Exp Lung Res*. 2006;32(5):201—214.

93. Stijn W, et al. Multiplex protein profiling of bronchoalveolar lavage in idiopathic pulmonary fibrosis and hypersensitivity pneumonitis. *Ann Thorac Med*. 2013;8(1):38—45.

94. Bauer Y, et al. MMP-7 is a predictive biomarker of disease progression in patients with idiopathic pulmonary fibrosis. *ERJ Open Res*. 2017;3(1):00074—2016.

95. Tzouvelekis A, et al. Validation of the prognostic value of MMP-7 in idiopathic pulmonary fibrosis. *Respirology*. 2017;22(3):486—493.

96. Yamashita CM, et al. Matrix metalloproteinase 3 is a mediator of pulmonary fibrosis. *Am J Pathol*. 2011; 179(4):1733—1745.

97. Zuo F, et al. Gene expression analysis reveals matrilysin as a key regulator of pulmonary fibrosis in mice and humans. *Proc Natl Acad Sci USA*. 2002;99(9):6292—6297.

98. Craig VJ, et al. Pro-fibrotic activities for matrix Metalloproteinase-8 during bleomycin-mediated lung injury. *J Immunol (Baltim Md 1950)*. 2013;190(8): 4283—4296.

99. Cabrera S, et al. Overexpression of MMP9 in macrophages attenuates pulmonary fibrosis induced by bleomycin. *Int J Biochem Cell Biol*. 2007;39(12): 2324—2338.

100. Degryse AL, et al. TGFβ signaling in lung epithelium regulates bleomycin-induced alveolar injury and fibroblast recruitment. *Am J Physiol Lung Cell Mol Physiol*. 2011; 300(6):L887—L897.

101. Eickelberg O, et al. Extracellular matrix deposition by primary human lung fibroblasts in response to TGF-β1 and TGF-β3. *Am J Physiol Lung Cell Mol Physiol*. 1999;276(5): L814—L824.

102. Aschner Y, et al. Protein tyrosine Phosphatase α mediates profibrotic signaling in lung fibroblasts through TGF-β responsiveness. *Am J Pathol*. 2014;184(5):1489—1502.

103. Lipson KE, et al. CTGF is a central mediator of tissue remodeling and fibrosis and its inhibition can reverse the process of fibrosis. *Fibrogenesis Tissue Repair*. 2012; 5(suppl 1):S24.

104. Allen JT, et al. Enhanced insulin-like growth factor binding protein—related protein 2 (connective tissue growth factor) expression in patients with idiopathic pulmonary fibrosis and pulmonary sarcoidosis. *Am J Respir Cell Mol Biol*. 1999;21(6):693—700.

105. Sonnylal S, et al. Selective expression of connective tissue growth factor in fibroblasts in vivo promotes systemic tissue fibrosis. *Arthritis Rheum*. 2010;62(5). https://doi.org/ 10.1002/art.27382.

106. Raghu G, et al. FG-3019 anti-connective tissue growth factor monoclonal antibody: results of an open-label clinical trial in idiopathic pulmonary fibrosis. *Eur Respir J*. 2016;47(5):1481—1491.

107. Noskovičová N, et al. Platelet-derived growth factor signaling in the lung. From lung development and disease to clinical studies. *Am J Respir Cell Mol Biol*. 2015; 52(3):263—284.

108. Grimminger F, Günther A, Vancheri C. The role of tyrosine kinases in the pathogenesis of idiopathic pulmonary fibrosis. *Eur Respir J*. 2015;45(5):1426—1433.

109. Antoniades HN, et al. Platelet-derived growth factor in idiopathic pulmonary fibrosis. *J Clin Investig*. 1990; 86(4):1055—1064.

110. Martinet Y, et al. Exaggerated spontaneous release of platelet-derived growth factor by alveolar macrophages from patients with idiopathic pulmonary fibrosis. *N Engl J Med*. 1987;317(4):202—209.

111. Hostettler KE, et al. Anti-fibrotic effects of nintedanib in lung fibroblasts derived from patients with idiopathic pulmonary fibrosis. *Respir Res*. 2014;15(1):157.

112. Aono Y, et al. Role of platelet-derived growth factor/ platelet-derived growth factor receptor axis in the trafficking of circulating fibrocytes in pulmonary fibrosis. *Am J Respir Cell Mol Biol*. 2014;51(6):793—801.

113. Re SL, et al. Platelet-derived growth factor—producing CD4+ Foxp3+ regulatory T lymphocytes promote lung fibrosis. *Am J Respir Crit Care Med*. 2011;184(11): 1270—1281.

114. Abdollahi A, et al. Inhibition of platelet-derived growth factor signaling attenuates pulmonary fibrosis. *J Exp Med.* 2005;201(6):925—935.

115. Inoue Y, et al. Human mast cell basic fibroblast growth factor in pulmonary fibrotic disorders. *Am J Pathol.* 1996;149(6):2037—2054.

116. Guzy RD, et al. Fibroblast growth factor 2 is required for epithelial recovery, but not for pulmonary fibrosis, in response to bleomycin. *Am J Respir Cell Mol Biol.* 2015; 52(1):116—128.

117. Peng X, et al. CD4+CD25+FoxP3+ regulatory Tregs inhibit fibrocyte recruitment and fibrosis via suppression of FGF-9 production in the TGF-β1 exposed murine lung. *Front Pharmacol.* 2014;5:80.

118. Shimbori C, et al. Fibroblast growth factor-1 attenuates TGF-β1-induced lung fibrosis. *J Pathol.* 2016;240(2): 197—210.

119. Sakamoto S, et al. Keratinocyte growth factor gene transduction ameliorates pulmonary fibrosis induced by bleomycin in mice. *Am J Respir Cell Mol Biol.* 2011;45(3): 489—497.

120. Gupte VV, et al. Overexpression of fibroblast growth factor-10 during both inflammatory and fibrotic phases attenuates bleomycin-induced pulmonary fibrosis in mice. *Am J Respir Crit Care Med.* 2009;180(5):424—436.

121. Murray LA, et al. Antifibrotic role of vascular endothelial growth factor in pulmonary fibrosis. *JCI Insight.* 2017; 2(16):e92192.

122. Stockmann C, et al. Loss of myeloid cell-derived vascular endothelial growth factor accelerates fibrosis. *Proc Natl Acad Sci USA.* 2010;107(9):4329—4334.

123. Farkas L, et al. VEGF ameliorates pulmonary hypertension through inhibition of endothelial apoptosis in experimental lung fibrosis in rats. *J Clin Investig.* 2009; 119(5):1298—1311.

124. Ando M, et al. Significance of serum vascular endothelial growth factor level in patients with idiopathic pulmonary fibrosis. *Lung.* 2010;188(3):247—252.

125. Barratt SL, et al. Differential expression of VEGF-Axxx isoforms is critical for development of pulmonary fibrosis. *Am J Respir Crit Care Med.* 2017;196(4):479—493.

126. Murray LA, et al. Targeting interleukin-13 with tralokinumab attenuates lung fibrosis and epithelial damage in a humanized SCID idiopathic pulmonary fibrosis model. *Am J Respir Cell Mol Biol.* 2014;50(5):985—994.

127. Jakubzick C, et al. Therapeutic attenuation of pulmonary fibrosis via targeting of IL-4- and IL-13-responsive cells. *J Immunol.* 2003;171(5):2684—2693.

128. Belperio JA, et al. Interaction of IL-13 and C10 in the pathogenesis of bleomycin-induced pulmonary fibrosis. *Am J Respir Cell Mol Biol.* 2002;27(4):419—427.

129. Lee CG, et al. Interleukin-13 induces tissue fibrosis by selectively stimulating and activating transforming growth factor β(1). *J Exp Med.* 2001;194(6):809—822.

130. Parker JM, et al. A phase 2 randomized controlled study of tralokinumab in subjects with idiopathic pulmonary fibrosis. *Am J Respir Crit Care Med.* 2018;197(1):94—103.

131. Aggarwal BB. Signalling pathways of the TNF superfamily: a double-edged sword. *Nat Rev Immunol.* 2003;3:745.

132. Piguet PF, et al. Expression and localization of tumor necrosis factor-alpha and its mRNA in idiopathic pulmonary fibrosis. *Am J Pathol.* 1993;143(3):651—655.

133. Whyte M, et al. Increased risk of fibrosing alveolitis associated with interleukin-1 receptor antagonist and tumor necrosis factor- α gene polymorphisms. *Am J Respir Crit Care Med.* 2000;162(2):755—758.

134. Sullivan DE, et al. TNF-α induces TGF-β(1) expression in lung fibroblasts at the transcriptional level via AP-1 activation. *J Cell Mol Med.* 2009;13(8b):1866—1876.

135. Miyazaki Y, et al. Expression of a tumor necrosis factor-alpha transgene in murine lung causes lymphocytic and fibrosing alveolitis. A mouse model of progressive pulmonary fibrosis. *J Clin Investig.* 1995;96(1):250—259.

136. Ortiz LA, et al. Upregulation of the p75 but not the p55 TNF-α receptor mRNA after silica and bleomycin exposure and protection from lung injury in double receptor knockout mice. *Am J Respir Cell Mol Biol.* 1999;20(4): 825—833.

137. Tumor necrosis factor/cachectin plays a key role in bleomycin-induced pneumopathy and fibrosis. *J Exp Med.* 1989;170(3):655—663.

138. Ortiz LA, et al. Expression of TNF and the necessity of TNF receptors in bleomycin-induced lung injury in mice. *Exp Lung Res.* 1998;24(6):721—743.

139. Raghu G, et al. Treatment of idiopathic pulmonary fibrosis with etanercept. *Am J Respir Crit Care Med.* 2008;178(9):948—955.

140. O'Flaherty BM, et al. CD8+ T cell response to gammaherpesvirus infection mediates inflammation and fibrosis in interferon gamma receptor-deficient mice. *PLoS One.* 2015;10(8):e0135719.

141. King TE, et al. Effect of interferon gamma-1b on survival in patients with idiopathic pulmonary fibrosis (INSPIRE): a multicentre, randomised, placebo-controlled trial. *Lancet.* 2009;374(9685):222—228.

142. Liang J, et al. A macrophage subpopulation recruited by CC chemokine ligand-2 clears apoptotic cells in noninfectious lung injury. *Am J Physiol Lung Cell Mol Physiol.* 2012;302(9):L933—L940.

143. Baran CP, et al. Important roles for macrophage colony-stimulating factor, CC chemokine ligand 2, and mononuclear phagocytes in the pathogenesis of pulmonary fibrosis. *Am J Respir Crit Care Med.* 2007;176(1): 78—89.

144. Moore BB, et al. Protection from pulmonary fibrosis in the absence of CCR2 signaling. *J Immunol.* 2001;167(8): 4368—4377.

145. Raghu G, et al. CC-chemokine ligand 2 inhibition in idiopathic pulmonary fibrosis: a phase 2 trial of carlumab. *Eur Respir J.* 2015;46(6):1740—1750.

146. Prasse A, et al. Serum CC-chemokine ligand 18 concentration predicts outcome in idiopathic pulmonary fibrosis. *Am J Respir Crit Care Med.* 2009;179(8): 717—723.

147. Guiot J, et al. Blood biomarkers in idiopathic pulmonary fibrosis. *Lung*. 2017;195(3):273–280.

148. Prasse A, et al. A vicious circle of alveolar macrophages and fibroblasts perpetuates pulmonary fibrosis via CCL18. *Am J Respir Crit Care Med*. 2006;173(7):781–792.

149. Atamas SP, et al. Pulmonary and activation-regulated chemokine stimulates collagen production in lung fibroblasts. *Am J Respir Cell Mol Biol*. 2003;29(6):743–749.

150. Carré PC, et al. Increased expression of the interleukin-8 gene by alveolar macrophages in idiopathic pulmonary fibrosis. A potential mechanism for the recruitment and activation of neutrophils in lung fibrosis. *J Clin Investig*. 1991;88(6):1802–1810.

151. Richards TJ, et al. Peripheral blood proteins predict mortality in idiopathic pulmonary fibrosis. *Am J Respir Crit Care Med*. 2012;185(1):67–76.

152. Choi ES, et al. Enhanced monocyte chemoattractant protein-3/CC chemokine Ligand-7 in usual interstitial pneumonia. *Am J Respir Crit Care Med*. 2004;170(5):508–515.

153. Moore BB, et al. The role of CCL12 in the recruitment of fibrocytes and lung fibrosis. *Am J Respir Cell Mol Biol*. 2006;35(2):175–181.

154. Collard HR, et al. Combined corticosteroid and cyclophosphamide therapy does not alter survival in idiopathic pulmonary fibrosis. *Chest*. 2004;125(6):2169–2174.

155. The Idiopathic Pulmonary Fibrosis Clinical Research Network. Prednisone, azathioprine, and *N*-acetylcysteine for pulmonary fibrosis. *N Engl J Med*. 2012;366(21):1968–1977.

156. Hussell T, Bell TJ. Alveolar macrophages: plasticity in a tissue-specific context. *Nat Rev Immunol*. 2014;14:81.

157. Gibbings SL, et al. Three unique interstitial macrophages in the murine lung at steady state. *Am J Respir Cell Mol Biol*. 2017;57(1):66–76.

158. Janssen WJ, et al. Fas determines differential fates of resident and recruited macrophages during resolution of acute lung injury. *Am J Respir Crit Care Med*. 2011;184(5):547–560.

159. McCubbrey DAL, et al. Deletion of c-FLIP from CD11bhi macrophages prevents development of bleomycin-induced lung fibrosis. *Am J Respir Cell Mol Biol*. 2018;58(1):66–78.

160. Misharin AV, et al. Monocyte-derived alveolar macrophages drive lung fibrosis and persist in the lung over the life span. *J Exp Med*. 2017;214(8):2387–2404.

161. Wynn TA, Vannella KM. Macrophages in tissue repair, regeneration, and fibrosis. *Immunity*. 2016;44(3):450–462.

162. Ballinger MN, et al. IRAK-M promotes alternative macrophage activation and fibroproliferation in bleomycin-induced lung injury. *J Immunol*. 2015;194(4):1894–1904.

163. Murray PJ, et al. Macrophage activation and polarization: nomenclature and experimental guidelines. *Immunity*. 2014;41(1):14–20.

164. Morimoto K, Janssen WJ, Terada M. Defective efferocytosis by alveolar macrophages in IPF patients. *Respir Med*. 2012;106(12):1800–1803.

165. Zemans RL, et al. Conceptual approaches to lung injury and repair. *Ann Am Thorac Soc*. 2015;12(suppl 1):S9–S15.

166. Luzina IG, et al. Roles of T lymphocytes in pulmonary fibrosis. *J Leukoc Biol*. 2008;83(2):237–244.

167. Birjandi SZ, et al. CD4(+)CD25(hi)Foxp3(+) cells exacerbate bleomycin-induced pulmonary fibrosis. *Am J Pathol*. 2016;186(8):2008–2020.

168. Gieseck 3rd RL, Wilson MS, Wynn TA. Type 2 immunity in tissue repair and fibrosis. *Nat Rev Immunol*. 2017;18(1):62.

169. Wilson MS, et al. Bleomycin and IL-1β–mediated pulmonary fibrosis is IL-17A dependent. *J Exp Med*. 2010;207(3):535–552.

170. Hoyne GF, et al. Idiopathic pulmonary fibrosis and a role for autoimmunity. *Immunol Cell Biol*. 2017;95:577.

171. Song JW, et al. Pathologic and radiologic differences between idiopathic and collagen vascular disease-related usual interstitial pneumonia. *Chest*. 2009;136(1):23–30.

172. Lee JS, et al. Prevalence and clinical significance of circulating autoantibodies in idiopathic pulmonary fibrosis. *Respir Med*. 2013;107(2):249–255.

173. Schiller HB, et al. Deep proteome profiling reveals common prevalence of MZB1-positive plasma B cells in human lung and skin fibrosis. *Am J Respir Crit Care Med*. 2017;196(10):1298–1310.

174. Vuga LJ, et al. C-X-C motif chemokine 13 (CXCL13) is a prognostic biomarker of idiopathic pulmonary fibrosis. *Am J Respir Crit Care Med*. 2014;189(8):966–974.

175. O'Donoghue RJJ, et al. Genetic partitioning of interleukin-6 signalling in mice dissociates Stat3 from Smad3-mediated lung fibrosis. *EMBO Mol Med*. 2012;4(9):939–951.

176. Kinder BW, et al. Baseline BAL neutrophilia predicts early mortality in idiopathic pulmonary fibrosis. *Chest*. 2008;133(1):226–232.

177. Obayashi Y, et al. The role of neutrophils in the pathogenesis of idiopathic pulmonary fibrosis. *Chest*. 1997;112(5):1338–1343.

178. Takemasa A, Ishii Y, Fukuda T. A neutrophil elastase inhibitor prevents bleomycin-induced pulmonary fibrosis in mice. *Eur Respir J*. 2012;40(6):1475–1482.

179. Chua F, et al. Mice lacking neutrophil elastase are resistant to bleomycin-induced pulmonary fibrosis. *Am J Pathol*. 2007;170(1):65–74.

180. Gregory AD, et al. Neutrophil elastase promotes myofibroblast differentiation in lung fibrosis. *J Leukoc Biol*. 2015;98(2):143–152.

181. Lee K-Y, et al. Neutrophil-derived elastase induces TGF-β1 secretion in human airway smooth muscle via NF-κB pathway. *Am J Respir Cell Mol Biol*. 2006;35(4):407–414.

182. Manoury B, et al. Influence of early neutrophil depletion on MMPs/TIMP-1 balance in bleomycin-induced lung fibrosis. *Int Immunopharmacol*. 2007;7(7):900–911.

183. Hasan SA, et al. Role of IL-17A and neutrophils in fibrosis in experimental hypersensitivity pneumonitis. *J Allergy Clin Immunol.* 2013;131(6):1663–1673.e5.

184. Chrysanthopoulou A, et al. Neutrophil extracellular traps promote differentiation and function of fibroblasts. *J Pathol.* 2014;233(3):294–307.

185. Mora AL, et al. Activation of alveolar macrophages via the alternative pathway in herpesvirus-induced lung fibrosis. *Am J Respir Cell Mol Biol.* 2006;35(4):466–473.

186. Lung infection with γ-herpesvirus induces progressive pulmonary fibrosis in Th2-biased mice. *Am J Physiol Lung Cell Mol Physiol.* 2005;289(5):L711–L721.

187. Mora AL, et al. Control of virus reactivation arrests pulmonary herpesvirus-induced fibrosis in IFN-γ receptor–deficient mice. *Am J Respir Crit Care Med.* 2007;175(11):1139–1150.

188. Williams KJ, et al. Experimental induction of pulmonary fibrosis in horses with the gammaherpesvirus equine herpesvirus 5. *PLoS One.* 2013;8(10):e77754.

189. Vannella KM, et al. Latent herpesvirus infection augments experimental pulmonary fibrosis. *Am J Respir Crit Care Med.* 2010;181(5):465–477.

190. Lok SS, et al. Murine gammaherpes virus as a cofactor in the development of pulmonary fibrosis in bleomycin resistant mice. *Eur Respir J.* 2002;20(5):1228–1232.

191. Tang Y-W, et al. Herpesvirus DNA is consistently detected in lungs of patients with idiopathic pulmonary fibrosis. *J Clin Microbiol.* 2003;41(6):2633–2640.

192. Bando M, et al. Infection of TT virus in patients with idiopathic pulmonary fibrosis. *Respir Med.* 2001;95(12):935–942.

193. Folcik VA, et al. Idiopathic pulmonary fibrosis is strongly associated with productive infection by herpesvirus saimiri. *Mod Pathol.* 2014;27(6):851–862.

194. Naik PN, et al. Pulmonary fibrosis induced by γ-herpesvirus in aged mice is associated with increased fibroblast responsiveness to transforming growth factor-β. *J Gerontol Ser A Biol Sci Med Sci.* 2012;67(7):714–725.

195. Wootton SC, et al. Viral infection in acute exacerbation of idiopathic pulmonary fibrosis. *Am J Respir Crit Care Med.* 2011;183(12):1698–1702.

196. Huie TJ, et al. A detailed evaluation of acute respiratory decline in patients with fibrotic lung disease: aetiology and outcomes. *Respirology.* 2010;15(6):909–917.

197. dos Santos GC, et al. Immunohistochemical detection of virus through its nuclear cytopathic effect in idiopathic interstitial pneumonia other than acute exacerbation. *Braz J Med Biol Res.* 2013;46(11):985–992.

198. Ushiki A, et al. Viral infections in patients with an acute exacerbation of idiopathic interstitial pneumonia. *Respir Investig.* 2014;52(1):65–70.

199. Han MK, et al. Association between lung microbiome and disease progression in IPF: a prospective cohort study. *Lancet Respir Med.* 2014;2(7):548–556.

200. Huang Y, et al. Microbes are associated with host innate immune response in idiopathic pulmonary fibrosis. *Am J Respir Crit Care Med.* 2017;196(2):208–219.

201. Molyneaux PL, et al. The role of bacteria in the pathogenesis and progression of idiopathic pulmonary fibrosis. *Am J Respir Crit Care Med.* 2014;190(8):906–913.

202. O'Dwyer DN, et al. The toll-like receptor 3 L412F polymorphism and disease progression in idiopathic pulmonary fibrosis. *Am J Respir Crit Care Med.* 2013;188(12):1442–1450.

203. Noth I, et al. Genetic variants associated with idiopathic pulmonary fibrosis susceptibility and mortality: a genome-wide association study. *Lancet Respir Med.* 2013;1(4):309–317.

204. Rangarajan S, et al. Targeted therapy for idiopathic pulmonary fibrosis: where to now? *Drugs.* 2016;76(3):291–300.

205. Fujii M, et al. Relevance of tissue factor and tissue factor pathway inhibitor for hypercoagulable state in the lungs of patients with idiopathic pulmonary fibrosis. *Thromb Res.* 2000;99(2):111–117.

206. Scotton CJ, et al. Increased local expression of coagulation factor X contributes to the fibrotic response in human and murine lung injury. *J Clin Investig.* 2009;119(9):2550–2563.

207. Kimura M, et al. The significance of cathepsins, thrombin and aminopeptidase in diffuse interstitial lung diseases. *J Med Investig.* 2005;52(1–2):93–100.

208. Kotani I, et al. Increased procoagulant and antifibrinolytic activities in the lungs with idiopathic pulmonary fibrosis. *Thromb Res.* 1995;77(6):493–504.

209. Chapman HA, Allen CL, Stone OL. Abnormalities in pathways of alveolar fibrin turnover among patients with interstitial lung disease. *Am Rev Respir Dis.* 1986;133(3):437–443.

210. Wygrecka M, et al. Role of protease-activated receptor-2 in idiopathic pulmonary fibrosis. *Am J Respir Crit Care Med.* 2011;183(12):1703–1714.

211. Mercer PF, et al. Pulmonary epithelium is a prominent source of proteinase-activated receptor-1–inducible CCL2 in pulmonary fibrosis. *Am J Respir Crit Care Med.* 2009;179(5):414–425.

212. Sprunger DB, et al. Pulmonary fibrosis is associated with an elevated risk of thromboembolic disease. *Eur Respir J.* 2012;39(1):125–132.

213. Sode BF, et al. Venous thromboembolism and risk of idiopathic interstitial pneumonia. *Am J Respir Crit Care Med.* 2010;181(10):1085–1092.

214. Günther A, et al. Prevention of bleomycin-induced lung fibrosis by aerosolization of heparin or urokinase in rabbits. *Am J Respir Crit Care Med.* 2003;168(11):1358–1365.

215. Yasui H, et al. Intratracheal administration of activated protein C inhibits bleomycin-induced lung fibrosis in the mouse. *Am J Respir Crit Care Med.* 2001;163(7):1660–1668.

216. Eitzman DT, et al. Bleomycin-induced pulmonary fibrosis in transgenic mice that either lack or overexpress the murine plasminogen activator inhibitor-1 gene. *J Clin Investig.* 1996;97(1):232–237.

217. Chambers RC, et al. Thrombin is a potent inducer of connective tissue growth factor production via proteolytic activation of protease-activated receptor-1. *J Biol Chem.* 2000;275(45):35584–35591.

218. Bogatkevich GS, et al. Thrombin differentiates normal lung fibroblasts to a myofibroblast phenotype via the proteolytically activated receptor-1 and a protein kinase C-dependent pathway. *J Biol Chem.* 2001;276(48): 45184–45192.

219. Borensztajn K, et al. Protease-activated receptor-2 induces myofibroblast differentiation and tissue factor upregulation during bleomycin-induced lung injury: potential role in pulmonary fibrosis. *Am J Pathol.* 2010;177(6): 2753–2764.

220. Blanc-Brude OP, et al. Factor Xa stimulates fibroblast procollagen production, proliferation, and calcium signaling via PAR1 activation. *Exp Cell Res.* 2005;304(1):16–27.

221. Noth I, et al. A placebo-controlled randomized trial of warfarin in idiopathic pulmonary fibrosis. *Am J Respir Crit Care Med.* 2012;186(1):88–95.

222. Bogatkevich GS, Ludwicka-Bradley A, Silver RM. Dabigatran, a direct thrombin inhibitor, blocks differentiation of normal fibroblasts to a myofibroblast phenotype and demonstrates anti-fibrotic effects on scleroderma lung fibroblasts. *Arthritis Rheum.* 2009;60(11):3455–3464.

223. Bogatkevich GS, et al. Anti-inflammatory and anti-fibrotic effects of the oral direct thrombin inhibitor dabigatran etexilate in a murine model of interstitial lung disease. *Arthritis Rheum.* 2011;63(5):1416–1425.

224. Shea BS, et al. Uncoupling of the profibrotic and hemostatic effects of thrombin in lung fibrosis. *JCI Insight.* 2017;2(9):e86608.

225. Annexin A2 contributes to lung injury and fibrosis by augmenting factor Xa fibrogenic activity. *Am J Physiol Lung Cell Mol Physiol.* 2017;312(5):L772–L782.

226. Peljto AL, et al. Association between the MUC5B promoter polymorphism and survival in patients with idiopathic pulmonary fibrosis. *JAMA.* 2013;309(21): 2232–2239.

227. Evans CM, et al. Idiopathic pulmonary fibrosis: a genetic disease that involves mucociliary dysfunction of the peripheral airways. *Physiol Rev.* 2016;96(4):1567–1591.

228. Fahy JV, Dickey BF. Airway mucus function and dysfunction. *N Engl J Med.* 2010;363(23):2233–2247.

229. Roy MG, et al. Muc5b is required for airway defense. *Nature.* 2014;505(7483):412–416.

230. Nakano Y, et al. MUC5B promoter variant rs35705950 affects MUC5B expression in the distal airways in idiopathic pulmonary fibrosis. *Am J Respir Crit Care Med.* 2016;193(4):464–466.

231. Yang IV, et al. Expression of cilium-associated genes defines novel molecular subtypes of idiopathic pulmonary fibrosis. *Thorax.* 2013;68(12):1114–1121.

232. Martino MB, et al. The ER stress transducer IRE1β is required for airway epithelial mucin production. *Mucosal Immunol.* 2013;6(3):639–654.

233. Tanjore H, Blackwell TS, Lawson WE. Emerging evidence for endoplasmic reticulum stress in the pathogenesis of idiopathic pulmonary fibrosis. *Am J Physiol Lung Cell Mol Physiol.* 2012;302(8):L721–L729.

234. Schafer MJ, et al. Cellular senescence mediates fibrotic pulmonary disease. *Nat Commun.* 2017;8:14532.

235. IPF lung fibroblasts have a senescent phenotype. *Am J Physiol Lung Cell Mol Physiol.* 2017;313(6):L1164–L1173.

236. Stuart BD, et al. Exome sequencing links mutations in PARN and RTEL1 with familial pulmonary fibrosis and telomere shortening. *Nat Genet.* 2015;47(5):512–517.

237. Kropski JA, et al. Rare genetic variants in PARN are associated with pulmonary fibrosis in families. *Am J Respir Crit Care Med.* 2017;196(11):1481–1484.

238. Cogan JD, et al. Rare variants in RTEL1 are associated with familial interstitial pneumonia. *Am J Respir Crit Care Med.* 2015;191(6):646–655.

239. Borie R, et al. Prevalence and characteristics of TERT and TERC mutations in suspected genetic pulmonary fibrosis. *Eur Respir J.* 2016;48(6):1721–1731.

240. Alder JK, et al. Short telomeres are a risk factor for idiopathic pulmonary fibrosis. *Proc Natl Acad Sci USA.* 2008;105(35):13051–13056.

241. Cronkhite JT, et al. Telomere shortening in familial and sporadic pulmonary fibrosis. *Am J Respir Crit Care Med.* 2008;178(7):729–737.

242. Stuart BD, et al. Effect of telomere length on survival in idiopathic pulmonary fibrosis: an observational study with independent validation. *Lancet Respir Med.* 2014; 2(7):557–565.

243. Degryse AL, et al. Telomerase deficiency does not alter bleomycin induced fibrosis in mice. *Exp Lung Res.* 2012; 38(3):124–134.

244. Calado RT, Dumitriu B. Telomere dynamics in mice and humans. *Semin Hematol.* 2013;50(2):165–174.

245. Noble PW, et al. Pirfenidone in patients with idiopathic pulmonary fibrosis (CAPACITY): two randomised trials. *Lancet.* 2011;377(9779):1760–1769.

246. King TEJ, et al. A phase 3 trial of pirfenidone in patients with idiopathic pulmonary fibrosis. *N Engl J Med.* 2014; 370(22):2083–2092.

247. Richeldi L, et al. Efficacy and safety of nintedanib in idiopathic pulmonary fibrosis. *N Engl J Med.* 2014;370(22): 2071–2082.

248. Richeldi L, et al. Efficacy of a tyrosine kinase inhibitor in idiopathic pulmonary fibrosis. *N Engl J Med.* 2011; 365(12):1079–1087.

249. Rangarajan S, et al. Novel mechanisms for the antifibrotic action of nintedanib. *Am J Respir Cell Mol Biol.* 2016; 54(1):51–59.

250. Knüppel L, et al. A novel antifibrotic mechanism of nintedanib and pirfenidone. Inhibition of collagen fibril assembly. *Am J Respir Cell Mol Biol.* 2017;57(1):77–90.

251. van den Blink B, et al. Recombinant human pentraxin-2 therapy in patients with idiopathic pulmonary fibrosis: safety, pharmacokinetics and exploratory efficacy. *Eur Respir J.* 2016;47(3):889–897.

252. Murray LA, et al. Serum amyloid P therapeutically attenuates murine bleomycin-induced pulmonary fibrosis via its effects on macrophages. *PLoS One.* 2010;5(3):e9683.

253. Murray LA, et al. TGF-beta driven lung fibrosis is macrophage dependent and blocked by serum amyloid P. *Int J Biochem Cell Biol.* 2011;43(1):154−162.

254. Horan GS, et al. Partial inhibition of integrin αvβ6 prevents pulmonary fibrosis without exacerbating inflammation. *Am J Respir Crit Care Med.* 2008;177(1):56−65.

255. Moshai EF, et al. Targeting the hedgehog−glioma-associated oncogene homolog pathway inhibits bleomycin-induced lung fibrosis in mice. *Am J Respir Cell Mol Biol.* 2014;51(1):11−25.

256. Knipe RS, et al. The rho kinase isoforms ROCK1 and ROCK2 each contribute to the development of experimental pulmonary fibrosis. *Am J Respir Cell Mol Biol.* 2018;58(4):471−481.

257. Ahluwalia N, Shea BS, Tager AM. New therapeutic targets in idiopathic pulmonary fibrosis. Aiming to rein in runaway wound-healing responses. *Am J Respir Crit Care Med.* 2014;190(8):867−878.

CHAPTER 4

Genetics of Pulmonary Fibrosis

REBECCA KEITH, MD • KEVIN K. BROWN, MD • TASHA FINGERLIN, PHD

INTRODUCTION

The development of clinically significant scarring in the lung, or pulmonary fibrosis, is known to be associated with a number of systemic disorders, environmental exposures, and infections. When it occurs in the absence of a known association, it is recognized as a fibrosing idiopathic interstitial pneumonia (fibrosing IIP), with idiopathic pulmonary fibrosis (IPF) being the most common and lethal form. More than 50,000 individuals are affected by pulmonary fibrosis annually in the United States,[1] and its prevalence is increasing.[1,2] A number of genetic mutations and variants have been identified as associated with the development of pulmonary fibrosis. Linkage studies in families and genome-wide association studies (GWAS), in both sporadic and familial cases of IIP, have identified several candidate genes that require further scientific inquiry. GWAS studies examine genetic variants between individuals over the entire genome to identify genetic variants which may be associated with disease. These types of unbiased genetic approaches provide a unique opportunity to identify unexpected genetic factors that contribute to disease development.[3–5] In this chapter, we will review the known, putative genetic determinants of pulmonary fibrosis.[6]

USING FAMILIAL PULMONARY FIBROSIS TO IDENTIFY RARE VARIANTS

Pulmonary fibrosis likely occurs in genetically susceptible individuals. The evidence for a genetic component to this disease includes its development in monozygotic twins raised apart[7] and genetically related members of several families[8,9] in both autosomal dominant[10,11] and recessive inheritance patterns.[12] Familial pulmonary fibrosis (FPF) is identified when two or more family members have evidence of a fibrosing IIP,[10] and 10%–19% of patients with a fibrosing IIP are reported to have a family history of interstitial lung disease (ILD).[13,14] Most studies to date have used a candidate gene approach or linkage studies in families to identify

genetic drivers, and mutations have been described in the following genes using this approach: surfactant protein C (SFTPC),[14–17] surfactant protein A2 (SFTPA2),[18] telomerase RNA component (TERC),[19,20] telomerase reverse transcriptase (TERT),[20,21] Mucin 5B (MUC5B),[5] ELMOD2,[22] Poly(A)-specific ribonuclease deadenylation nuclease (PARN),[23] and regulator of telomere elongation helicase 1 (RTEL1).[23]

SURFACTANT PROTEIN C MUTATIONS

Pulmonary surfactant is a mixture of phospholipids and proteins secreted by alveolar type II epithelial cells. It acts to reduce the surface tension at the air-liquid interface to prevent alveolar collapse. In 2001, Amin and colleagues first reported a case of familial interstitial pneumonia in a mother and her two daughters related to surfactant protein C (SPC) deficiency.[24] That same year, Nogee et al. described a family with a full-term infant who presented with neonatal respiratory distress, due to nonspecific interstitial pneumonia (NSIP), born to a woman with desquamative interstitial pneumonia.[24] Sequencing identified a mutation in the SFTPC gene. In 2002, Thomas and colleagues used a candidate gene approach to identify a mutation in the same gene in one large family that was associated with pathologic usual interstitial pneumonia (UIP) pattern in the adults and an NSIP pattern in the children.[16] The mutation was associated with accumulation of pro-SPC within alveolar epithelial cells, and electron microscopy revealed abnormal lamellar bodies within atypical alveolar type II cells (AEC II). In 2004, Chibbar and colleagues also described a family with a mutation in SFTPC in which the adults had UIP and the children NSIP.[25] In 2010, van Moorsel reported SFTPC mutations in 5 of 20 FPF cases and none of the sporadic IPF cases in a Dutch cohort.[14] SFTPC mutations have thus far not been associated with the much more common, nonfamilial (or sporadic) IPF.[19,26]

In 2008, Lawson and colleagues evaluated lung biopsies from individuals in a family carrying an

SFTPC mutation and noted that unfolded protein response (UPR) pathway markers were upregulated in the alveolar epithelium lining areas of fibrosis.[27] Evidence of a similar endoplasmic reticulum (ER) stress response has also been identified in AECII cells from patients with sporadic IPF, i.e., unrelated to SPFTC mutations. This suggests that ER stress and UPR pathways may play a role in the pathogenesis of IPF.[27,28]

SURFACTANT PROTEIN A MUTATIONS

In 2009, Wang and colleagues used whole genome linkage analysis and sequencing to describe a missense mutation in SFTPA2 in two families with pulmonary fibrosis and lung cancer.[18] Surfactant protein A is an innate immune system collection that has two isoforms encoded by different genes.[29] Wang and colleagues showed how this mutation caused accumulation of misfolded SFTPA2 in the ER, possibly leading to an ER stress response. Mutant SFTPA2 protein has also been shown to induce secretion of the profibrotic cytokine TGF-β1.[30] Patients with SFTPA2 mutation had two- to threefold higher levels of TGF-β1 in their alveolar lavage fluid than family members without the mutation. Taken together, these findings implicate mutations in surfactant proteins in both ER stress and the TGF-β autocrine feedback loop in pulmonary fibrosis.

TELOMERASE MUTATIONS

Telomeres are a series of tandem repeated DNA sequences found at the end of chromosomes that serve to prevent chromosomal deterioration during DNA replication and cell division. Without telomeres, the genome would progressively lose information with each cell division. Telomeres are shortened with each cell division, and shortened telomeres have been linked to aging, general cell senescence, cancer, anemia, and pulmonary fibrosis.[31] Telomerase is a specialized reverse transcriptase that can add tandem repeats to the 3' end of the chromosome to counteract telomere shortening.[32] The telomerase complex consists of TERT, TERC, and several additional factors, such as dyskerin, that are required for telomerase assembly, trafficking, and recruitment to telomeres.[32] When telomerase fails to perform its critical functions, telomeres will progressively shorten with each cell division, important genetic information is subsequently lost, and cellular dysfunction ultimately occurs.[33]

Dyskeratosis congenita (DC) is a rare genetic disorder at the severe end of the spectrum of telomerase disorders; it manifests with oral leukoplakia, abnormal skin pigmentation, and nail dystrophy.[32] Bone marrow failure is common, with a more than 90% penetrance by age 30.[32] There are nine genes reported to be associated with DC and short telomeres including TERT, TERC, and DKC1.[34–38] Individuals with DC are at high risk of developing various cancers, pulmonary fibrosis, and liver disease. In 2007, Armanios and colleagues evaluated 73 families in the Vandervilt Familial Pulmonary Fibrosis Registry for mutations in TERT or TERC to determine if these genes could be involved in the development of familial pulmonary fibrosis.[21] Five families had heterozygous mutations in TERT, and one had a mutation in TERC, all in the absence of other clinical evidence of DC. Other familial studies have revealed mutations in TERT and TERC associated with adult-onset IPF,[20,38–40] and short telomeres have been described as associated with IPF independent of mutations in telomerase genes.[41]

More recently, whole exome sequencing and linkage analysis have identified mutations in PARN and RTEL1 associated with FPF and shortened telomeres.[23] Stuart et al., performed exome sequencing and linkage analysis on individuals with FPF of unknown cause and identified two candidate genes: PARN and RTEL1. Both genes were associated with shortened telomere length in genomic DNA from circulating leukocytes when compared with controls, implicating both genes in telomere dysfunction associated with FPF.[23] The mechanism linking PARN, and endoribonuclease, to telomere length remains unknown.[23]

ELMOD2

In 2006, Hodgson and colleagues reported the identification of ELMOD2 as a novel candidate gene in FPF.[22] Using a genome-wide scan followed by hierarchical fine mapping, they identified a shared haplotype in 8 of 24 Finnish families on chromosome 4q31, harboring two functionally uncharacterized genes, ELMOD2 and LOC152586. Expression analysis revealed that LOC152568 was expressed only in the testis, whereas ELMOD2 was expressed in all tissues, including the human lung and IPF-derived fibroblast cell lines. ELMOD2 is thought to be involved in regulation of antiviral responses via Toll-like receptor 3.[42] All nine exons of the ELMOD2 gene were sequenced from one affected patient in each family, but no mutations in coding regions were identified.

MUCIN 5B

In 2011, a promoter polymorphism (rs35705950) located 3 kb upstream of the transcription start site in the *MUC5B* gene was identified via a linkage and fine mapping study of patients with FPF.[5] This was the first common promoter polymorphism to be associated with pulmonary fibrosis. The MUC5B SNP has now been validated in seven independent cohorts and appears to be specific to FPF and IPF, as the SNP was not associated with scleroderma-associated ILD, asbestosis, chronic obstructive pulmonary disease, asthma, or lung cancer.[4,6,43−48] The minor allele was present at a frequency of 34% among individuals with FPF, 38% among subjects with sporadic IPF, and 9% among controls.[5] The odds ratio for disease development in those heterozygous for the minor allele was 6.8 and 20.8 for individuals who were homozygous.[5] The odds ratio for disease development in IPF was 9.0 and 21.8, respectively.[5] There was a 14.1-fold higher MUC5B expression in the lung of subjects with IPF compared with controls, and in control lungs, there was a 37.4-fold higher expression in individuals carrying the minor allele compared with those with the wild-type allele.[5] Immunohistochemical staining identifies accumulation of MUC5B in the honeycomb cyst in IPF and in the distal airways of normal lung.[49]

The MUC5B promoter polymorphism has been associated with chest computerized tomographic (CT) imaging evidence of lung abnormalities in a study of the general Framingham population.[50] Interstitial lung abnormalities were identified in 7% of all individuals studied.[50] Carriers of the minor allele had a 2.7-fold increase in the odds of imaging abnormalities and a 6.3-fold increase in the odds of definite chest CT evidence of pulmonary fibrosis.[50] Taken together, these data suggest that ILD associated with the *MUC5B* promoter SNP may be more common than previously considered, and in the future, it may be able to identify individuals with preclinical forms of IPF. Interestingly, although the MUC5B promoter polymorphism is associated with disease development, paradoxically, it has also been shown to be associated with improved survival, independent of age, sex, forced vital capacity, diffusing capacity of carbon monoxide, metalloproteinase-7 (MMP-7), or treatment status [26]. Because the minor allele of *MUC5B* is present in either the heterozygous or homozygous state in an estimated 19% of the general population,[5] and clinically apparent IPF occurs in less than 0.5% of the population,[1,2] other factors must play a role in disease development.

GENOME-WIDE ASSOCIATION STUDIES IDENTIFY COMMON VARIANTS

To date, three GWAS have been completed in IIP.[3−5] The first GWAS, conducted by Mushiroda and colleagues in 2008, studied 159 patients with IPF and 934 controls in a Japanese population. They identified an SNP in intron 2 of the TERT gene. In 2013, two additional studies were published using IIP subjects of European descent. Noth and colleagues evaluated 542 patients with IPF and 542 controls and identified five SNPs that reached genome-wide significance, including three SNPs in TOLLIP at 11p15.5, one MUC5B SNP at 11p15.5, and one SNP in SPPL2C at 17q21.31. Fingerlin and colleagues conducted a study of 1616 non-Hispanic white subjects with IIP and 4683 controls which confirmed genetic association with *TERT*, *TERC*, and *MUC5B*.[6] They also identified seven new loci, including *FAM13A, DSP, OBFC1, ATP11A, DPP9*, and chromosomal regions 7q22 and 15q14-15.[6] The *MUC5B* promoter SNP (rs35705950) remained the strongest genetic signal associated with IIP, with an odds ratio for disease development of 4.51 for a single risk allele compared with none.[6]

Like Noth and colleagues, Fingerlin and colleagues found several SNPs at the 17q21 locus that were significantly associated with IIP. However, Fingerlin and coauthors reported that the 17q21 region contains a common inversion polymorphism, and the haplotypes (referred to as H2) that contain the inversion show marked frequency differences across European populations.[51,52] When they stratified their GWAS discovery and replication samples, by carriage of the H2 haplotypes, and tested for association across the genome in those without the H2 haplotypes to assess the potential for confounding by local ancestry in the chromosome 17q21 region, the association signal at chromosome 17q21 was completely confounded by carriage of an H2 haplotype. This raises the possibility that SPPL2C could also be confounded by carriage of the H2 haplotypes. Fingerlin and colleagues also found 11 additional SNPs in the 11p15.5 region that were genome-wide significant. However, after adjustment for the MUC5B SNP (rs35705950), only one of the SNPs at 11p15 near MUC2 (rs4077759) remained associated with IIP ($P = .03$), suggesting that the associations observed with other SNPs, including TOLLIP, at 11p15.5 may be due to weak linkage disequilibrium with rs35705950. Interestingly, the risk estimates from the Fingerlin GWAS[6] and the *MUC5B* promoter SNP[5] are similar for both familial and sporadic forms of IPF, suggesting a common genetic etiology of both conditions.

Fingerlin and colleagues went on to perform a genome-wide genotype imputation analysis using data from their GWAS study to identify two HLA alleles associated with fibrosing IIP (DRB*15:01 and DQB1*06: 02).[53] These alleles were associated with increased lung tissue expression of DQB1 in fibrosing IIP.[53] Taken together, this may suggest a remaining role for autoimmunity in a subset of fibrosing IIP.

TRANSCRIPTIONAL PROFILING

In 2013, Yang and colleagues analyzed transcriptional profiles of lung tissue from 119 patients with IPF and 50 nondiseased controls using comparative RNA microarray data analysis.[54] Their analysis identified two distinct subsets of IPF based on gene expression patterns, suggesting that the disease we currently identify as IPF likely represents more than one disease process.[54] Elevated expression of cilium genes (DNAH6, DNAH7, DNAI1, and RPGRIP1L) were associated with more microscopic honeycombing and higher expression of both MUC5B and MMP-7 in adjacent lung tissue to that analyzed in the array.[54] These findings were validated in an independent cohort of 111 patients with IPF and 39 nondisease controls. Expression of cilium genes seems to identify two unique clinical IPF phenotypes, but it remains unclear if these different molecular profiles are associated with divergent outcomes or responses to therapy.

GENETIC SYNDROMES

Pulmonary fibrosis is known to complicate a number of genetic disorders, including Hermanski-Pudlak syndrome (HPS),[55] neurofibromatosis,[56] Niemann-Pick disease,[57,58] and Gaucher's disease.[59] Of these diseases, HPS is most similar to IPF. HPS is characterized by ocular albinism, platelet dysfunction, granulomatous colitis, and pulmonary fibrosis[60] and is thought to occur because of disturbed trafficking of intracellular secretory vesicles and lysosome-related organelles.[61] There are nine genetic loci associated with HPS, but only a few are associated with the development of pulmonary fibrosis.[61,62] Lung histology is suggested to bear similarities to the UIP pattern seen in IPF.[61] Impaired intracellular trafficking may result in alveolar epithelial dysfunction and a lower threshold for apoptosis leading to fibrosis.[62]

MOVING FORWARD

The recently conducted GWAS studies provide several new and interesting candidate genes. Each will require confirmation by sequencing and further testing. The genetics of pulmonary fibrosis provide novel pathways of interest that will require years of basic research before we understand the mechanisms by which these genes interact with the environment or each other to result in the development of pulmonary fibrosis. Individuals may be eager to use genetic profiling to provide risk estimates for disease development and/or prognosis; however, there are currently no data to support these types of estimates. The odds ratios for disease development apply at a population level. Prospective studies are needed to determine whether and how accurately such mutations predict what will happen to individuals who carry one or more of them.

REFERENCES

1. Raghu G, Collard HR, Egan JJ, et al. An official ATS/ERS/JRS/ALAT statement: idiopathic pulmonary fibrosis: evidence-based guidelines for diagnosis and management. *Am J Respir Crit Care Med.* 2011;183(6):788–824.
2. Olson AL, Swigris JJ, Lezotte DC, Norris JM, Wilson CG, Brown KK. Mortality from pulmonary fibrosis increased in the United States from 1992 to 2003. *Am J Respir Crit Care Med.* 2007;176(3):277–284.
3. Mushiroda T, Wattanapokayakit S, Takahashi A, et al. A genome-wide association study identifies an association of a common variant in TERT with susceptibility to idiopathic pulmonary fibrosis. *J Med Genet.* 2008;45(10):654–656.
4. Noth I. Genetic variants associated with idiopathic pulmonary fibrosis susceptibility and mortality: a genome-wide association study. *Lancet Respir Med.* 2013;1(4):309–317.
5. Seibold MA, Wise AL, Speer MC, et al. A common MUC5B promoter polymorphism and pulmonary fibrosis. *N Engl J Med.* 2011;364(16):1503–1512.
6. Fingerlin TE, Murphy E, Zhang W, et al. Genome-wide association study identifies multiple susceptibility loci for pulmonary fibrosis. *Nat Genet.* 2013;45(11):1409.
7. Javaheri S, Lederer DH, Pella JA, Mark GJ, Levine BW. Idiopathic pulmonary fibrosis in monozygotic twins. The importance of genetic predisposition. *Chest.* 1980;78(4):591–594.
8. Bitterman PB, Rennard SI, Keogh BA, Wewers MD, Adelberg S, Crystal RG. Familial idiopathic pulmonary fibrosis. Evidence of lung inflammation in unaffected family members. *N Engl J Med.* 1986;314(21):1343–1347.
9. Lee HL, Ryu JH, Wittmer MH, et al. Familial idiopathic pulmonary fibrosis: clinical features and outcome. *Chest.* 2005;127(6):2034–2041.
10. Steele MP, Speer MC, Loyd JE, et al. Clinical and pathologic features of familial interstitial pneumonia. *Am J Respir Crit Care Med.* 2005;172(9):1146–1152.
11. Adelman AG, Chertkow G, Hayton RC. Familial fibrocystic pulmonary dysplasia: a detailed family study. *Can Med Assoc J.* 1966;95(12):603–610.

12. Tsukahara M, Kajii T. Interstitial pulmonary fibrosis in two sisters. Possible autosomal recessive inheritance. *Jinrui Idengaku Zasshi.* 1983;28(4):263–267. Jpn J Hum Genet.

13. Loyd JE. Pulmonary fibrosis in families. *Am J Respir Cell Mol Biol.* 2003;29(Suppl 3):S47–S50.

14. van Moorsel CH, van Oosterhout MF, Barlo NP, et al. Surfactant protein C mutations are the basis of a significant portion of adult familial pulmonary fibrosis in a Dutch cohort. *Am J Respir Crit Care Med.* 2010;182(11): 1419–1425.

15. Ono S, Tanaka T, Ishida M, et al. Surfactant protein C G100S mutation causes familial pulmonary fibrosis in Japanese kindred. *Eur Respir J.* 2011;38(4):861–869.

16. Thomas AQ, Lane K, Phillips 3rd J, et al. Heterozygosity for a surfactant protein C gene mutation associated with usual interstitial pneumonitis and cellular nonspecific interstitial pneumonitis in one kindred. *Am J Respir Crit Care Med.* 2002;165(9):1322–1328.

17. Crossno PF, Polosukhin VV, Blackwell TS, et al. Identification of early interstitial lung disease in an individual with genetic variations in ABCA3 and SFTPC. *Chest.* 2010; 137(4):969–973.

18. Wang Y, Kuan PJ, Xing C, et al. Genetic defects in surfactant protein A2 are associated with pulmonary fibrosis and lung cancer. *Am J Hum Genet.* 2009;84(1):52–59.

19. Aalbers AM, Kajigaya S, van den Heuvel-Eibrink MM, van der Velden VH, Calado RT, Young NS. Human telomere disease due to disruption of the CCAAT box of the TERC promoter. *Blood.* 2012;119(13):3060–3063.

20. Tsakiri KD, Cronkhite JT, Kuan PJ, et al. Adult-onset pulmonary fibrosis caused by mutations in telomerase. *Proc Natl Acad Sci USA.* 2007;104(18):7552–7557.

21. Armanios MY, Chen JJ, Cogan JD, et al. Telomerase mutations in families with idiopathic pulmonary fibrosis. *N Engl J Med.* 2007;356(13):1317–1326.

22. Hodgson U, Pulkkinen V, Dixon M, et al. ELMOD2 is a candidate gene for familial idiopathic pulmonary fibrosis. *Am J Hum Genet.* 2006;79(1):149–154.

23. Stuart BD, Choi J, Zaidi S, et al. Exome sequencing links mutations in PARN and RTEL1 with familial pulmonary fibrosis and telomere shortening. *Nat Genet.* 2015;47(5): 512–517.

24. Amin RS, Wert SE, Baughman RP, et al. Surfactant protein deficiency in familial interstitial lung disease. *J Pediatr.* 2001;139(1):85–92.

25. Chibbar R, Shih F, Baga M, et al. Nonspecific interstitial pneumonia and usual interstitial pneumonia with mutation in surfactant protein C in familial pulmonary fibrosis. *Mod Pathol.* 2004;17(8):973–980.

26. Markart P, Ruppert C, Wygrecka M, et al. Surfactant protein C mutations in sporadic forms of idiopathic interstitial pneumonias. *Eur Respir J.* 2007;29(1):134–137.

27. Lawson WE, Crossno PF, Polosukhin VV, et al. Endoplasmic reticulum stress in alveolar epithelial cells is prominent in IPF: association with altered surfactant protein processing and herpesvirus infection. *Am J Physiol Lung Cell Mol Physiol.* 2008;294(6):L1119–L1126.

28. Korfei M, Ruppert C, Mahavadi P, et al. Epithelial endoplasmic reticulum stress and apoptosis in sporadic idiopathic pulmonary fibrosis. *Am J Respir Crit Care Med.* 2008;178(8):838–846.

29. Scavo LM, Ertsey R, Gao BQ. Human surfactant proteins A1 and A2 are differentially regulated during development and by soluble factors. *Am J Physiol.* 1998;275(4 Pt 1): L653–L669.

30. Maitra M, Cano CA, Garcia CK. Mutant surfactant A2 proteins associated with familial pulmonary fibrosis and lung cancer induce TGF-beta1 secretion. *Proc Natl Acad Sci USA.* 2012;109(51):21064–21069.

31. Kong CM, Lee XW, Wang X. Telomere shortening in human diseases. *FEBS J.* 2013;280(14):3180–3193.

32. Gramatges MM, Bertuch AA. Short telomeres: from dyskeratosis congenita to sporadic aplastic anemia and malignancy. *Transl Res.* 2013;162(6):353–363.

33. Wong JM, Collins K. Telomere maintenance and disease. *Lancet.* 2003;362(9388):983–988.

34. Vulliamy T, Marrone A, Goldman F, et al. The RNA component of telomerase is mutated in autosomal dominant dyskeratosis congenita. *Nature.* 2001;413(6854): 432–435.

35. Armanios M, Chen JL, Chang YP, et al. Haploinsufficiency of telomerase reverse transcriptase leads to anticipation in autosomal dominant dyskeratosis congenita. *Proc Natl Acad Sci USA.* 2005;102(44):15960–15964.

36. Vulliamy TJ, Walne A, Baskaradas A, Mason PJ, Marrone A, Dokal I. Mutations in the reverse transcriptase component of telomerase (TERT) in patients with bone marrow failure. *Blood Cells Mol Dis.* 2005;34(3):257–263.

37. Walne AJ, Vulliamy T, Marrone A, et al. Genetic heterogeneity in autosomal recessive dyskeratosis congenita with one subtype due to mutations in the telomerase-associated protein NOP10. *Hum Mol Genet.* 2007;16(13): 1619–1629.

38. Fernandez BA, Fox G, Bhatia R, et al. A Newfoundland cohort of familial and sporadic idiopathic pulmonary fibrosis patients: clinical and genetic features. *Respir Res.* 2012;13:64.

39. Cronkhite JT, Xing C, Raghu G, et al. Telomere shortening in familial and sporadic pulmonary fibrosis. *Am J Respir Crit Care Med.* 2008;178(7):729–737.

40. Diaz de Leon A, Cronkhite JT, Yilmaz C, et al. Subclinical lung disease, macrocytosis, and premature graying in kindreds with telomerase (TERT) mutations. *Chest.* 2011; 140(3):753–763.

41. Alder JK, Chen JJ, Lancaster L, et al. Short telomeres are a risk factor for idiopathic pulmonary fibrosis. *Proc Natl Acad Sci USA.* 2008;105(35):13051–13056.

42. Pulkkinen V, Bruce S, Rintahaka J, et al. ELMOD2, a candidate gene for idiopathic pulmonary fibrosis, regulates antiviral responses. *FASEB J.* 2010;24(4):1167–1177.

43. Borie R, Crestani B, Dieude P, et al. The MUC5B variant is associated with idiopathic pulmonary fibrosis but not with systemic sclerosis interstitial lung disease in the European Caucasian population. *PLoS One.* 2013;8(8):e70621.

44. Peljto AL, Steele MP, Fingerlin TE, et al. The pulmonary fibrosis-associated MUC5B promoter polymorphism does not influence the development of interstitial pneumonia in systemic sclerosis. *Chest.* 2012;142(6):1584–1588.

45. Stock CJ, Sato H, Fonseca C, et al. Mucin 5B promoter polymorphism is associated with idiopathic pulmonary fibrosis but not with development of lung fibrosis in systemic sclerosis or sarcoidosis. *Thorax.* 2013;68(5):436–441.

46. Zhang Y, Noth I, Garcia JG, Kaminski N. A variant in the promoter of MUC5B and idiopathic pulmonary fibrosis. *N Engl J Med.* 2011;364(16):1576–1577.

47. Horimasu Y, Ohshimo S, Bonella F, et al. MUC5B promoter polymorphism in Japanese patients with idiopathic pulmonary fibrosis. *Respirology.* 2015;20(3):439–444.

48. Wei R, Li C, Zhang M, et al. Association between MUC5B and TERT polymorphisms and different interstitial lung disease phenotypes. *Transl Res.* 2014;163(5):494–502.

49. Seibold MA, Smith RW, Urbanek C, et al. The idiopathic pulmonary fibrosis honeycomb cyst contains a mucociliary pseudostratified epithelium. *PLoS One.* 2013;8(3):e58658.

50. Hunninghake GM, Hatabu H, Okajima Y, et al. MUC5B promoter polymorphism and interstitial lung abnormalities. *N Engl J Med.* 2013;368(23):2192–2200.

51. Boettger LM, Handsaker RE, Zody MC, McCarroll SA. Structural haplotypes and recent evolution of the human 17q21.31 region. *Nat Genet.* 2012;44(8):881–885.

52. Steinberg KM, Antonacci F, Sudmant PH, et al. Structural diversity and African origin of the 17q21.31 inversion polymorphism. *Nat Genet.* 2012;44(8):872–880.

53. Fingerlin TE, Zhang W, Yang IV, et al. Genome-wide imputation study identifies novel HLA locus for pulmonary fibrosis and potential role for auto-immunity in fibrotic idiopathic interstitial pneumonia. *BMC Genet.* 2016;17(1):74.

54. Yang IV, Coldren CD, Leach SM, et al. Expression of cilium-associated genes defines novel molecular subtypes of idiopathic pulmonary fibrosis. *Thorax.* 2013;68(12):1114–1121.

55. Hermansky F, Pudlak P. Albinism associated with hemorrhagic diathesis and unusual pigmented reticular cells in the bone marrow: report of two cases with histochemical studies. *Blood.* 1959;14(2):162–169.

56. Trisolini R, Livi V, Lazzari Agli L, Patelli M. Diffuse lung disease in neurofibromatosis. *Lung.* 2012;190(2):249–250.

57. Nicholson AG, Florio R, Hansell DM, et al. Pulmonary involvement by Niemann-Pick disease. A report of six cases. *Histopathology.* 2006;48(5):596–603.

58. Gonzalez-Reimers E, Sanchez-Perez MJ, Bonilla-Arjona A, et al. Case report. Pulmonary involvement in an adult male affected by type B Niemann-Pick disease. *Br J Radiol.* 2003;76(911):838–840.

59. Jarnvig IL, Milman N, Jacobsen GK, Kassis E. Adult Gaucher's disease with pulmonary involvement. *Ugeskrift Laeger.* 1991;153(40):2832–2834.

60. Gahl WA, Brantly M, Kaiser-Kupfer MI, et al. Genetic defects and clinical characteristics of patients with a form of oculocutaneous albinism (Hermansky-Pudlak syndrome). *N Engl J Med.* 1998;338(18):1258–1264.

61. Pierson DM, Ionescu D, Qing G, et al. Pulmonary fibrosis in hermansky-pudlak syndrome. A case report and review. *Respir Int Rev Thorac Dis.* 2006;73(3):382–395.

62. Young LR, Gulleman PM, Bridges JP, et al. The alveolar epithelium determines susceptibility to lung fibrosis in Hermansky-Pudlak syndrome. *Am J Respir Crit Care Med.* 2012;186(10):1014–1024.

CHAPTER 5

Imaging of Idiopathic Pulmonary Fibrosis

J. CALEB RICHARDS, MD • TILMAN KOELSCH, MD

INTRODUCTION

Imaging plays an important role in the diagnosis of idiopathic pulmonary fibrosis (IPF). The radiologic and histologic pattern that correlates with IPF is usual interstitial pneumonia (UIP). Several studies have shown that a confident UIP pattern determined by high-resolution computed tomography (HRCT) confers a positive predictive value of 95%−100% for histologic UIP.[1−7] This means that, in the appropriate clinical setting, patients with a UIP pattern at HRCT do not need to undergo surgical lung biopsy to establish the diagnosis of IPF. However, a confident HRCT pattern of UIP cannot be achieved in a substantial portion of patients who are ultimately diagnosed with IPF.[8−10] Additionally, a UIP pattern of fibrosis does not necessarily indicate IPF, as several other entities can result in a UIP pattern. When clinical suspicion and the imaging diagnosis do not coincide, multidisciplinary discussion should take place to work through causes of diagnostic uncertainty. The clear impact of imaging in the diagnosis of IPF stresses the importance of a firm understanding of the computed tomography (CT) features of fibrotic lung disease and evolving classification scheme for UIP. Additionally, imaging can provide information on prognosis, identify complications, and give clues to alternative diagnoses in the differential.

COMPUTED TOMOGRAPHY FEATURES OF FIBROTIC LUNG DISEASE

Honeycombing

The Fleischner Society defines honeycombing as clustered, cystic air spaces with well-defined walls, subpleural location, and nearly uniform diameter, usually 3−10 mm, although can measure up to 25 mm[11] (Fig. 5.1). Although often cited as multilayered, a single layer of subpleural cysts is sufficient to establish honeycombing.[12] It is important to note that the radiologic and histologic definitions of honeycombing differ. The histologic definition of honeycombing is "destroyed and fibrotic lung tissue with numerous cystic air spaces with thick fibrous walls representing the late stage of various lung diseases, with complete loss of acinar architecture," measuring 1−2 mm and below resolution of HRCT.[13−15] Histologic honeycombing may be absent in patients with honeycombing on CT and vice versa.[16] Despite this contrast, radiologic honeycombing plays a very important role classifying fibrosing lung disease and is the requisite feature of a typical UIP pattern.

Reticulation

Reticular abnormality is often seen in fibrotic lung disease, manifesting at HRCT as fine or coarse netlike linear opacity (Fig. 5.2). As defined by the Fleischner Society, reticular abnormality represents interlobular septal thickening, intralobular lines, or the walls of honeycomb cysts.[11] In UIP, the reticular abnormality is heterogeneous, showing variable thickening of the lines and irregular spacing. In contrast, reticular abnormality in nonspecific interstitial pneumonia (NSIP) is more evenly spaced and homogenous in appearance.[17]

Hunninghake et al. showed that the combination of upper lung irregular lines and honeycombing were the CT findings most predictive of histologic UIP.[18] This upper lung reticulation should not be misinterpreted to imply upper lung predominance of fibrosis. Rather, an overall craniocaudal gradient of fibrosis is maintained, but reticulation often involves all lung zones and extends into the upper lungs.

Traction Bronchiectasis

Traction bronchiectasis or bronchiolectasis represents bronchial or bronchiolar irregularity and dilation due to adjacent fibrotic and distorted lung parenchyma[11] (Fig. 5.3). The presence of background fibrosis is key in distinguishing traction bronchiectasis from free-standing bronchiectasis.[12] Traction bronchiolectasis can be challenging to distinguish from honeycombing and may have been a source of disagreement regarding the presence or absence of honeycombing in previous studies.[19] Using multiplanar and contiguous images can be helpful in distinguishing between honeycombing and traction bronchiectasis. Traction bronchiectasis has been shown to be reversible in cases of nitrofurantoin-induced lung toxicity.[20] In the setting of UIP, however, reversibility is not noted, and traction bronchiectasis actually has poor prognostic significance.

Ground Glass

Ground glass opacity is defined as hazy increased lung density that does not obscure underlying bronchovascular structures[11] (Fig. 5.4). In patients with fibrotic lung disease, it is common to see ground glass abnormality superimposed on background reticular abnormality or associated with traction bronchiectasis and should not be regarded as inconsistent with a UIP pattern. However, if the ground glass is diffuse or separate from areas of fibrosis, other etiologies should be considered, such as an acute exacerbation or infection.[17]

CLASSIFICATION OF USUAL INTERSTITIAL PNEUMONIA

In 2011, the American Thoracic Society, European Respiratory Society, Japanese Respiratory Society, and Latin American Thoracic Association issued a joint statement on evidence-based guidelines for the diagnosis and management of IPF.[21] The importance of HRCT in the diagnosis of IPF was emphasized, requiring a UIP pattern on HRCT in patients who do not undergo surgical lung biopsy or specific HRCT and surgical lung biopsy patterns in patients who do undergo biopsy. The guideline outlines three categories for the HRCT diagnosis of UIP: UIP, possible UIP, and inconsistent with UIP.

More recently, the Fleischner Society issued a White Paper on the diagnostic criteria for IPF with HRCT categories of typical UIP, probable UIP, indeterminate

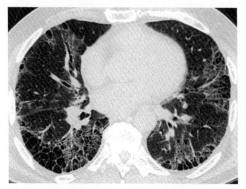

FIG. 5.1

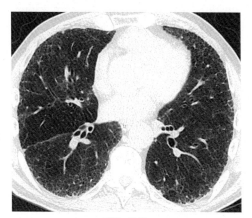

FIG. 5.2

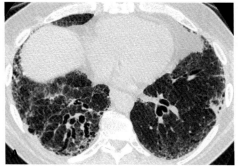

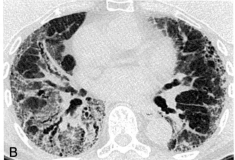

FIG. 5.3

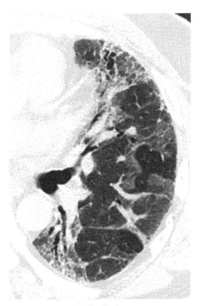

FIG. 5.4

for UIP, and CT features most suggestive of a non-IPF diagnosis.[17] These updated diagnostic criteria reflect important advances in knowledge since the 2011 guidelines. Specifically, a confident diagnosis of IPF can be made if a CT pattern of typical or probable UIP is present and the clinical context is appropriate. The implication is that patients with probable UIP may not have to undergo surgical lung biopsy. This is contrary to the 2011 guidelines, which would have classified a probable UIP pattern as possible UIP, conferring the recommendation of surgical lung biopsy. Second, it is now recognized that some CT features previously regarded as "inconsistent with UIP" (e.g., mosaic attenuation and air trapping) may be found in subjects with histologic UIP; after lung biopsy and multidisciplinary evaluation, these cases may be diagnosed with IPF.

In the updated classification scheme, a **typical** UIP pattern of fibrosis must show a distribution that is peripheral in the axial plane and diffuse to lower lung predominant in the craniocaudal plane. Honeycombing is a requisite finding for the diagnosis of a typical UIP pattern. Reticulation and traction bronchiectasis are often present but not required. Features from the "most consistent with a non-IPF diagnosis" category are absent. The **probable** UIP pattern does not have honeycombing but is otherwise similar to typical UIP. The **indeterminate** UIP pattern shows evidence of fibrosis with some inconspicuous features that might suggest a non-UIP pattern (e.g., peribronchovascular

extension of fibrosis, pure ground glass attenuation, mosaic attenuation, air trapping). **CT features most consistent with a non-IPF diagnosis** include any of the following features: an upper or midlung predominant fibrosis, peribronchovascular predominance with subpleural sparing, predominant consolidation, extensive ground glass opacity, diffuse nodules or cysts, or extensive mosaic attenuation with extensive sharply defined lobular air trapping on expiration (Fig. 5.5).

PROGNOSTIC VALUE OF COMPUTED TOMOGRAPHY IN USUAL INTERSTITIAL PNEUMONIA

It is clear that the overall extent of visually evident fibrosis is an important predictor of mortality in IPF.[22,23] However, studies evaluating the prognostic value of individual CT features show mixed results. Sumikawa et al. showed that in patients with IPF and histologic UIP, traction bronchiectasis and the overall percentage of parenchymal involvement of fibrosis were most influential predictors of prognosis, while the pattern did not statistically influence prognosis.[24] Edey et al. studied the findings of 146 patients with fibrotic idiopathic interstitial pneumonia and found the severity score of traction bronchiectasis was the greatest predictor of poor prognosis, no matter the background pattern.[25]

CHALLENGES IN CLASSIFYING USUAL INTERSTITIAL PNEUMONIA

Diagnostic Dilemma of Honeycombing

Honeycombing is a requisite feature for a UIP pattern, but the agreement on its presence can be challenging. Watadani et al. showed only moderate agreement on the identification of honeycombing among radiologists.[19] Disagreement may partly be related to mimics of honeycombing, such as traction bronchiectasis, thin-walled cysts, and complicated emphysema. Careful evaluation of multiplanar images can help resolve these dilemmas. Another potential cause for disagreement is lack of consistency regarding the definition of honeycombing, particularly whether honeycombing should be multilayered or whether a single layer would suffice. Most authors now agree that a single layer of subpleural honeycomb cysts is adequate for diagnosis.[17] However, several recent papers have emphasized that the diagnosis of UIP can be made in the absence of honeycombing. For example, Gruden studied 38 patients with a clinical diagnosis of IPF and HRCT without honeycombing but otherwise meeting criteria for UIP.[26] Heterogeneity of fibrosis and upper lung involvement were

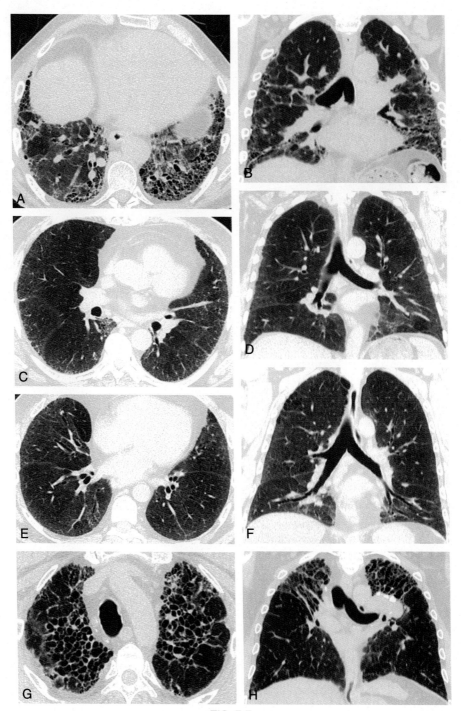

FIG. 5.5

shown to be helpful features in characterizing UIP. Chung et al. showed that CT features of probable UIP had an 82% predictive value for the presence of histologic UIP.[16]

Mosaic Pattern and Air Trapping

The 2011 guideline suggests that a mosaic pattern or air trapping in three or more lobes is inconsistent with UIP. The intent is that air trapping may suggest an alternative diagnosis, such as hypersensitivity pneumonitis (HP). However, the requirement of three lobes seems arbitrary and rigid. Additionally, recent studies suggest that a mosaic pattern or air trapping is not uncommon in IPF. Silva et al. showed mosaic attenuation in 43% of cases with biopsy-proven UIP.[6] In a separate study of patients with IPF from the IPFNet cohort, a mosaic pattern or air trapping was present in 21.3% of patients with histologic UIP. Although there is a likely selection bias in this study, the suggestion is that the 2011 guideline's criteria for "inconsistent with UIP" are too restrictive.[27] For this reason, the recent Fleischner Society criteria indicate that "extensive mosaic attenuation with extensive sharply defined lobular air trapping" is required to suggest a non-IPF diagnosis.[17]

Asymmetric Fibrosis

Asymmetric distribution of fibrosis should not sway one away from UIP or IPF and indeed may support this diagnosis. Interestingly, patients with asymmetric fibrosis showed higher rates of gastroesophageal reflux (GER) (62.5% vs. 31.3%) and acute exacerbation (46.9% vs. 17.2%) compared with patients with symmetric disease.[28]

Atypical Appearance of Idiopathic Pulmonary Fibrosis

Although imaging can help diagnose IPF when typical UIP findings are present, the absence of such findings does not exclude IPF. A confident diagnosis of UIP on HRCT coinciding with a strong clinical suspicion has a very high positive predictive value for IPF, reported over 95%.[1–4,18] However, it is important to recognize that a significant portion of patients that are ultimately diagnosed with IPF may not have a UIP pattern of pulmonary fibrosis on HRCT. This is often secondary to the inability to characterize the pattern of fibrosis as UIP with a high degree of confidence. Many recent studies highlight this issue. For example, in a recent trial of 1061 patients with IPF, only 567 (53%) had typical UIP findings.[29] A separate trial of 428 patients with IPF revealed only 141 (32.9%) had a confident HRCT diagnosis of UIP.[30] Additional studies have shown

that up to 60% of patients with typical histologic UIP do not have typical HRCT findings of UIP.[8,24,27] Hence, IPF should not be excluded if a confident HRCT pattern of UIP is not established.

Patients with IPF may present with imaging features "inconsistent with UIP" by the 2011 guidelines, or "suggestive of an alternative diagnosis" by the Fleischner Society criteria, such as chronic HP, NSIP, sarcoidosis, or organizing pneumonia.[4,6,8,24,27] If such features are present, an alternative diagnosis must be strongly considered.

Familial Pulmonary Fibrosis

IPF may cluster in families and is thought to often have a strong genetic component. Nearly 20% of patients undergoing lung transplant for IPF have a family history of pulmonary fibrosis.[31] Several genetic loci have been linked to pulmonary fibrosis.[32–36] The most likely mode of genetic inheritance is autosomal dominant transmission with incomplete penetrance,[37–39] which helps explain why such patients often have not only one, but several family members with interstitial lung disease (ILD).

Individuals with familial pulmonary fibrosis are still considered to be idiopathic for management purposes. Many cases of familial IPF are indistinguishable from IPF. However, familial IPF does have some radiologic differences, with a higher prevalence of diffuse or upper lung involvement.[38,40] In our experience, family members may have dissimilar patterns of fibrosis. In patients with a family history of pulmonary fibrosis but do not meet the criteria for typical UIP, careful multidisciplinary discussion is needed, as a diagnosis of IPF can still be made.

MULTIDISCIPLINARY EVALUATION

Multidisciplinary discussion and dynamic interaction among expert pulmonologists, radiologists, and pathologists is essential in establishing the correct diagnosis of IPF. In a study by Flaherty et al.,[41] 58 consecutive patients with suspected idiopathic interstitial pneumonia were evaluated by clinicians, radiologists, and pathologists. In sequential steps, increasing information was provided, and each expert recorded their diagnosis and level of confidence with each step. The level of confidence in the diagnosis increased with each step. On disclosure of histology, radiologists were shown to change their final diagnosis more than clinicians. Final histologic diagnosis was "IPF" in 30 cases. Clinicians identified 75% of these cases before histology was revealed, whereas radiologists identified

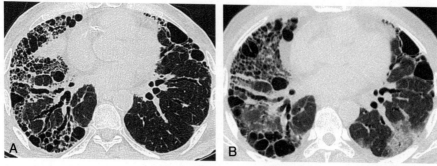

FIG. 5.6

48%.[41] Importantly, in 11 (19%) of the 58 cases, the histologic diagnosis was changed following multidisciplinary discussion. This suggests that histologic diagnosis can no longer be regarded as a gold standard for clinical diagnosis.

COMPLICATIONS

Acute Exacerbation

The natural history of IPF has been described as a steady, progressive decline in lung function, although recent evidence suggests that the clinical course may be less predictable, with some patients experiencing acute respiratory deterioration.[42,43] These acute episodes have been labeled acute exacerbations of IPF. The main histologic finding associated with an acute exacerbation is diffuse alveolar damage, especially in the organizing phase, while organizing pneumonia is the next most common pattern.[43,44] At HRCT, bilateral ground glass and consolidative opacities are commonly seen superimposed on the background fibrosis[43,44] (Fig. 5.6). Distribution of the opacities is most commonly diffuse but can also be multifocal or peripheral.[45] Multifocal and peripheral patterns have better survival; although, interestingly, the multifocal pattern is thought to be a precursor to the diffuse pattern.[46] Before attributing the ground glass opacity and consolidation to an acute exacerbation, other acute entities, such as infection and pulmonary edema, should be excluded.

Lung Cancer

The risk of lung cancer is markedly increased in patients with IPF, particularly older male smokers.[47,48] Lung cancer in patients with IPF shows lower lobe predominance and commonly arises in the periphery of the lung in areas of fibrosis[49–51] (Fig. 5.7). A recent study of 63 patients with lung cancer in the setting of an idiopathic interstitial pneumonia showed that 53% of tumors occurred at the interface of fibrotic and normal lung parenchyma.[51] The morphologic appearance is variable and has been reported as well defined or lobulated nodules, as well as areas of mass-like consolidation. While the appearance is variable, this information should encourage the radiologist to carefully scrutinize the peripheral fibrotic parenchyma for any new or progressing abnormality, especially because there can be a delay of the initial diagnosis of lung cancer in the setting of idiopathic interstitial pneumonia.[51] Adenocarcinoma and squamous cell carcinoma are the two most common histologic types of lung cancer in IPF.[47,51]

Pulmonary Hypertension

Patients with IPF are at increased risk to develop pulmonary hypertension (PH), which is associated with worse outcomes.[52] Transthoracic echocardiography is a frequently used screening tool for PH, but its accuracy is diminished in patients with fibrotic lung disease.[53] Measurement of the main pulmonary artery (PA) diameter and assessment of the main PA to ascending aorta ratio are two methods used in assessment of PH on HRCT and are attractive options as they are noninvasive. However, the results are conflicting as to how reliable these measurements are in actually predicting PH. One study found that a main PA diameter greater than or equal to 29 mm and segmental artery to bronchus ratio >1.1 in three or four lobes has 100% specificity for PH.[54] The same study showed that using a main PA diameter ≥29 mm alone in patients with parenchymal lung disease has an 84% specificity and 75% specificity for PH. McCall et al. showed using a main PA diameter >30 mm in patients with scleroderma yielded a sensitivity of 81.3% and specificity of 87.5%.[55] The main PA:AA ratio >1 has been shown to be associated with worse outcomes in patients with IPF and may be more reliable than using the absolute PA diameter.[56] It has been hypothesized that PA

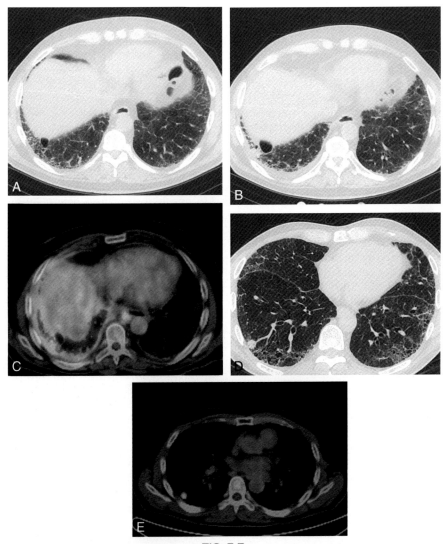

FIG. 5.7

diameter may be increased in patients with fibrosis because of traction-related effects, further leading to hesitancy in using this as a reliable marker for PH.[56] Further work is needed, although using the PA:AA ratio may provide more prognostic value.

Gastroesophageal Reflux

GER occurs in a high number of patients with IPF. Raghu et al. showed a prevalence of GER in 87% of patients with IPF as measured by 24 h pH probe, although less than half actually described symptoms of GER.[57] GER is thought to contribute to disease progression in IPF, and studies have shown antiacid

treatment may be beneficial.[58] The prevalence of hiatal hernia on CT in IPF is about 39%, substantially higher than in COPD or asthma.[59]

Combined Pulmonary Fibrosis and Emphysema

Combined pulmonary fibrosis and emphysema (CPFE) is a distinct phenotype of IPF, but it is still regarded as IPF in the idiopathic interstitial pneumonia classification system.[60] Recognition of this abnormality is important as the prognosis is worse than IPF alone, which is driven by the increased risk of PH and lung cancer. Patients who are typically older men who present with severe dyspnea and relatively preserved lung volumes (mildly subnormal spirometry), however, have severely impaired carbon monoxide diffusion capacity and marked hypoxemia during exercise. This contrasts with a typical IPF patient who shows reduced lung volumes and restrictive spirometry with advanced disease.[61-65]

The presence of emphysema can influence the correct diagnosis of the HRCT pattern. Akira et al. showed the difficulty in distinguishing between UIP and NSIP in individuals with superimposed emphysema, with the correct diagnosis being made in only 44% of readings (30 of 68). The difficulty may partly be related to increased coarseness of the parenchyma and emphysema or cysts being mistaken for honeycombing.[66]

On HRCT in patients with both UIP and emphysema, it is important that radiologists specifically describe the severity and extent of emphysema. Currently, there is no clear consensus definition of CPFE. Smoking is a risk factor for the development of both IPF and emphysema, and up to one-third of patients with IPF have emphysema. However, many of these patients do not have the characteristics associated with CPFE.[10,63,64,67,68] Given the lack of consensus diagnostic criteria, a clear description of the severity of emphysema may help the clinician evaluate if a patient with UIP has features that suggest the distinct phenotype of CPFE.

DIFFERENTIAL DIAGNOSIS
A UIP pattern on HRCT or histology does not always equate a firm clinical diagnosis of IPF. A variety of other conditions can result in a UIP pattern of fibrosis, including connective tissue disease (CTD), chronic HP, and drug reactions. Therefore, it is important to evaluate for other secondary causes of a UIP pattern of fibrosis even if the clinical situation is appropriate for IPF. For example, potential exposures that could result in chronic HP should be discussed even if the clinical situation is appropriate for IPF,[39,69] including in elderly male patients that have a much higher likelihood of having IPF based on age and gender alone.[70-72] The importance of this is not only to determine an accurate diagnosis, but there are also prognostic and treatment implications for different causes of a UIP pattern on HRCT.

Nonspecific Interstitial Pneumonia
NSIP is the second most common idiopathic interstitial pneumonia and carries a much better prognosis than

UIP.[60] Unfortunately, NSIP is the least agreed upon pattern by radiologists, largely due to significant overlap with other idiopathic interstitial pneumonias, including UIP.[5,73] There are features that are helpful in distinguishing NSIP from UIP. Particularly, subpleural sparing has a high specificity for NSIP (Fig. 5.8) but is only present in up to 63% of patients.[73,74] Other unique features are the confluent appearance of the fibrosis in the axial plane and areas of peribronchovascular extension and minimal or no involvement of the upper lungs. Mildly extensive NSIP and UIP can have a similar appearance, with both often presenting as basilar predominant fibrosis without honeycombing.[21,74-78] Up to one-third of patients with NSIP progress to a UIP pattern.[60,79-82] Typical features (peribronchovascular fibrosis with traction bronchiectasis, subpleural sparing, and little involvement of the upper lungs) permit a confident diagnosis of NSIP, when present. However, the overlap of NSIP and UIP should be recognized. If there is clinical uncertainty, surgical lung biopsy may be required for a more definitive diagnosis.

Chronic Hypersensitivity Pneumonitis
Chronic HP is classically described as upper lung predominant pulmonary fibrosis.[6,10,83] Interestingly, a significant portion of patients with chronic HP present with mid to lower lung distribution of fibrosis, and approximately 30% of patients show a UIP pattern.[6,39,84] Various clues can help suggest chronic HP, the most important being lobular air trapping (Fig. 5.9). Lobular air trapping is present in three or more lobes. If all lobes are involved, chronic HP is strongly suggested.[38,85,86] This stresses the importance of routinely obtaining expiratory images as part of the HRCT protocol. Other findings that may suggest HP include profuse centrilobular ground glass nodules, extensive ground glass opacity, or mosaic attenuation.[78,84,85] Unfortunately, these findings are often absent, and patients with chronic HP may present with a UIP pattern and no other imaging features to suggest HP.[84,86] Although a thorough history is important in identifying potential exposures that may cause HP, no causal antigen is identified in up to 50%−60% of patients ultimately diagnosed with HP,[87,88] many of who are likely related to an unrecognized antigen. Bronchoalveolar lavage (BAL) may be helpful. Lymphocytes often account for greater than 40% of white blood cells on BAL. Lymphocytosis may resolve or be absent in some cases. As one can see, the diagnosis of chronic HP is often difficult to make, and no universally accepted criteria exist.[17,83]

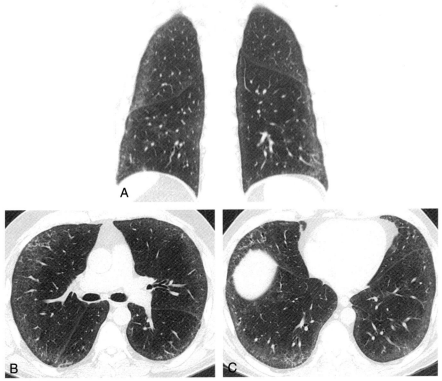

FIG. 5.8

Connective Tissue Disease

Patients with CTD can develop ILDs, including UIP. The presence of esophageal dilatation, pleural effusion, or pericardial abnormality should raise the possibility of an underlying CTD. Recently, Chung et al. described signs that suggest a UIP pattern related to underlying CTD. This includes the "straight edge" (sharp horizontal demarcation between fibrotic and normal lung, without substantial extension along the lateral chest wall), "exuberant honeycomb" (honeycomb cysts involving more than 70% of the fibrotic parts of the lung), and "anterior upper lobe" signs (lower lobe fibrosis, with relatively focal fibrosis in the anterior upper lobes).[89] Otherwise, there is significant overlap between HRCT findings of UIP related to CTD and IPF,[17,90,91] and it is often very difficult to distinguish an underlying cause.

UIP is the most common pattern in rheumatoid arthritis associated interstitial lung disease (RA-ILD) (Fig. 5.10). Lee et al. found UIP (56%) to be the most common pattern in RA-ILD, followed by NSIP (33%), and organizing pneumonia (11%).[92] Given that rheumatoid arthritis is diagnosed in 1% of the population,

and 7% of those develop RA-ILD, this is clearly an important cause of a UIP pattern of fibrosis.[90,93–95]

Other forms of CTD manifest as UIP less frequently. In scleroderma, NSIP is the most common pattern, followed by a smaller, but substantial, number of patients with UIP.[96–98] NSIP is also the most common pattern in dermatomyositis/polymyositis and mixed CTD, although a UIP pattern can be seen. Sjögren syndrome—related ILD typically manifests as lymphocytic interstitial pneumonia, with UIP rarely seen.[95,99] ILD is uncommon in systemic lupus erythematosus, manifesting in 3% of patients, with NSIP and UIP potentially seen.[95,100–103] A UIP pattern in CTD often has a poorer prognosis compared with CTD with a non-UIP pattern.[90,99,104–106]

A popular topic related to CTD is interstitial pneumonia with autoimmune features IPAF. This refers to patients with ILD who do not meet the criteria for any specific CTD but have some autoimmune features or nonspecific but suggestive serology.[91,107–112] Many of these patients have a UIP pattern, and outcomes similar to IPF.[69] Recent criteria have been proposed to identify

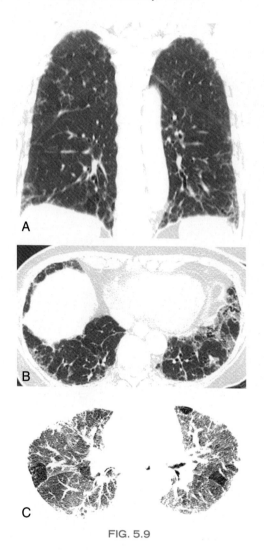

FIG. 5.9

patients with IPAF but have not yet been validated in their ability to differentiate from IPF. Patients with IPAF should be considered to have IPF if they otherwise would fit this diagnosis.[17]

Drug-Related Pulmonary Fibrosis

A large number of medications can result in lung injury and ILD.[113] Most cases of drug toxicity demonstrate an organizing pneumonia or NSIP pattern rather than UIP. Methotrexate and nitrofurantoin are among the drugs most commonly presenting as UIP, although the pattern of lung injury can vary.[78,114] If present, superimposed organizing pneumonia may be helpful in suggesting drug toxicity as a secondary cause of UIP. Establishing a temporal relationship may be helpful in suggesting drug toxicity as the cause of the ILD, but pulmonary manifestations may be delayed weeks or months,[115] making the diagnosis more difficult. Multidisciplinary discussion should address the relevance of any medication exposures that could result in lung injury.

Asbestosis and Occupational Lung Disease

Asbestosis (i.e., asbestos-induced pulmonary fibrosis) has an imaging pattern similar to that seen in IPF. Asbestos-related pleural disease is more common than asbestosis and manifests as bilateral pleural plaques, pleural calcifications, and/or significant pleural thickening. Therefore, the majority of patients with asbestosis also have asbestos-related pleural disease, which is very useful in differentiating asbestosis from IPF (Fig. 5.11). Asbestosis rarely presents without pleural disease.[46,116,117] Asbestosis typically develops at least 20–40 years after exposure. Acquiring history, severity, and latency of any prior asbestos exposure history is necessary in evaluating patients with pulmonary fibrosis.[117,118]

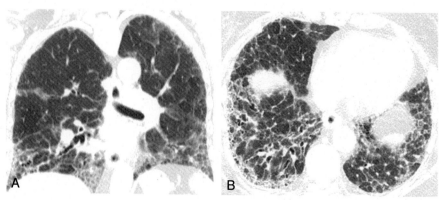

FIG. 5.10

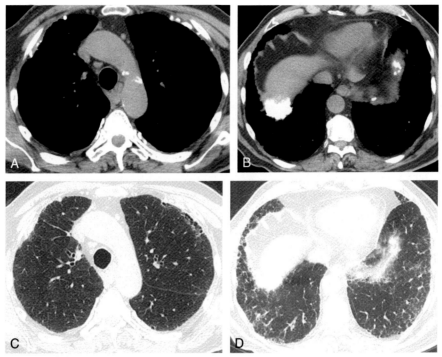

FIG. 5.11

Other occupational exposures that can result in pulmonary fibrosis include dust and mining.[119,120] An IPF-like condition can be seen in up to 10% of coal miners and those with silicosis.[119,121] Such patients tend to be older with a longer exposure history.[122] Uranium miners may also develop pulmonary fibrosis, including UIP, which is thought to be radiation induced. Although such patients also often have concomitant silica exposure, fibrosis may develop without evidence of silicosis, as determined by biopsy or autopsy.[123]

CONCLUSION

Imaging not only plays a critical role in the diagnosis of IPF but also provides input on the prognosis and identifies complications. Recognition of definite or probable patterns of UIP on CT, in the correct clinical context, permits a confident diagnosis without biopsy. However, biopsy and multidisciplinary evaluation remain important in establishing the diagnosis in those with less typical CT features and in those with potentially significant exposures or CTD.

REFERENCES

1. Hunninghake GW, Zimmerman MB, Schwartz DA, et al. Utility of a lung biopsy for the diagnosis of idiopathic pulmonary fibrosis. *Am J Respir Crit Care Med.* 2001;164(2): 193–196. https://doi.org/10.1164/ajrccm.164.2.2101090.
2. Lee KS, Primack SL, Staples CA, Mayo JR, Aldrich JE, Müller NL. Chronic infiltrative lung disease: comparison of diagnostic accuracies of radiography and low- and conventional-dose thin-section CT. *Radiology.* 1994;191(3):669–673. https://doi.org/10.1148/radiology.191.3.8184044.
3. Grenier P, Valeyre D, Cluzel P, Brauner MW, Lenoir S, Chastang C. Chronic diffuse interstitial lung disease: diagnostic value of chest radiography and high-resolution CT. *Radiology.* 1991;179(1):123–132. https://doi.org/10.1148/radiology.179.1.2006262.
4. Swensen SJ, Aughenbaugh GL, Myers JL. Diffuse lung disease: diagnostic accuracy of CT in patients undergoing surgical biopsy of the lung. *Radiology.* 1997;205(1):229–234. https://doi.org/10.1148/radiology.205.1.9314990.
5. Flaherty KR, Thwaite EL, Kazerooni EA, et al. Radiological versus histological diagnosis in UIP and NSIP: survival implications. *Thorax.* 2003;58(2):143–148. https://doi.org/10.1136/thorax.58.2.143.

6. Silva CIS, Müller NL, Lynch DA, et al. Chronic hypersensitivity pneumonitis: differentiation from idiopathic pulmonary fibrosis and nonspecific interstitial pneumonia by using thin-section CT. *Radiology*. 2008;246(1):288–297. https://doi.org/10.1148/radiol.2453061881.

7. Johkoh T, Müller NL, Cartier Y, et al. Idiopathic interstitial pneumonias: diagnostic accuracy of thin-section CT in 129 patients. *Radiology*. 1999;211(2):555–560. https://doi.org/10.1148/radiology.211.2.r99ma01555.

8. Sverzellati N, Wells AU, Tomassetti S, et al. Biopsy-proved idiopathic pulmonary fibrosis: spectrum of nondiagnostic thin-section CT diagnoses. *Radiology*. 2010;254(3):957–964. https://doi.org/10.1148/radiol.0990898.

9. Nicholson AG, Addis BJ, Bharucha H, et al. Inter-observer variation between pathologists in diffuse parenchymal lung disease. *Thorax*. 2004;59(6):500–505. https://doi.org/10.1136/thx.2003.011734.

10. Martin MD, Chung JH, Kanne JP. Idiopathic pulmonary fibrosis. *J Thorac Imaging*. 2016;31(3):127–139. https://doi.org/10.1097/RTI.0000000000000204.

11. Hansell DM, Bankier AA, MacMahon H, McLoud TC, Müller NL, Remy J. Fleischner society: glossary of terms for thoracic imaging. *Radiology*. 2008;246(3):697–722. https://doi.org/10.1148/radiol.2462070712.

12. Jacob J, Hansell DM. HRCT of fibrosing lung disease. *Respirology*. 2015;20(6):859–872. https://doi.org/10.1111/resp.12531.

13. Arakawa H, Honma K. Honeycomb lung: history and current concepts. *AJR Am J Roentgenol*. 2011;196(4):773–782. https://doi.org/10.2214/AJR.10.4873.

14. Genereux GP. The end-stage lung: pathogenesis, pathology, and radiology. *Radiology*. 1975;116(02):279–289. https://doi.org/10.1148/116.2.279.

15. Nishimura K, Kitaichi M, Izumi T, Nagai S, Kanaoka M, Itoh H. Usual interstitial pneumonia: histologic correlation with high-resolution CT. *Radiology*. 1992;182(2):337–342. https://doi.org/10.1148/radiology.182.2.1732946.

16. Chung JH, Chawla A, Peljto AL, et al. CT scan findings of probable usual interstitial pneumonitis have a high predictive value for histologic usual interstitial pneumonitis. *Chest*. 2015;147(2):450–459. https://doi.org/10.1378/chest.14-0976.

17. Lynch DA, Sverzellati N, Travis WD, et al. Diagnostic criteria for idiopathic pulmonary fibrosis: a Fleischner society white paper. *Lancet Respir Med*. November 2017. https://doi.org/10.1016/S2213-2600(17)30433-2.

18. Hunninghake GW, Lynch DA, Galvin JR, et al. Radiologic findings are strongly associated with a pathologic diagnosis of usual interstitial pneumonia. *Chest*. 2003;124(4):1215–1223.

19. Watadani T, Sakai F, Johkoh T, et al. Interobserver variability in the CT assessment of honeycombing in the lungs. *Radiology*. 2013;266(3):936–944. https://doi.org/10.1148/radiol.12112516.

20. Sheehan RE, Wells AU, Milne DG, Hansell DM. Nitrofurantoin-induced lung disease: two cases demonstrating resolution of apparently irreversible CT abnormalities. *J Comput Assist Tomogr*. 2000;24(2):259–261.

21. Raghu G, Collard HR, Egan JJ, et al. An official ATS/ERS/JRS/ALAT statement: idiopathic pulmonary fibrosis: evidence-based guidelines for diagnosis and management. *Am J Respir Crit Care Med*. 2011;183(6):788–824. https://doi.org/10.1164/rccm.2009-040GL.

22. Best AC, Meng J, Lynch AM, et al. Idiopathic pulmonary fibrosis: physiologic tests, quantitative CT indexes, and CT visual scores as predictors of mortality. *Radiology*. 2008;246(3):935–940. https://doi.org/10.1148/radiol.2463062200.

23. Lynch DA, Godwin JD, Safrin S, et al. High-resolution computed tomography in idiopathic pulmonary fibrosis: diagnosis and prognosis. *Am J Respir Crit Care Med*. 2005;172(4):488–493. https://doi.org/10.1164/rccm.200412-1756OC.

24. Sumikawa H, Johkoh T, Colby TV, et al. Computed tomography findings in pathological usual interstitial pneumonia: relationship to survival. *Am J Respir Crit Care Med*. 2008;177(4):433–439. https://doi.org/10.1164/rccm.200611-1696OC.

25. Edey AJ, Devaraj AA, Barker RP, Nicholson AG, Wells AU, Hansell DM. Fibrotic idiopathic interstitial pneumonias: HRCT findings that predict mortality. *Eur Radiol*. 2011;21(8):1586–1593. https://doi.org/10.1007/s00330-011-2098-2.

26. Gruden JF, Panse PM, Gotway MB, Jensen EA, Wellnitz CV, Wesselius L. Diagnosis of usual interstitial pneumonitis in the absence of honeycombing: evaluation of specific CT criteria with clinical follow-up in 38 patients. *AJR Am J Roentgenol*. 2016;206(3):472–480. https://doi.org/10.2214/AJR.15.14525.

27. Yagihashi K, Huckleberry J, Colby TV, et al. Radiologic-pathologic discordance in biopsy-proven usual interstitial pneumonia. *Eur Respir J*. 2016;47(4):1189–1197. https://doi.org/10.1183/13993003.01680-2015.

28. Tcherakian C, Cottin V, Brillet P-Y, et al. Progression of idiopathic pulmonary fibrosis: lessons from asymmetrical disease. *Thorax*. 2011;66(3):226–231. https://doi.org/10.1136/thx.2010.137190.

29. Raghu G, Wells AU, Nicholson AG, et al. Effect of nintedanib in subgroups of idiopathic pulmonary fibrosis by diagnostic criteria. *Am J Respir Crit Care Med*. 2017;195(1):78–85. https://doi.org/10.1164/rccm.201602-0402OC.

30. Richeldi L, Costabel U, Selman M, et al. Efficacy of a tyrosine kinase inhibitor in idiopathic pulmonary fibrosis. *N Engl J Med*. 2011;365(12):1079–1087. https://doi.org/10.1056/NEJMoa1103690.

31. Tomiyama N, Müller NL, Johkoh T, et al. Acute respiratory distress syndrome and acute interstitial pneumonia: comparison of thin-section CT findings. *J Comput Assist Tomogr.* 2001;25(1):28–33.

32. Borie R, Kannengiesser C, Nathan N, Tabèze L, Pradère P, Crestani B. Familial pulmonary fibrosis. *Rev Mal Respir.* 2015;32(4):413–434. https://doi.org/10.1016/j.rmr.2014.07.017.

33. Fingerlin TE, Murphy E, Zhang W, et al. Genome-wide association study identifies multiple susceptibility loci for pulmonary fibrosis. *Nat Genet.* 2013;45(6):613–620. https://doi.org/10.1038/ng.2609.

34. Alder JK, Chen JJ-L, Lancaster L, et al. Short telomeres are a risk factor for idiopathic pulmonary fibrosis. *Proc Natl Acad Sci USA.* 2008;105(35):13051–13056. https://doi.org/10.1073/pnas.0804280105.

35. Hunninghake GM, Hatabu H, Okajima Y, et al. MUC5B promoter polymorphism and interstitial lung abnormalities. *N Engl J Med.* 2013;368(23):2192–2200. https://doi.org/10.1056/NEJMoa1216076.

36. Barlo NP, van Moorsel CHM, Ruven HJT, Zanen P, van den Bosch JMM, Grutters JC. Surfactant protein-D predicts survival in patients with idiopathic pulmonary fibrosis. *Sarcoidosis Vasc Diffus Lung Dis.* 2009;26(2):155–161.

37. Lee H-L, Ryu JH, Wittmer MH, et al. Familial idiopathic pulmonary fibrosis: clinical features and outcome. *Chest.* 2005;127(6):2034–2041. https://doi.org/10.1378/chest.127.6.2034.

38. Lee HY, Seo JB, Steele MP, et al. High-resolution CT scan findings in familial interstitial pneumonia do not conform to those of idiopathic interstitial pneumonia. *Chest.* 2012;142(6):1577–1583. https://doi.org/10.1378/chest.11-2812.

39. Chung JH, Montner SM, Adegunsoye A, et al. CT findings associated with survival in chronic hypersensitivity pneumonitis. *Eur Radiol.* 2017;27(12):5127–5135. https://doi.org/10.1007/s00330-017-4936-3.

40. Nishiyama O, Taniguchi H, Kondoh Y, et al. Familial idiopathic pulmonary fibrosis: serial high-resolution computed tomography findings in 9 patients. *J Comput Assist Tomogr.* 2004;28(4):443–448.

41. Flaherty KR, King TE, Raghu G, et al. Idiopathic interstitial pneumonia: what is the effect of a multidisciplinary approach to diagnosis? *Am J Respir Crit Care Med.* 2004;170(8):904–910. https://doi.org/10.1164/rccm.200402-147OC.

42. Collard HR, Moore BB, Flaherty KR, et al. Acute exacerbations of idiopathic pulmonary fibrosis. *Am J Respir Crit Care Med.* 2007;176(7):636–643. https://doi.org/10.1164/rccm.200703-463PP.

43. Kim DS, Park JH, Park BK, Lee JS, Nicholson AG, Colby T. Acute exacerbation of idiopathic pulmonary fibrosis: frequency and clinical features. *Eur Respir J.* 2006;27(1):143–150. https://doi.org/10.1183/09031936.06.00114004.

44. Parambil JG, Myers JL, Ryu JH. Histopathologic features and outcome of patients with acute exacerbation of idiopathic pulmonary fibrosis undergoing surgical lung biopsy. *Chest.* 2005;128(5):3310–3315. https://doi.org/10.1378/chest.128.5.3310.

45. Silva CIS, Müller NL, Fujimoto K, et al. Acute exacerbation of chronic interstitial pneumonia: high-resolution computed tomography and pathologic findings. *J Thorac Imaging.* 2007;22(3):221–229. https://doi.org/10.1097/01.rti.0000213588.52343.13.

46. Akira M, Kozuka T, Yamamoto S, Sakatani M. Computed tomography findings in acute exacerbation of idiopathic pulmonary fibrosis. *Am J Respir Crit Care Med.* 2008;178(4):372–378. https://doi.org/10.1164/rccm.200709-1365OC.

47. Aubry M-C, Myers JL, Douglas WW, et al. Primary pulmonary carcinoma in patients with idiopathic pulmonary fibrosis. *Mayo Clin Proc.* 2002;77(8):763–770.

48. Hubbard R, Venn A, Lewis S, Britton J. Lung cancer and cryptogenic fibrosing alveolitis. A population-based cohort study. *Am J Respir Crit Care Med.* 2000;161(1):5–8. https://doi.org/10.1164/ajrccm.161.1.9906062.

49. Kishi K, Homma S, Kurosaki A, Motoi N, Yoshimura K. High-resolution computed tomography findings of lung cancer associated with idiopathic pulmonary fibrosis. *J Comput Assist Tomogr.* 2006;30(1):95–99.

50. Lee HJ, Im JG, Ahn JM, Yeon KM. Lung cancer in patients with idiopathic pulmonary fibrosis: CT findings. *J Comput Assist Tomogr.* 1996;20(6):979–982.

51. Oh SY, Kim MY, Kim J-E, et al. Evolving early lung cancers detected during follow-up of idiopathic interstitial pneumonia: serial CT features. *AJR Am J Roentgenol.* 2015;204(6):1190–1196. https://doi.org/10.2214/AJR.14.13587.

52. Shorr AF, Wainright JL, Cors CS, Lettieri CJ, Nathan SD. Pulmonary hypertension in patients with pulmonary fibrosis awaiting lung transplant. *Eur Respir J.* 2007;30(4):715–721. https://doi.org/10.1183/09031936.00107206.

53. Nathan SD, Shlobin OA, Barnett SD, et al. Right ventricular systolic pressure by echocardiography as a predictor of pulmonary hypertension in idiopathic pulmonary fibrosis. *Respir Med.* 2008;102(9):1305–1310. https://doi.org/10.1016/j.rmed.2008.03.022.

54. Tan RT, Kuzo R, Goodman LR, Siegel R, Haasler GB, Presberg KW. Utility of CT scan evaluation for predicting pulmonary hypertension in patients with parenchymal lung disease. Medical College of Wisconsin Lung Transplant Group. *Chest.* 1998;113(5):1250–1256.

55. McCall RK, Ravenel JG, Nietert PJ, Granath A, Silver RM. Relationship of main pulmonary artery diameter to pulmonary arterial pressure in scleroderma patients with and without interstitial fibrosis. *J Comput Assist Tomogr.* 2014;38(2):163–168. https://doi.org/10.1097/RCT.0b013e3182aa7fc5.

56. Shin S, King CS, Puri N, et al. Pulmonary artery size as a predictor of outcomes in idiopathic pulmonary fibrosis. *Eur Respir J.* 2016;47(5):1445–1451. https://doi.org/10.1183/13993003.01532-2015.

57. Raghu G, Freudenberger TD, Yang S, et al. High prevalence of abnormal acid gastro-oesophageal reflux in idiopathic pulmonary fibrosis. *Eur Respir J.* 2006;27(1):136–142. https://doi.org/10.1183/09031936.06.00037005.

58. Lee JS, Collard HR, Anstrom KJ, et al. Anti-acid treatment and disease progression in idiopathic pulmonary fibrosis: an analysis of data from three randomised controlled trials. *Lancet Respir Med.* 2013;1(5):369–376. https://doi.org/10.1016/S2213-2600(13)70105-X.

59. Noth I, Zangan SM, Soares RV, et al. Prevalence of hiatal hernia by blinded multidetector CT in patients with idiopathic pulmonary fibrosis. *Eur Respir J.* 2012;39(2):344–351. https://doi.org/10.1183/09031936.00099910.

60. Travis WD, Costabel U, Hansell DM, et al. An official American Thoracic Society/European Respiratory Society statement: update of the international multidisciplinary classification of the idiopathic interstitial pneumonias. *Am J Respir Crit Care Med.* 2013;188(6):733–748. https://doi.org/10.1164/rccm.201308-1483ST.

61. Cottin V, Nunes H, Brillet P-Y, et al. Combined pulmonary fibrosis and emphysema: a distinct underrecognised entity. *Eur Respir J.* 2005;26(4):586–593. https://doi.org/10.1183/09031936.05.00021005.

62. Margaritopoulos GA, Harari S, Caminati A, Antoniou KM. Smoking-related idiopathic interstitial pneumonia: a review. *Respirology.* 2016;21(1):57–64. https://doi.org/10.1111/resp.12576.

63. Jankowich MD, Rounds SIS. Combined pulmonary fibrosis and emphysema syndrome: a review. *Chest.* 2012;141(1):222–231. https://doi.org/10.1378/chest.11-1062.

64. Mejía M, Carrillo G, Rojas-Serrano J, et al. Idiopathic pulmonary fibrosis and emphysema: decreased survival associated with severe pulmonary arterial hypertension. *Chest.* 2009;136(1):10–15. https://doi.org/10.1378/chest.08-2306.

65. Ryerson CJ, Hartman T, Elicker BM, et al. Clinical features and outcomes in combined pulmonary fibrosis and emphysema in idiopathic pulmonary fibrosis. *Chest.* 2013;144(1):234–240. https://doi.org/10.1378/chest.12-2403.

66. Akira M, Inoue Y, Kitaichi M, Yamamoto S, Arai T, Toyokawa K. Usual interstitial pneumonia and nonspecific interstitial pneumonia with and without concurrent emphysema: thin-section CT findings. *Radiology.* 2009;251(1):271–279. https://doi.org/10.1148/radiol.2511080917.

67. Wells AU, Desai SR, Rubens MB, et al. Idiopathic pulmonary fibrosis: a composite physiologic index derived from disease extent observed by computed tomography. *Am J Respir Crit Care Med.* 2003;167(7):962–969. https://doi.org/10.1164/rccm.2111053.

68. Mura M, Zompatori M, Pacilli AMG, Fasano L, Schiavina M, Fabbri M. The presence of emphysema further impairs physiologic function in patients with idiopathic pulmonary fibrosis. *Respir Care.* 2006;51(3):257–265.

69. Chung JH, Montner SM, Adegunsoye A, et al. CT findings, radiologic-pathologic correlation, and imaging predictors of survival for patients with interstitial pneumonia with autoimmune features. *AJR Am J Roentgenol.* 2017;208(6):1229–1236. https://doi.org/10.2214/AJR.16.17121.

70. Nalysnyk L, Cid-Ruzafa J, Rotella P, Esser D. Incidence and prevalence of idiopathic pulmonary fibrosis: review of the literature. *Eur Respir Rev.* 2012;21(126):355–361. https://doi.org/10.1183/09059180.00002512.

71. Fell CD, Martinez FJ, Liu LX, et al. Clinical predictors of a diagnosis of idiopathic pulmonary fibrosis. *Am J Respir Crit Care Med.* 2010;181(8):832–837. https://doi.org/10.1164/rccm.200906-0959OC.

72. Salisbury ML, Xia M, Murray S, et al. Predictors of idiopathic pulmonary fibrosis in absence of radiologic honeycombing: a cross sectional analysis in ILD patients undergoing lung tissue sampling. *Respir Med.* 2016;118:88–95. https://doi.org/10.1016/j.rmed.2016.07.016.

73. Kusmirek JE, Martin MD, Kanne JP. Imaging of idiopathic pulmonary fibrosis. *Radiol Clin North Am.* 2016;54(6):997–1014. https://doi.org/10.1016/j.rcl.2016.05.004.

74. Elliot TL, Lynch DA, Newell JD, et al. High-resolution computed tomography features of nonspecific interstitial pneumonia and usual interstitial pneumonia. *J Comput Assist Tomogr.* 2005;29(3):339–345.

75. Kligerman SJ, Groshong S, Brown KK, Lynch DA. Nonspecific interstitial pneumonia: radiologic, clinical, and pathologic considerations. *Radiographics.* 2009;29(1):73–87. https://doi.org/10.1148/rg.291085096.

76. Jeong YJ, Lee KS, Müller NL, et al. Usual interstitial pneumonia and non-specific interstitial pneumonia: serial thin-section CT findings correlated with pulmonary function. *Korean J Radiol.* 2005;6(3):143–152. https://doi.org/10.3348/kjr.2005.6.3.143.

77. Sumikawa H, Johkoh T, Fujimoto K, et al. Pathologically proved nonspecific interstitial pneumonia: CT pattern analysis as compared with usual interstitial pneumonia CT pattern. *Radiology.* 2014;272(2):549–556. https://doi.org/10.1148/radiol.14130853.

78. Lynch DA, Huckleberry JM. Usual interstitial pneumonia: typical and atypical high-resolution computed tomography features. *Semin Ultrasound CT MR.* 2014;35(1):12–23. https://doi.org/10.1053/j.sult.2013.10.003.

79. Kim H-C, Ji W, Kim MY, et al. Interstitial pneumonia related to undifferentiated connective tissue disease: pathologic pattern and prognosis. *Chest.* 2015;147(1):165–172. https://doi.org/10.1378/chest.14-0272.

80. Franks TJ, Galvin JR. Hypersensitivity pneumonitis: essential radiologic and pathologic findings. *Surg Pathol Clin.* 2010;3(1):187–198. https://doi.org/10.1016/j.path.2010.03.005.

81. Silva CIS, Müller NL, Hansell DM, Lee KS, Nicholson AG, Wells AU. Nonspecific interstitial pneumonia and idiopathic pulmonary fibrosis: changes in pattern and distribution of disease over time. *Radiology*. 2008;247(1): 251–259. https://doi.org/10.1148/radiol.2471070369.

82. MacDonald SL, Rubens MB, Hansell DM, et al. Nonspecific interstitial pneumonia and usual interstitial pneumonia: comparative appearances at and diagnostic accuracy of thin-section CT. *Radiology*. 2001;221(3): 600–605. https://doi.org/10.1148/radiol.2213010158.

83. Hirschmann JV, Pipavath SNJ, Godwin JD. Hypersensitivity pneumonitis: a historical, clinical, and radiologic review. *Radiographics*. 2009;29(7):1921–1938. https://doi.org/10.1148/rg.297095707.

84. Chung JH, Zhan X, Cao M, et al. Presence of air trapping and mosaic attenuation on chest computed tomography predicts survival in chronic hypersensitivity pneumonitis. *Ann Am Thorac Soc*. 2017;14(10):1533–1538. https://doi.org/10.1513/AnnalsATS.201701-035OC.

85. Hansell DM, Wells AU, Padley SP, Müller NL. Hypersensitivity pneumonitis: correlation of individual CT patterns with functional abnormalities. *Radiology*. 1996;199(1):123–128. https://doi.org/10.1148/radiology.199.1.8633133.

86. Sahin H, Brown KK, Curran-Everett D, et al. Chronic hypersensitivity pneumonitis: CT features comparison with pathologic evidence of fibrosis and survival. *Radiology*. 2007;244(2):591–598. https://doi.org/10.1148/radiol.2442060640.

87. Fernández Pérez ER, Swigris JJ, Forssén AV, et al. Identifying an inciting antigen is associated with improved survival in patients with chronic hypersensitivity pneumonitis. *Chest*. 2013;144(5):1644–1651. https://doi.org/10.1378/chest.12-2685.

88. Mooney JJ, Elicker BM, Urbania TH, et al. Radiographic fibrosis score predicts survival in hypersensitivity pneumonitis. *Chest*. 2013;144(2):586–592. https://doi.org/10.1378/chest.12-2623.

89. Chung JH, Cox CW, Montner SM, et al. CT features of the usual interstitial pneumonia pattern: differentiating connective tissue disease-associated interstitial lung disease from idiopathic pulmonary fibrosis. *AJR Am J Roentgenol*. November 2017:1–7. https://doi.org/10.2214/AJR.17.18384.

90. Hwang J-H, Misumi S, Sahin H, Brown KK, Newell JD, Lynch DA. Computed tomographic features of idiopathic fibrosing interstitial pneumonia: comparison with pulmonary fibrosis related to collagen vascular disease. *J Comput Assist Tomogr*. 2009;33(3):410–415. https://doi.org/10.1097/RCT.0b013e318181d551.

91. Fischer A, Antoniou KM, Brown KK, et al. An official European Respiratory Society/American Thoracic Society research statement: interstitial pneumonia with autoimmune features. *Eur Respir J*. 2015;46(4):976–987. https://doi.org/10.1183/13993003.00150-2015.

92. Lee H-K, Kim DS, Yoo B, et al. Histopathologic pattern and clinical features of rheumatoid arthritis-associated interstitial lung disease. *Chest*. 2005;127(6):2019–2027. https://doi.org/10.1378/chest.127.6.2019.

93. Vogel MNA, Kreuter M, Kauczor H-U, Heußel C-P. Pulmonary manifestations in collagen vascular diseases. *Radiologe*. 2016;56(10):910–916. https://doi.org/10.1007/s00117-016-0157-z.

94. Mittoo S, Gelber AC, Christopher-Stine L, Horton MR, Lechtzin N, Danoff SK. Ascertainment of collagen vascular disease in patients presenting with interstitial lung disease. *Respir Med*. 2009;103(8):1152–1158. https://doi.org/10.1016/j.rmed.2009.02.009.

95. Jokerst C, Purdy H, Bhalla S. An overview of collagen vascular disease-associated interstitial lung disease. *Semin Roentgenol*. 2015;50(1):31–39. https://doi.org/10.1053/j.ro.2014.04.006.

96. Bouros D, Wells AU, Nicholson AG, et al. Histopathologic subsets of fibrosing alveolitis in patients with systemic sclerosis and their relationship to outcome. *Am J Respir Crit Care Med*. 2002;165(12):1581–1586. https://doi.org/10.1164/rccm.2106012.

97. Kim DS, Yoo B, Lee JS, et al. The major histopathologic pattern of pulmonary fibrosis in scleroderma is nonspecific interstitial pneumonia. *Sarcoidosis Vasc Diffuse Lung Dis*. 2002;19(2):121–127.

98. Fischer A, Swigris JJ, Groshong SD, et al. Clinically significant interstitial lung disease in limited scleroderma: histopathology, clinical features, and survival. *Chest*. 2008; 134(3):601–605. https://doi.org/10.1378/chest.08-0053.

99. Parambil JG, Myers JL, Lindell RM, Matteson EL, Ryu JH. Interstitial lung disease in primary Sjögren syndrome. *Chest*. 2006;130(5):1489–1495. https://doi.org/10.1378/chest.130.5.1489.

100. Haupt HM, Moore GW, Hutchins GM. The lung in systemic lupus erythematosus. Analysis of the pathologic changes in 120 patients. *Am J Med*. 1981;71(5):791–798.

101. Quadrelli SA, Alvarez C, Arce SC, et al. Pulmonary involvement of systemic lupus erythematosus: analysis of 90 necropsies. *Lupus*. 2009;18(12):1053–1060. https://doi.org/10.1177/0961203309106601.

102. Tansey D, Wells AU, Colby TV, et al. Variations in histological patterns of interstitial pneumonia between connective tissue disorders and their relationship to prognosis. *Histopathology*. 2004;44(6):585–596. https://doi.org/10.1111/j.1365-2559.2004.01896.x.

103. Capobianco J, Grimberg A, Thompson BM, Antunes VB, Jasinowodolinski D, Meirelles GSP. Thoracic manifestations of collagen vascular diseases. *Radiographics*. 2012; 32(1):33–50. https://doi.org/10.1148/rg.321105058.

104. Park JH, Kim DS, Park I-N, et al. Prognosis of fibrotic interstitial pneumonia: idiopathic versus collagen vascular disease-related subtypes. *Am J Respir Crit Care Med*. 2007;175(7):705–711. https://doi.org/10.1164/rccm.200607-912OC.

105. Kim EJ, Collard HR, King TE. Rheumatoid arthritis-associated interstitial lung disease: the relevance of histopathologic and radiographic pattern. *Chest*. 2009;136(5): 1397–1405. https://doi.org/10.1378/chest.09-0444.

106. Bongartz T, Nannini C, Medina-Velasquez YF, et al. Incidence and mortality of interstitial lung disease in rheumatoid arthritis: a population-based study. *Arthritis Rheum*. 2010;62(6):1583–1591. https://doi.org/10.1002/art.27405.

107. Vij R, Noth I, Strek ME. Autoimmune-featured interstitial lung disease: a distinct entity. *Chest*. 2011;140(5): 1292–1299. https://doi.org/10.1378/chest.10-2662.

108. Kinder BW, Collard HR, Koth L, et al. Idiopathic nonspecific interstitial pneumonia: lung manifestation of undifferentiated connective tissue disease? *Am J Respir Crit Care Med*. 2007;176(7):691–697. https://doi.org/10.1164/rccm.200702-220OC.

109. Corte TJ, Copley SJ, Desai SR, et al. Significance of connective tissue disease features in idiopathic interstitial pneumonia. *Eur Respir J*. 2012;39(3):661–668. https://doi.org/10.1183/09031936.00174910.

110. Alhamad EH, Cal JG, AlBoukai AA, Shaik SA, Omair MA. Autoimmune symptoms in idiopathic pulmonary fibrosis: clinical significance. *Clin Respir J*. 2016;10(3): 350–358. https://doi.org/10.1111/crj.12224.

111. Ahmad K, Barba T, Gamondes D, et al. Interstitial pneumonia with autoimmune features: clinical, radiologic, and histological characteristics and outcome in a series of 57 patients. *Respir Med*. 2017;123:56–62. https://doi.org/10.1016/j.rmed.2016.10.017.

112. Vij R, Strek ME. Diagnosis and treatment of connective tissue disease-associated interstitial lung disease. *Chest*. 2013; 143(3):814–824. https://doi.org/10.1378/chest.12-0741.

113. Prasad R, Gupta P, Singh A, Goel N. Drug induced pulmonary parenchymal disease. *Drug Discov Ther*. 2014; 8(6):232–237. https://doi.org/10.5582/ddt.2014.01046.

114. Padley SP, Adler B, Hansell DM, Müller NL. High-resolution computed tomography of drug-induced lung disease. *Clin Radiol*. 1992;46(4):232–236.

115. Cleverley JR, Screaton NJ, Hiorns MP, Flint JDA, Müller NL. Drug-induced lung disease: high-resolution CT and histological findings. *Clin Radiol*. 2002;57(4): 292–299. https://doi.org/10.1053/crad.2001.0792.

116. Akira M, Yamamoto S, Inoue Y, Sakatani M. High-resolution CT of asbestosis and idiopathic pulmonary fibrosis. *Am J Roentgenol*. 2003;181(1):163–169. https://doi.org/10.2214/ajr.181.1.1810163.

117. Roach HD, Davies GJ, Attanoos R, Crane M, Adams H, Phillips S. Asbestos: when the dust settles an imaging review of asbestos-related disease. *Radiographics*. 2002; 22 Spec No(suppl 1):S167–S184. https://doi.org/10.1148/radiographics.22.suppl_1.g02oc10s167.

118. Cha YK, Kim JS, Kim Y, Kim YK. Radiologic diagnosis of asbestosis in Korea. *Korean J Radiol*. 2016;17(5): 674–683. https://doi.org/10.3348/kjr.2016.17.5.674.

119. Brichet A, Tonnel AB, Brambilla E, et al. Chronic interstitial pneumonia with honeycombing in coal workers. *Sarcoidosis Vasc Diffus Lung Dis*. 2002;19(3):211–219.

120. Katabami M, Dosaka-Akita H, Honma K, et al. Pneumoconiosis-related lung cancers: preferential occurrence from diffuse interstitial fibrosis-type pneumoconiosis. *Am J Respir Crit Care Med*. 2000;162(1):295–300. https://doi.org/10.1164/ajrccm.162.1.9906138.

121. Arakawa H, Johkoh T, Honma K, et al. Chronic interstitial pneumonia in silicosis and mix-dust pneumoconiosis: its prevalence and comparison of CT findings with idiopathic pulmonary fibrosis. *Chest*. 2007;131(6): 1870–1876. https://doi.org/10.1378/chest.06-2553.

122. Honma K, Chiyotani K. Diffuse interstitial fibrosis in nonasbestos pneumoconiosis — a pathological study. *Respiration*. 1993;60(2):120–126.

123. Archer VE, Renzetti AD, Doggett RS, Jarvis JQ, Colby TV. Chronic diffuse interstitial fibrosis of the lung in uranium miners. *J Occup Environ Med*. 1998;40(5): 460–474.

The Pathology of Usual Interstitial Pneumonia

ROSANE DUARTE ACHCAR, MD

HISTOLOGIC FEATURES OF USUAL INTERSTITIAL PNEUMONIA

Usual interstitial pneumonia (UIP) is a nonuniform pattern of chronic lung injury defined by a combination of morphologic features, including remodeling of the pulmonary parenchyma architecture (architectural distortion). Architectural distortion is required for the diagnosis of the UIP pattern. UIP characteristically involves the basilar regions of the lungs bilaterally. The UIP pattern cannot be reliably identified with transbronchial biopsy specimens. Surgical wedge lung biopsies obtained through open thoracotomy or video-assisted thoracoscopic surgery are the most appropriate samples for diagnosis. More than one biopsy site should be sampled. If possible, samples should be obtained from all lobes on the biopsied side to reduce the possibility of sampling error. Samples from the lower lobes should be taken above the most advanced area of fibrosis.

GEOGRAPHIC HETEROGENEITY AND FIBROBLASTIC ACTIVITY

UIP is characterized by the presence of patchy interstitial fibrosis admixed with areas of normal or near-normal lung (geographic heterogeneity) (Fig. 6.1). The pattern of interstitial fibrosis is typically temporally heterogeneous, characterized by the presence of chronic, inactive, dense, pink, mature ("old") interstitial scarring/fibrosis and active, loosely arranged, light blue, immature ("recent") interstitial foci of fibroblastic activity (Fig. 6.2). Fibroblastic foci are usually seen within honeycombed or scarred areas or at the transition zones between dense fibrosis and normal lung. They are composed of loosely arranged fibroblasts and myofibroblasts, embedded within a myxoid stroma, located in the interstitium, and lined by flattened or hyperplastic bronchiolar epithelium or pneumocytes (Fig. 6.3).

With pentachrome (Movat) special stain, foci of fibroblastic activity stain green, whereas dense fibrosis stains a characteristic yellow (Fig. 6.4).

Foci of fibroblastic activity are areas of recent organization and are believed to represent the initial event in UIP. It has been proposed that multiple foci of fibroblastic activity recurring over many years account for the chronic progressive course of the disease with eventual scarring and honeycombing. Accordingly, cases with increased number of fibroblastic foci tend to be associated with worse clinical course and shorter survival. Fibroblastic foci of UIP should not be confused with the fibroblastic tissue of organizing pneumonia (OP); although sometimes it may be challenging to make the distinction. Fibroblastic foci in UIP are located within the interstitium (Figs. 6.2 and 6.3), whereas fibroblastic tissue (plugs) in OP are located within airspaces. Fibroblastic foci of UIP are usually single and randomly distributed, whereas fibroblastic plugs in OP are usually bunched within the airspaces. While occasional foci of OP may be seen in UIP, the presence of significant OP is unusual and may indicate a superimposed process such as infection, aspiration, or acute exacerbation (AEx). AEx of UIP is clinically unrelated to infection or heart failure and is characterized microscopically by features of diffuse alveolar damage (DAD) superimposed on UIP (Fig. 6.5A and B) with its characteristic, patchy, or end-stage interstitial scarring (old fibrosis) and honeycomb change. In AEx of UIP, if more than one lobe is biopsied, UIP morphology may be identified in one lobe, whereas DAD is noted in another lobe.

HONEYCOMB CHANGE

Besides being basilar predominant, UIP has a subpleural and paraseptal distribution and contains areas of honeycomb change. It is unclear how microscopic honeycomb cysts form, but some authors have suggested

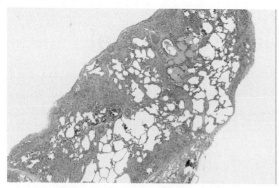

FIG. 6.1 At low power, usual interstitial pneumonia (UIP) has a variegated appearance with subpleural and paraseptal areas of interstitial fibrosis, peripheral honeycomb change, and areas of uninvolved lung. Architectural distortion is *required* for the diagnosis of UIP.

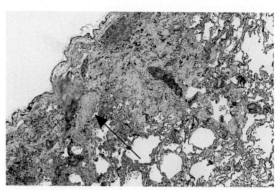

FIG. 6.4 The immature interstitial subepithelial focus of fibroblastic activity (*arrow*) stains green with pentachrome (Movat) special stain, whereas the mature dense fibrosis stains yellow.

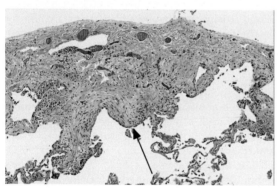

FIG. 6.2 The temporally heterogeneous process is characterized by the presence of chronic, inactive, dense, pink, mature ("old") interstitial fibrosis (upper field) and active, loosely arranged, light blue/myxoid, immature ("recent") foci of fibroblastic activity (*arrow*).

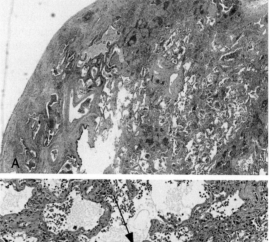

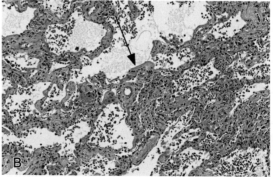

FIG. 6.5 **(A)** Acute exacerbation of usual interstitial pneumonia (UIP): There is acute and organizing lung injury (right fields) superimposed on underlying lung parenchyma showing subpleural dense fibrosis with honeycomb change of UIP (left fields). **(B)** High power view of (A) (from right fields) showing superimposed acute diffuse alveolar damage with focal fibrinous exudate and numerous hyaline membranes (*arrow*) located along the alveolar septa, which are expanded by a sparse, mononuclear inflammatory cell infiltrate.

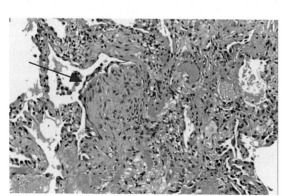

FIG. 6.3 Fibroblastic foci (*arrow*) are located in the interstitium and lined by flattened or hyperplastic epithelium. They should not be confused with foci of OP, which are located within the airspaces.

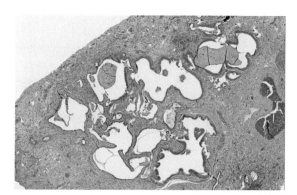

FIG. 6.6 Peripheral microscopic honeycomb change is characterized by the presence of enlarged, irregular spaces lined at least partially by bronchiolar type of epithelium. Notice the honeycomb cysts are surrounded by dense fibrosis and chronic inflammation and contain a mucinous exudate composed of macrophages and mixed inflammatory cells.

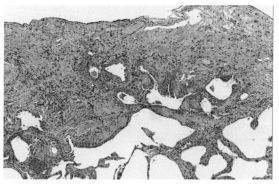

FIG. 6.7 Squamous cell metaplasia: metaplastic squamous epithelium may be seen associated with usual interstitial pneumonia and should not be confused with squamous cell carcinoma.

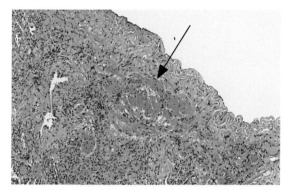

FIG. 6.8 Peripheral smooth muscle hyperplasia (*arrow*) is another finding commonly seen in usual interstitial pneumonia.

that they represent centrilobular airways trapped within fibrous remodeling that pulls them to the periphery of the lobule. This hypothesis would explain the presence of peripheral/subpleural fibrosis with smooth muscle prominence. Microscopic honeycombing is characterized by the presence of enlarged, irregular spaces (usually 1–3 mm), lined at least partially, by bronchiolar-type epithelium, surrounded by dense fibrosis and chronic inflammation, and often filled with a mucinous exudate that contains macrophages and mixed inflammatory cells (Fig. 6.6). Architectural distortion is required for the diagnosis of UIP, and honeycomb change is generally present. However, in rare cases, honeycomb change may be absent, and scarring may be the only manifestation of architectural distortion. Interstitial inflammation, if present, is typically patchy and mild, mostly noted in the areas of honeycombing. Usually there is little or no interstitial inflammation away from the areas of fibrosis. Interstitial chronic inflammation, located away from areas of fibrosis, may be seen in patients with underlying collagen vascular disease, fibrotic phase of chronic hypersensitivity pneumonia (HP), or in familial forms of UIP.

VASCULAR CHANGES
In UIP, traction bronchi-/bronchiolectasis, peribronchiolar metaplasia, squamous cell metaplasia, and smooth muscle hyperplasia (Figs. 6.7–6.9) may be present. Vascular changes, including intimal and medial hypertrophy, are usually present within areas of honeycombing (Fig. 6.10) and are secondary to local parenchymal destruction. Such vascular changes away from areas of honeycombing are unusual and should raise

suspicion for pulmonary hypertension, particularly if the patient has an underlying connective tissue disease, such as scleroderma.

UIP AND NSIP-LIKE AREAS
Temporally uniform, fibrotic nonspecific interstitial pneumonia (fibrotic NSIP)-like areas may be present in UIP. However, the final histologic diagnosis should be based on the pattern present in the histologically most severely affected area(s) (Fig. 6.11). Prominent (start a new sentence) architectural distortion, honeycomb change, and fibroblastic activity are usually absent and never prominent in fibrotic NSIP. If there is incongruence between imaging studies (showing a UIP pattern with honeycombing) and pathology findings (showing only fibrotic NSIP-like areas), the possibility of sampling error should be considered. Sampling error is less likely to occur if more than one lobe is biopsied, and the lower lobe is always included.

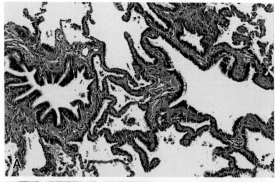

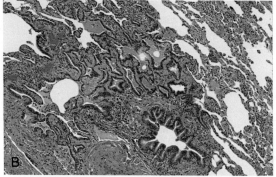

FIG. 6.9 Peribronchiolar metaplasia **(A)** may be seen in usual interstitial pneumonia and when prominent **(B)**, although nonspecific, raises the possibility of underlying chronic hypersensitivity pneumonia.

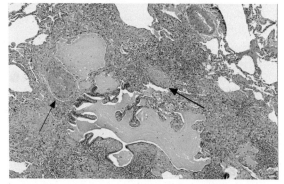

FIG. 6.10 Thickened pulmonary artery (*left arrow*) within an area of honeycombing. Note the foci of fibroblastic activity (*right arrow*).

FEATURES SUGGESTING THE CAUSES OF USUAL INTERSTITIAL PNEUMONIA

Potential etiologies for histologic UIP include systemic autoimmune/connective tissue diseases, familial pulmonary fibrosis, pneumoconiosis (e.g., asbestosis), fibrotic phase of chronic HP, and possible drug toxicity. All must be clinically excluded before

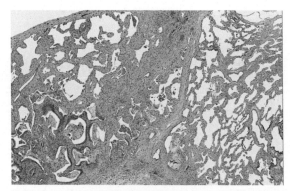

FIG. 6.11 Nonspecific interstitial pneumonia-like areas (right) may be present in usual interstitial pneumonia, but the final diagnosis should be based on the pattern in the most severely affected areas. In this picture, in the most severely affected area, there is honeycomb change and fibroblastic activity (left), characteristic of UIP.

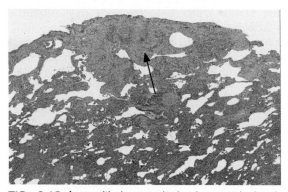

FIG. 6.12 Area with increased alveolar septal chronic inflammation away from areas with typical features of usual interstitial pneumonia (UIP). Note subpleural smooth muscle hyperplasia (*arrow*). The presence of increased interstitial inflammation away from the areas of honeycombing should raise the possibility of underlying connective tissue disease, chronic hypersensitivity pneumonia, or possibly familial forms of UIP.

diagnosing idiopathic pulmonary fibrosis (IPF) in a patient with histologic UIP.

Besides increased interstitial chronic inflammation away from the areas of honeycombing, the presence of numerous prominent lymphoid follicles with reactive germinal centers and chronic pleuritis should also raise suspicion for underlying connective tissue disease, particularly rheumatoid arthritis (Figs. 6.12 and 6.13). Similar morphology may be also seen in cases of chronic hypersensitivity pneumonia or familial forms of UIP. The presence of pleural plaques may be associated with asbestosis, and their presence should

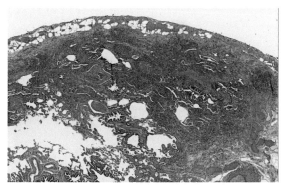

FIG. 6.13 Prominent lymphoid follicles with reactive germinal centers, although nonspecific, are suggestive of underlying connective tissue disease.

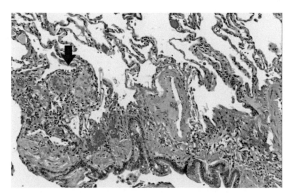

FIG. 6.14 The presence of frequent, poorly formed, nonnecrotizing granulomas (*arrow*) should raise the possibility of underlying chronic hypersensitivity pneumonia.

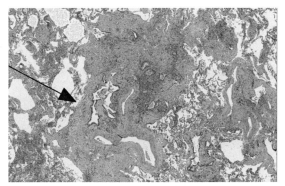

FIG. 6.15 Small airway (*arrow*) with peribronchiolar fibrosis. Peribronchiolar fibrosis, although nonspecific, may be seen associated with fibrotic phase of chronic hypersensitivity pneumonia.

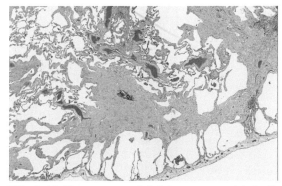

FIG. 6.16 The presence of stellate scars associated with adjacent traction emphysema and respiratory bronchiolitis should raise the possibility of fibrotic phase of pulmonary Langerhans cell histiocytosis.

prompt a search for ferruginous bodies and clinical investigation into asbestos exposure.

DIFFERENTIATING USUAL INTERSTITIAL PNEUMONIA FROM OTHER FORMS OF PULMONARY FIBROSIS

Unlike cases of idiopathic UIP in which interstitial fibroblastic activity is located in subpleural areas or at the interface between scarred and normal lung, in the fibrotic phase of HP, fibroblastic activity may be located in peribronchiolar areas. Fibrotic phase of chronic HP should be considered when there is prominent cellular bronchiolitis, prominent peribronchiolar metaplasia (Fig. 6.9), peribronchiolar nonnecrotizing poorly formed granulomas (Fig. 6.14) or multinucleated giant cells, peribronchiolar fibrosis (Fig. 6.15), peribronchiolar fibroblastic activity, or residual areas of bronchiolocentric cellular interstitial pneumonia with few foci of OP. Histologically, HP is typically a predominantly centrilobular/bronchiolocentric process involving the middle and upper lung zones, while the classic UIP pattern in IPF usually involves subpleural and paraseptal zones in lung basilar regions bilaterally.

Other diseases that can mimic UIP include fibrotic phase of pulmonary Langerhans cell histiocytosis (PLCH), pleuroparenchymal fibroelastosis (PPFE), bronchiectasis with scarring, and end-stage honeycomb lung. A comparison of the histopathologic findings is presented in Table 6.1. In severe cases of PLCH, interstitial fibrosis with honeycomb change may develop, and Langerhans cell clusters may not be readily identified. However, in PLCH, bronchiolocentric fibrotic scars are usually associated with traction emphysema and often maintain the stellate shape of the cellular lesions. This can be a clue that suggests PLCH in cases where only fibrotic lesions are sampled (Fig. 6.16). In addition, because PLCH classically occurs in patients who smoke, although

TABLE 6.1
Comparison of Histopathologic Findings In Interstitial Fibrosing Processes

Morphologic Findings/ Disease	Idiopathic UIP	CVD/ UIP	HP-Fibrotic Phase/UIP	Asbestosis/ UIP	PLCH-Fibrotic Phase/UIP	SRIF	PPFE	End-Stage Honeycomb Lung
Variegated temporal and geographic heterogeneous	X	X	X	X	X			
Honeycomb change with fibrosis	X	X	X	X	X			X
No significant fibroblastic activity						X	X	
Occasional foci of OP	X	X	X		X			
Increased interstitial inflammation away from areas of honeycomb fibrosis		X	X					
Prominent lymphoid follicles with reactive germinal center		X						
Chronic pleuritis		X						
Pleural plaques and ferruginous bodies				X				
Prominent peribronchiolar metaplasia			X					
Poorly formed nonnecrotizing granulomas			X					
Multinucleated giant cells			X					
Centrilobular/peribronchial fibroblastic activity			X					
Prominent airway—centered interstitial fibrosis			X		X			

Feature						
Bronchiolocentric distribution						
Predominant lower lobes involvement	X					
Predominant upper lobes involvement		X	X	X		
Stellate scar and paracicatricial emphysema		X				
Significant respiratory bronchiolitis		X	X			
Subpleural distinct hyalinized collagen and marked emphysema			X			
Subpleural fibroelastotic scarring				X		

CVD, collagen vascular disease; HP, hypersensitivity pneumonia; OP, organizing pneumonia; PLCH, pulmonary Langerhans cell histiocytosis; PPFE, pleuroparenchymal fibroelastosis; SRIF, Smoking-related interstitial fibrosis; UIP, usual interstitial pneumonia.

nonspecific, the finding of pigmented macrophages (of the smoker's type) filling airspaces (respiratory bronchiolitis), or within scars, provides a useful clue to the diagnosis. As in HP, PLCH usually involves mid- and upper zones in a predominantly centrilobular/peribronchiolar distribution. Smoking-related interstitial fibrosis (SRIF) may also be associated with severe, subpleural fibrosis. However, the hyalinized quality of the collagen deposition associated with marked emphysema seen in SRIF (Figs. 6.17 and 6.18) is not typical of UIP. In addition, SRIF rarely shows fibroblastic activity and lacks significant honeycomb change typical of UIP.

PPFE shows marked thickening of the visceral pleura and remodeling of the subpleural parenchymal architecture by a homogeneous mixture of dense collagen and elastic tissue (fibroelastotic scarring) (Fig. 6.19). PPFE affects upper lobes and does not have the variegated temporal heterogeneous pattern of fibrosis seen in UIP. Fibroblastic activity is unusual in PPFE.

In rare cases, parenchymal scarring from bronchiectasis may mimic the interstitial fibrosis of UIP with features of honeycomb change, metaplastic epithelium, and mucous pooling in airspaces. Clinical and radiologic features and the presence of airway centered centered scarring (seen in bronchiectasis) rather than temporal heterogeneous process with peripheral honeycombing (seen in UIP), are helpful in making the distinction between these diagnoses.

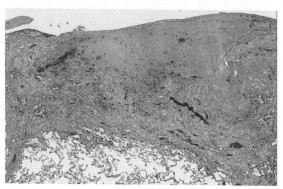

FIG. 6.19 Pleuroparenchymal fibroelastosis (PPFE): There is subpleural thickening of the visceral pleura and remodeling of the subpleural parenchyma by homogeneous, fibroelastotic scarring. Note the abrupt transition between fibroelastotic and normal lung parenchyma. Temporal heterogeneity with fibroblastic activity and honeycombing are not features typical of PPFE.

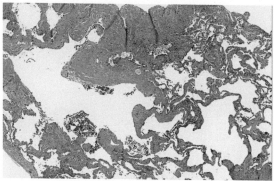

FIG. 6.17 Smoking-related interstitial fibrosis: There is subpleural, characteristic, hyalinized collagen deposition associated with emphysema and respiratory bronchiolitis. Note the absence of temporal heterogeneity or honeycombing that characterizes usual interstitial pneumonia.

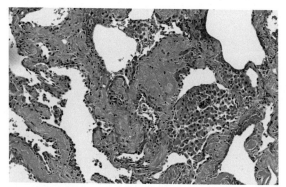

FIG. 6.18 Smoking-related interstitial fibrosis: high power view of Fig. 6.17 showing marked alveolar septal expansion by distinct, hyalinized collagen bundles. Respiratory bronchiolitis is characterized by the presence of clusters of pigmented macrophages within the alveolar spaces.

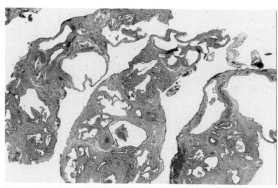

FIG. 6.20 End-stage honeycomb lung showing diffuse and dramatic remodeling of the lung parenchymal architecture. It is similar to the honeycombing seen in usual interstitial pneumonia (UIP), but it lacks the temporal heterogeneous pattern of fibrosis characteristic of UIP.

End-stage honeycomb lung represents an end-stage pattern of injury that may result from a variety of inflammatory and fibrosing interstitial processes, including UIP, desquamative interstitial pneumonia, interstitial granulomatous disease (e.g., infections, HP, sarcoidosis, chronic beryllium disease), PLCH, and pneumoconiosis (e.g., asbestosis and hard metal lung disease/giant cell pneumoconiosis). Although most cases take many years to develop, end-stage honeycomb lung may arise within a few weeks in patients with DAD from severe and acute injurious processes such as acute interstitial pneumonia. The microscopic appearance of end-stage honeycomb lung (Fig. 6.20) is nonspecific and similar to the honeycombing seen in UIP. Regardless of the etiology, end-stage honeycomb lung lacks the temporally heterogenous pattern of interstitial fibrosis characteristic of UIP. Clinical and radiologic correlation and review of previously obtained biopsies (if available) may be required to determine the cause. End-stage honeycomb lung is often identified in cases where only a single biopsy is taken from the most scarred area of the lung.

ACKNOWLEDGMENTS

I gratefully acknowledge my colleagues Dr. Carlyne Cool and Dr. Steve Groshong at National Jewish Health, Denver, Colorado, for their generous review and constructive comments.

SELECTED REFERENCES

Churg A, Hall R, Bilawich A. Respiratory bronchiolitis with fibrosis-interstitial lung disease: a new form of smoking-induced interstitial lung disease. *Arch Pathol Med.* 2015; 139(4):437−440.

Churg A, Muller NL, Silva CI, et al. Acute exacerbation (acute lung injury of unknown cause) in UIP and other forms of fibrotic interstitial lung pneumonias. *Am J Surg Pathol.* 2007;31(2):277−284.

Churg A, Muller J, Suarez T, et al. Airway-centered interstitial fibrosis: a distinct form of aggressive diffuse lung disease. *Am J Surg Pathol.* 2004;28(1):62−68.

Duarte Achcar R, Groshong S, Cool C. *Pulmonary Pathology, Differential Diagnosis in Surgical Pathology Series.* 1st ed. Philadelphia, PA: Wolters Kluer Heatlh Series; 2016.

English JC, Mayi JR, Levy R, et al. Pleuroparenchymal fibroelastosis: a rare interstitial lung disease. *Respirol Case Rep.* 2015; 3(2):82−84.

Frankel SK, Cool CD, Lynch DA, Brown KK. Idiopathic pleuroparenchymal fibroelastosis. Description of a novel clinicopathologic entity. *Chest.* 2004;126:2007.

Fukuoka J, Franks TJ, Colby TV, et al. Peribronchiolar metaplasia: a common histologic lesion in diffuse lung disease and rare cause of interstitial lung disease: clinocopathologic features of 15 cases. *Am J Surg Pathol.* 2005;29(7): 948.

Katzentein AL, Mukhopadhyay S, Myers JL. Diagnosis of usual interstitial pneumonia and distinction from other fibrosing interstitial lung diseases. *Hum Pathol.* 2008;39(11): 1275−1294.

Katzenstein AL. Smoking-related interstitial fibrosis (SRIF): pathologic findings and distinction from other chronic fibrosing diseases. *J Clin Pathol.* 2013;66(10):882.

Katzenstein AL. *Diagnostic Atlas of Non-Neoplastic Lung Disease: A Practical Guide for Surgical Pathologists.* New York, NY: Springer Publishing Company; 2016.

Kim HC, Ji W, Kim MY, et al. Interstitial pneumonia related to undifferentiated connective tissue disease: pathologic pattern and prognosid. *Chest.* 2015;147:165.

Leslie KO, Wick MR. *Practical Pulmonary Pathology: A Diagnostic Approach.* 2nd ed. Philadelphia, PA: Elsevier Saunders; 2011.

Reddy TL, Tominaga M, Hasell DM, et al. Pleuroparenchymal fibroelastosis: a spectrum of histopathological and imaging phenotypes. *Eur Respir J.* 2012;40(2):377.

Smith M, Dalurzo M, Panse P, et al. Usual interstitial pneumonia-pattern fibrosis in surgical lung biopsies. Clinical, radiologic, and histopathological clues to etiology. *J Clin Pathol.* 2013;66(10):896.

Takemura T, Akashi T, Kamiya H, et al. Pathological differentiation of chronic hypersensitivity pneumonitis from idiopathic pulmonary fibrosis/usual interstitial pneumonia. *Histopathology.* 2012;61(6):1020−1035.

Trahan S, Hanak V, Ryu JH, et al. Rloe of surgical lung biopsy in separating chronic hypersensitivity pneumonia from usual interstitial pneumonia/idiopathic pulmonary fibrosis: analysis of 31 biopsies from 15 pateints. *Chest.* 2008;134: 126−132.

Travis WD, Colby TV, Koss MN, et al. *Non-Neoplastic Disorders of the Lower Respiratory Tract. AFIP Atlas of Nontumor Pathology Series.* Washington DC: Armec Forces Institute of Pathology; 2002.

Traviz WD, Costabel U, Hansell DM, et al. ATS/ERS Committee on Idiopathic Interstitial Pneumonias. Respiratory Society statement: update of the international multidisciplinary classification of the idiopathic interstitial pneumonias. *Am J Res Crit Care Med.* 2013;188(6):733.

Yousem SA, Dacic S. Idiopathic bronchiolocentric interstitial pneumonia. *Mod Pathol.* 2002;15(11):1148.

CHAPTER 7

Making the Diagnosis

TRISTAN HUIE, MD • STEPHEN K. FRANKEL, MD, FCCM, FCCP

INTRODUCTION

Idiopathic pulmonary fibrosis (IPF) is the most common form of interstitial lung disease (ILD).[1] ILD is a broad category of more than 200 diseases characterized by inflammation, scarring, or both that affect lung parenchyma. Most forms of ILD present with respiratory symptoms, restrictive physiology, and diffuse abnormalities on imaging. Many forms of ILD result in pulmonary fibrosis. Also, many ILDs have identifiable causes and are treated with exposure avoidance or immunosuppressive drugs. The idiopathic interstitial pneumonias (IIPs) are a subset of ILD without an identifiable etiology that are classified according to the histologic pattern of lung injury.[2,3] IPF is the most common IIP (Fig. 7.1).

IPF is a progressive, scarring lung disease with a median survival of 3–5 years from the time of diagnosis.[1] Unlike many other forms of ILD, IPF does not respond to immunosuppressive therapy, and the combination of prednisone, azathioprine, and N-acetylcysteine has been shown to be harmful.[1,4] Two antifibrotic therapies were approved for the treatment of IPF in 2014.[5] An accurate diagnosis of ILD is necessary to convey accurate information about prognosis and to tailor appropriate therapy.

CATEGORIZATION OF ILD BY ETIOLOGY AND PATTERN

A practical approach to the diagnosis of IPF requires a clinician to carefully consider the broader differential of ILD. We advocate a process that identifies the *context* and *pattern* for a given case. Context refers to the potential etiology and the risk factors for ILD. The etiology of ILD falls into several categories as follows: systemic disease, inhalational exposures, drug exposure, familial disease, or idiopathic disease.[2] Systemic diseases primarily include connective tissues diseases or immunodeficiency. Inhalational exposures may be further divided into inorganic dust exposures and organic exposures. Inorganic dust exposures such as asbestos,

silica, and coal dust lead to pneumoconioses. Organic exposures such as avian proteins, mold, or thermophilic bacteria may result in hypersensitivity pneumonitis (HP). Exposures to medications, illicit drugs, or radiation may cause ILD. ILD may run in families. If a detailed evaluation identifies no cause, the disease should be categorized as idiopathic.

There are a limited number of named patterns of lung injury that occur in ILD. Most of these patterns are characterized in the joint international statements on IIPs.[2,3] In addition to the injury patterns that occur in the IIP, granulomatous lung disease may occur.[6,7] Specific, additional findings may suggest an underlying diagnosis due to connective tissue disease or HP. Chapter 6 provides additional details.

The combination of context and pattern is essential to consider because a given clinical context may result in various patterns of lung injury with differing prognoses. A useful example is the case of rheumatoid arthritis (RA)-associated lung involvement. Parenchymal injury due to RA most commonly results in a usual interstitial pneumonia (UIP) pattern of fibrosis, but nonspecific interstitial pneumonia (NSIP) or organizing pneumonia (OP) are not uncommon.[8] Furthermore, diffuse alveolar damage (DAD) may occur in patients with RA. Similarly, HP may result in a pattern of UIP, cellular or fibrotic NSIP, or a pattern of OP.[9,10] Thus, etiology alone is thus insufficient to characterize an ILD. The prognosis of RA-associated ILD or HP depends in part on the underlying pattern of injury.[11]

The pattern of lung disease is similarly insufficient to fully characterize an ILD. Most lung injury patterns are not specific for any one entity; thus, each pattern may occur in idiopathic clinical contexts or in the setting of various secondary causes. The pattern of UIP is illustrative of this point. Histologic UIP may occur in the setting of autoimmune diseases, such as RA; inhalational exposures, such as asbestosis or HP; drug exposure, such as chemotherapy; or an idiopathic clinical context. There are data to suggest that UIP due to an identifiable cause has a better prognosis than IPF,

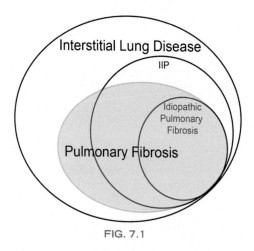

FIG. 7.1

although other data suggest similar outcomes between patients with IPF and those with secondary (or known-cause) UIP.[12,13] This may be particularly true if a culpable exposure can be eliminated.[14]

CLINICAL EVALUATION

The process of excluding known causes of ILD requires a detailed evaluation based on history, physical examination, and laboratory testing.

History

A structured approach to the history will ensure relevant systemic diseases and exposures are considered.[1] A rigorous occupational and environmental history is necessary. Occupational history should look for triggers of pneumoconioses—recognizing that pneumoconiosis may present decades after an exposure. The history should clarify specific duties at work and quantification of any relevant exposures. Exposure to fungi or thermophilic bacteria should be sought. This includes prior episodes of water damage in the home or at work and exposure to water sources such as swimming pools, hot tubs, or humidifiers. It should include an evaluation for exposure to avian antigens, including pet bird use and exposure to down bedding or other feather-containing products.

Family history should seek the presence of ILD and extrathoracic diagnoses associated with familial forms of pulmonary fibrosis, including cryptogenic cirrhosis, bone marrow failure syndromes, macrocytosis, premature osteoporosis, and premature graying of the hair (typically in the 1920s).[15,16] Prescription and nonprescription medication use, over-the-counter dietary supplement use, and illicit drug use must be considered.

A comprehensive online database of pulmonary complications of drug use is available at pnemotox.com.[17] Questionnaires may facilitate the efficient collection of relevant historical information. Examples are available online.[18]

The evaluation should establish the clinical probability of IPF. A diagnosis of IPF is more likely than other IIPs with increasing age (particularly age > 60 years old), male gender, and a history of smoking.[19,20] Available data primarily relate to the risk of IPF relative to other IIPs. Elderly patients may present with other forms of ILD, including those due to connective tissue disease or exposure to inhalational antigens or drug use.[21–24]

Physical Examination

The physical examination should confirm the presence of the expected pulmonary findings of basilar predominant end-expiratory crackles. The examination must be comprehensive and include an investigation for evidence of extrapulmonary manifestations that suggest an underlying systemic disease. A detailed joint and skin examination, particularly including an evaluation of the hands, may identify subtle changes of connective tissue disease.[1] The examination also seeks to identify complications such as pulmonary hypertension that warrant additional evaluation and treatment.

Laboratory Testing

A serologic evaluation screens for underlying connective tissue disease. Specific tests should be guided primarily by clinical suspicion. An important caveat is that the first manifestation of a systemic autoimmune disease may be ILD.[25–27] There is no consensus regarding the appropriate laboratories to be ordered as screening tests. International guidelines recommend antinuclear antibody titer and pattern, rheumatoid factor, and anti-cyclic citrullinated peptide.[1] A rheumatologist may assist in identifying subtle coexisting connective tissue disease.

RADIOGRAPHIC EVALUATION

The initial assessment of the pattern of ILD relies on high-resolution computed tomography (HRCT). Radiologists should interpret the presence or absence of UIP pattern and the confidence of this finding. Technical aspects of HRCT and a detailed discussion of the imaging of IPF are reviewed in Chapter 5.

Joint international guidelines from 2011 recognize three radiographic patterns as follows: definite UIP, possible UIP, and inconsistent with UIP.[1] A definite UIP pattern requires a reticular pattern with traction bronchiectasis and bronchiolectasis in peripheral predominant and basilar predominant distribution. Honeycombing (clustered subpleural cysts) should be present, and atypical features should be absent. Atypical features include the wrong distribution of abnormality (upper or midlung predominance or peribronchovascular predominance), ground glass that is greater than the reticular abnormality, profuse micronodules, cystic lung disease, diffuse mosaic attenuation or air trapping, or areas of consolidation.[1] A possible UIP pattern differs from a definite UIP pattern only by the absence of honeycomb cysts. Inconsistency with UIP applies to fibrotic lung disease with any of the atypical abovementioned features listed. Diagnostic and radiological guidelines will continue to be updated as new information becomes available.

It is widely accepted that a (definite) UIP radiographic pattern does not require a surgical lung biopsy.[1] The specificity of a UIP radiographic pattern is between 94% and 100% in most studies.[1,28–30] Additional information is unlikely to be obtained with a surgical lung biopsy in these patients. The joint international guidelines recommended surgical lung biopsy for a definitive diagnosis of IPF for all patients that did not have a definite UIP pattern on imaging. More recent data suggest that the absence of honeycombing does not substantially lower the likelihood of a histologic UIP pattern (82%–94% specificity).[31,32] A proposed CT pattern of probable UIP should replace the previously described possible UIP pattern.[16,33] It should be emphasized that the CT patterns are not sensitive to the presence of histologic UIP: more than half of patients with a radiographic pattern of inconsistency with UIP will have a UIP pattern on biopsy.[33]

PATHOLOGIC EVALUATION

A pathologic pattern of UIP is characterized by temporal and spatial heterogeneity of fibrosis. Areas of fibrosis are intermixed with areas of less involved or normal lung. International guidelines recognize four patterns as follows: definite UIP, probable UIP, possible UIP, or not UIP. A UIP pattern requires marked fibrosis with or without microscopic honeycombing, patchy involvement of abnormality, the presence of fibroblastic foci, and the absence of features that suggest an alternative diagnosis (hyaline membranes, OP, extensive granulomas, marked interstitial inflammation, airway-centered changes, or other features that suggest an alternative diagnosis). A probable UIP pattern has marked fibrosis with no features to suggest an alternative diagnosis and lacks either the patchy involvement

of abnormality or fibroblastic foci. It may also demonstrate honeycomb change only (which is assumed to reflect end-stage lung disease). A possible UIP pattern has patchy or diffuse involvement with fibrosis without the other features that argue for or against a UIP pattern. The not UIP pattern has any of the features that suggest an alternative diagnosis. Additional details are provided in Chapter 6.

A surgical lung biopsy should obtain tissue from the upper, middle, and lower lung zone.[34,35] Areas of end-stage fibrosis should be avoided as these are likely to be nondiagnostic.[1] Multiple biopsies are useful as more than one pattern of injury may be present in the same patient (e.g., UIP and fibrotic NSIP in the same patient). In patients with discordant pathologic patterns, the presence of UIP dictates the prognosis and thus diagnosis.[34,35]

DIAGNOSIS

The 2011 joint international guidelines require the absence of an identifiable etiology and the presence of a UIP pattern on HRCT or a specific combination of findings on imaging and surgical lung biopsy.[1] The diagnosis requires a multidisciplinary approach to evaluate the clinical context and pattern of injury. A multidisciplinary discussion between clinicians, radiologists, and pathologists has been shown to result in better agreement in the final diagnosis, and this is viewed as the gold standard approach.[1,36,37] This approach requires experienced participants, else the diagnosis is likely to default to IPF.[37,38]

This proposed approach presents several pitfalls. A surgical lung biopsy is required for any patient without a definite UIP pattern on HRCT. As noted earlier, many patients (those with a probable UIP pattern) would undergo a lung biopsy that is unlikely to provide additional useful information. It also results in a large number of patients that may be unclassifiable without a surgical lung biopsy, as the 2011 guidelines do not provide guidance on how to proceed in the absence of a surgical lung biopsy for patients without a definite UIP pattern on HRCT.

We enthusiastically endorse the approach to the diagnosis proposed by a working group on behalf of the Fleischner Society published in 2018.[16] This review revises the proposed radiographic patterns, formalizes an approach that takes into account the clinical likelihood of IPF, provides guidance to a multidisciplinary discussion, and introduces a working diagnosis of IPF. The Fleischner Society review proposes revised imaging categories that include definite

UIP, probable UIP, indeterminate for UIP, and CT features most consistent with non-IPF diagnosis. They encourage consideration into whether the clinical context is likely to reflect IPF. If no identifiable cause for pulmonary fibrosis can be identified in a patient older than 60 years, this reflects a likely clinical context of IPF. The authors advocate patients with a compatible clinical context, and either a definite or probable UIP pattern on imaging does not require a biopsy for a confident diagnosis of IPF. Patients who are younger than 60 years, who have potentially relevant environmental or medication exposures, or who have evidence of a connective tissue disease are considered to have an indeterminate clinical context for IPF. In patients with an indeterminate clinical context or indeterminate imaging, surgical lung biopsy is more likely to be informative.

The Fleischner Society review recognizes that an incomplete evaluation may occur in some patients, either because of safety concerns regarding surgical lung biopsy or patient preference. Such patients will benefit from a working diagnosis to guide ongoing management.[16] This working diagnosis should be obtained through multidisciplinary discussion and should take into account the clinical likelihood of IPF; available imaging; nonstandard testing, including bronchoscopy if performed; and longitudinal disease behavior.

The Fleischner Society review recommends a multidisciplinary discussion for cases with either an indeterminate clinical context or imaging pattern. This discussion is intended to assist with recommendations regarding further diagnostic steps, including bronchoscopy or surgical lung biopsy, and to incorporate these results into the diagnostic process. Multidisciplinary discussion is used to establish a working diagnosis based on available information.[16]

SPECIAL CONSIDERATIONS

The role of bronchoscopy in the diagnosis of suspected IPF is unclear. Transbrachial biopsy obtains very small samples of lung tissue that are generally inadequate to evaluate the architectural involvement of the given ILD.[39] It may assist in the diagnosis of airway-centered ILDs such as HP or sarcoidosis. Bronchoalveolar lavage (BAL) may be used to demonstrate a lymphocytosis that argues in favor of HP, cellular NSIP, or other forms of inflammatory ILD that may respond to immunosuppression.[40] The threshold value of lymphocytosis that strongly suggests these diagnoses has not been determined. Lymphocyte percentages greater than 25%–50% have been cited.[40]

Transbronchial cryobiopsy has been proposed as an alternative to surgical lung biopsy.[41-45] This approach involves using a cryoprobe that cools tissue from −85 to −95 °C. The frozen lung tissue obtained by this approach is substantially larger than traditional transbronchial biopsies but smaller than those obtained by surgical lung biopsy.[41] Various case series have demonstrated a diagnostic yield that may approach 80%.[44] Drawbacks to this approach include the relatively smaller samples obtained and the more central location (vs. peripheral) of the biopsies. It has not been shown that this technique can be safely applied outside centers with extensive experience.

Disease behavior may provide a practical clue to the diagnosis.[16,46] IPF is characterized by a natural history of inexorable progression. In cases with an indeterminate clinical context or imaging pattern but with a natural history consistent with IPF, a working diagnosis of IPF is suggested. It must be recognized that fibrosing HP and UIP due to connective tissue diseases also have a natural history of progressive fibrosis. Optimal therapies for these patients have not been well studied.

ADDITIONAL CHALLENGES

Many patients will have exposures of unclear significance (e.g., remote occupational exposure or a potential inhaled exposure). The specific dose and timing of exposures in relation to the onset of ILD is helpful in assessing the potential relevance. A multidisciplinary discussion may inform the utility of further testing (such as bronchoscopy with BAL) or a surgical biopsy. Disease behavior may be informative in establishing a working diagnosis of IPF.[16]

Familial forms of pulmonary fibrosis are characterized by two or more relatives with ILD.[47] Familial interstitial pneumonia may be associated with common genetic variants (e.g., a promoter variant that leads to increased MUC5B mucin production) or rare mutations in genes associated with telomere maintenance or surfactant production.[48] Affected families with familial interstitial pneumonia may have family members with various patterns of injury including UIP, NSIP, or granulomatous lung disease resembling HP.[47] Family members may have identifiable causes of lung disease, including autoimmune disease or inhalational exposures. Imaging patterns in familial forms of UIP are more commonly upper lung predominant or diffuse in the axial and craniocaudal plane than sporadic IPF.[49] Unclassifiable patterns of pulmonary fibrosis may be more commonly seen in familial interstitial pneumonia than in sporadic IIP.[47] Risk of familial pulmonary fibrosis is associated with male sex, advanced age, and tobacco exposure.[47] A multidisciplinary discussion may provide useful guidance regarding the potential utility of a biopsy and result in a working diagnosis of familial IPF without a biopsy.

As noted earlier, various patterns of lung injury may result from established autoimmune disease. Although lung biopsy may provide additional prognostic information, it is often not pursued because is it unlikely to change management. It is well recognized that many patients will have features that suggest an underlying CTD but that do not meet formal diagnostic criteria. Interstitial pneumonia with autoimmune features (IPAFs) was introduced as a research concept to evaluate questions regarding prognosis and appropriate management of these patients. Many patients with IPAF have a UIP pattern of lung injury. We currently advocate treating patients with IPAF and a suspected pattern of UIP as IPF.

Combined pulmonary fibrosis and emphysema (CPFE) has been proposed as a distinct phenotype of IPF, while some experts view it as simply two smoking-related lung diseases in the same patient.[50–53,54] Substantial emphysema may distort the radiographic pattern of interstitial changes and make it more difficult to assess for a definitive pattern. Initial reports suggested that the fibrosis of CPFE always represented a pattern of UIP; however, additional reports have now demonstrated that NSIP and unclassifiable patterns of fibrosis may also be seen.[52] Furthermore, CPFE has been recognized to frequently occur in patients with RA-associated pulmonary fibrosis.[55] Therefore, the usual detailed, multidisciplinary evaluation into the context and pattern of injury should occur in patients with evidence of fibrosis and emphysema. Clinicians need to determine if the emphysema or the fibrosis is the dominant process and should target appropriate therapy to each component.

Pleuroparenchymal fibroelastosis (PPFE) is a newly recognized pattern of upper lobe predominant fibrosis characterized by an exuberant deposition of elastin in the pleura. Increasing recognition of this entity led to its inclusion as a rare pattern of IIP.[3,56–60] Case series have shown that patients with PPFE may also frequently have UIP present.[60,61] In addition, PPFE has been recognized to be idiopathic in some cases and to occur in the context of drug exposure (especially certain forms of chemotherapy) and autoimmune disease. The rarity of this entity limits the current understanding of appropriate therapies. Until more is known about the overlap of UIP and PPFE, patients who would otherwise meet criteria for IPF should be classified as IPF, regardless of the presence of superimposed features of PPFE.[16]

SUMMARY

- The diagnosis of a specific ILD requires a detailed evaluation of the context in which the disease arose and evaluation of the pattern of lung involvement.
- IPF requires a multidisciplinary approach to diagnosis.
- A working diagnosis may provide a practical approach for patients who do not meet current diagnostic criteria.

REFERENCES

1. Raghu G, et al. An official ATS/ERS/JRS/ALAT statement: idiopathic pulmonary fibrosis: evidence-based guidelines for diagnosis and management. *Am J Respir Crit Care Med.* 2011;183(6):788–824.
2. American Thoracic Society/European Respiratory Society International Multidisciplinary Consensus Classification of the Idiopathic Interstitial Pneumonias. This joint statement of the American Thoracic Society (ATS), and the European Respiratory Society (ERS) was adopted by the ATS board of directors, June 2001 and by the ERS executive committee, June 2001. *Am J Respir Crit Care Med.* 2002; 165(2):277–304.
3. Travis WD, et al. An official American Thoracic Society/European Respiratory Society statement: update of the international multidisciplinary classification of the idiopathic interstitial pneumonias. *Am J Respir Crit Care Med.* 2013; 188(6):733–748.
4. Idiopathic Pulmonary Fibrosis Clinical Research N, et al. Randomized trial of acetylcysteine in idiopathic pulmonary fibrosis. *N Engl J Med.* 2014;370(22):2093–2101.
5. Raghu G, et al. An official ATS/ERS/JRS/ALAT clinical practice guideline: treatment of idiopathic pulmonary fibrosis. An update of the 2011 clinical practice guideline. *Am J Respir Crit Care Med.* 2015;192(2):e3–19.
6. Myers JL. Hypersensitivity pneumonia: the role of lung biopsy in diagnosis and management. *Mod Pathol.* 2012; 25(suppl 1):S58–S67.
7. Morell F, et al. Chronic hypersensitivity pneumonitis in patients diagnosed with idiopathic pulmonary fibrosis: a prospective case-cohort study. *Lancet Respir Med.* 2013; 1(9):685–694.
8. Tsuchiya Y, et al. Lung diseases directly associated with rheumatoid arthritis and their relationship to outcome. *Eur Respir J.* 2011;37(6):1411–1417.
9. Selman M, et al. Hypersensitivity pneumonitis caused by fungi. *Proc Am Thorac Soc.* 2010;7(3):229–236.
10. Lacasse Y, et al. Clinical diagnosis of hypersensitivity pneumonitis [see comment]. *Am J Respir Crit Care Med.* 2003; 168(8):952–958.

11. Yunt ZX, et al. High resolution computed tomography pattern of usual interstitial pneumonia in rheumatoid arthritis-associated interstitial lung disease: relationship to survival. *Respir Med.* 2017;126:100−104.

12. Park JH, et al. Prognosis of fibrotic interstitial pneumonia: idiopathic versus collagen vascular disease-related subtypes. *Am J Respir Crit Care Med.* 2007;175(7):705−711.

13. Kim EJ, et al. Usual interstitial pneumonia in rheumatoid arthritis-associated interstitial lung disease. *Eur Respir J.* 2010;35(6):1322−1328.

14. Fernandez Perez ER, et al. Identifying an inciting antigen is associated with improved survival in patients with chronic hypersensitivity pneumonitis. *Chest.* 2013;144(5):1644−1651.

15. Garcia CK, Wright WE, Shay JW. Human diseases of telomerase dysfunction: insights into tissue aging. *Nucl Acids Res.* 2007;35(22):7406−7416.

16. Lynch DA, et al. Diagnostic criteria for idiopathic pulmonary fibrosis: a Fleischner Society White Paper. *Lancet Respir Med.* 2018;6(2):138−153.

17. The Drug-induced Respiratory Disease Website. Available from: www.pneumotox.com.

18. CHEST Interstitial and Diffuse Lung Disease Patient Questionnaire. Available from: http://www.chestnet.org/sitecore modules/web/~/media/chesnetorg/Foundation/Documents/Lung Disease Questionaire.ashx.

19. Brownell R, et al. The use of pretest probability increases the value of high-resolution CT in diagnosing usual interstitial pneumonia. *Thorax.* 2017;72(5):424−429.

20. Fell CD, et al. Clinical predictors of a diagnosis of idiopathic pulmonary fibrosis. *Am J Respir Crit Care Med.* 2010;181(8):832−837.

21. Patterson KC, et al. Interstitial lung disease in the elderly. *Chest.* 2017;151(4):838−844.

22. Spagnolo P, Cordier JF, Cottin V. Connective tissue diseases, multimorbidity and the ageing lung. *Eur Respir J.* 2016;47(5):1535−1558.

23. Zamora-Legoff JA, et al. Patterns of interstitial lung disease and mortality in rheumatoid arthritis. *Rheumatology.* 2017;56(3):344−350.

24. Woge MJ, Ryu JH, Moua T. Diagnostic implications of positive avian serology in suspected hypersensitivity pneumonitis. *Respir Med.* 2017;129:173−178.

25. Raghu G, et al. Incidence and prevalence of idiopathic pulmonary fibrosis. *Am J Respir Crit Care Med.* 2006;174(7):810−816.

26. Nadrous HF, et al. Idiopathic pulmonary fibrosis in patients younger than 50 years. *Mayo Clin Proc.* 2005;80(1):37−40.

27. Homma Y, et al. Can interstitial pneumonia as the sole presentation of collagen vascular diseases be differentiated from idiopathic interstitial pneumonia? *Respiration.* 1995;62(5):248−251.

28. Silva CI, et al. Chronic hypersensitivity pneumonitis: differentiation from idiopathic pulmonary fibrosis and nonspecific interstitial pneumonia by using thin-section CT. *Radiology.* 2008;246(1):288−297.

29. Hunninghake GW, et al. Utility of a lung biopsy for the diagnosis of idiopathic pulmonary fibrosis. *Am J Respir Crit Care Med.* 2001;164(2):193−196.

30. Raghu G, et al. The accuracy of the clinical diagnosis of new-onset idiopathic pulmonary fibrosis and other interstitial lung disease: a prospective study. *Chest.* 1999;116(5):1168−1174.

31. Chung JH, et al. CT scan findings of probable usual interstitial pneumonitis have a high predictive value for histologic usual interstitial pneumonitis. *Chest.* 2015;147(2):450−459.

32. Raghu G, et al. Diagnosis of idiopathic pulmonary fibrosis with high-resolution CT in patients with little or no radiological evidence of honeycombing: secondary analysis of a randomised, controlled trial. *Lancet Respir Med.* 2014;2(4):277−284.

33. Chung JH, et al. CT-pathologic correlation of major types of pulmonary fibrosis: insights for revisions to current guidelines. *Am J Roentgenol.* 2018;210(5):1034−1041.

34. Flaherty KR, et al. Histopathologic variability in usual and nonspecific interstitial pneumonias. *Am J Respir Crit Care Med.* 2001;164(9):1722−1727.

35. Monaghan H, et al. Prognostic implications of histologic patterns in multiple surgical lung biopsies from patients with idiopathic interstitial pneumonias. *Chest.* 2004;125(2):522−526.

36. Flaherty KR, et al. Idiopathic interstitial pneumonia: what is the effect of a multidisciplinary approach to diagnosis? *Am J Respir Crit Care Med.* 2004;170(8):904−910.

37. Flaherty KR, et al. Idiopathic interstitial pneumonia: do community and academic physicians agree on diagnosis? *Am J Respir Crit Care Med.* 2007;175(10):1054−1060.

38. Walsh SLF, et al. Diagnostic accuracy of a clinical diagnosis of idiopathic pulmonary fibrosis: an international case−cohort study. *Eur Respir J.* 2017;50(2).

39. Sheth JS, et al. Utility of transbronchial vs surgical lung biopsy in the diagnosis of suspected fibrotic interstitial lung disease. *Chest.* 2017;151(2):389−399.

40. Meyer KC, et al. An official American Thoracic Society clinical practice guideline: the clinical utility of bronchoalveolar lavage cellular analysis in interstitial lung disease. *Am J Respir Crit Care Med.* 2012;185(9):1004−1014.

41. Johannson KA, et al. Diagnostic yield and complications of transbronchial lung cryobiopsy for interstitial lung disease. A systematic review and metaanalysis. *Ann Am Thorac Soc.* 2016;13(10):1828−1838.

42. Ravaglia C, et al. Safety and diagnostic yield of transbronchial lung cryobiopsy in diffuse parenchymal lung diseases: a comparative study versus video-assisted thoracoscopic lung biopsy and a systematic review of the literature. *Respiration.* 2016;91(3):215−227.

43. Tomassetti S, et al. Bronchoscopic lung cryobiopsy increases diagnostic confidence in the multidisciplinary diagnosis of idiopathic pulmonary fibrosis. *Am J Respir Crit Care Med.* 2016;193(7):745−752.

44. Colby TV, et al. Transbronchial cryobiopsy in diffuse lung disease: update for the pathologist. *Arch Pathol Lab Med.* 2017;141(7):891−900.

45. Casoni GL, et al. Transbronchial lung cryobiopsy in the diagnosis of fibrotic interstitial lung diseases. *PLoS One Electron Resour.* 2014;9(2):e86716.
46. Wells AU. The revised ATS/ERS/JRS/ALAT diagnostic criteria for idiopathic pulmonary fibrosis (IPF)—practical implications. *Respir Res.* 2013;14(suppl 1):S2.
47. Steele MP, et al. Clinical and pathologic features of familial interstitial pneumonia. *Am J Respir Crit Care Med.* 2005;172(9):1146–1152.
48. Mathai SK, et al. Pulmonary fibrosis in the era of stratified medicine. *Thorax.* 2016;71(12):1154–1160.
49. Lee HL, et al. Familial idiopathic pulmonary fibrosis: clinical features and outcome. *Chest.* 2005;127(6):2034–2041.
50. Mejia M, et al. Idiopathic pulmonary fibrosis and emphysema: decreased survival associated with severe pulmonary arterial hypertension. *Chest.* 2009;136(1):10–15.
51. Mura M, et al. The presence of emphysema further impairs physiologic function in patients with idiopathic pulmonary fibrosis. *Respir Care.* 2006;51(3):257–265.
52. Akira M, et al. Usual interstitial pneumonia and nonspecific interstitial pneumonia with and without concurrent emphysema: thin-section CT findings. *Radiology.* 2009;251(1):271–279.
53. Cottin V. The impact of emphysema in pulmonary fibrosis. *Eur Respir Rev.* 2013;22(128):153–157.
54. Ryerson CJ, et al. CLinical features and outcomes in combined pulmonary fibrosis and emphysema in idiopathic pulmonary fibrosis. *Chest J.* 2013;144(1):234–240.
55. Antoniou K. Smoking-related emphysema is associated with idiopathic pulmonary fibrosis and rheumatoid lung. *Respirology.* 2013.
56. Frankel SK, et al. Idiopathic pleuroparenchymal fibroelastosis: description of a novel clinicopathologic entity. *Chest.* 2004;126(6):2007–2013.
57. von der Thusen JH, et al. Pleuroparenchymal fibroelastosis in patients with pulmonary disease secondary to bone marrow transplantation. *Mod Pathol.* 2011;24(12):1633–1639.
58. Piciucchi S, et al. High resolution CT and histological findings in idiopathic pleuroparenchymal fibroelastosis: features and differential diagnosis. *Respir Res.* 2011;12:111.
59. Reddy TL, et al. Pleuroparenchymal fibroelastosis: a spectrum of histopathological and imaging phenotypes. *Eur Respir J.* 2012;40(2):377–385.
60. Khiroya R, et al. Pleuroparenchymal fibroelastosis: a review of histopathologic features and the relationship between histologic parameters and survival. *Am J Surg Pathol.* 2017;41(12):1683–1689.
61. Oda T, et al. Distinct characteristics of pleuroparenchymal fibroelastosis with usual interstitial pneumonia compared with idiopathic pulmonary fibrosis. *Chest.* 2014;146(5):1248–1255.

IPF Look-Alikes: Chronic Hypersensitivity Pneumonitis, Connective Tissue Disorder—Related Pulmonary Fibrosis, and Other Fibrosing Interstitial Pneumonias

EVANS R. FERNÁNDEZ PÉREZ, MD, MS, FCCP • ISABELLE AMIGUES, MD • JOSHUA J. SOLOMON, MD

A crucial component of the diagnosis of idiopathic pulmonary fibrosis (IPF) is the radiographic pattern on high-resolution computed tomography (HRCT). After exclusion of other known causes of pulmonary fibrosis, a pattern of usual interstitial pneumonia (UIP) can lead to a diagnosis of IPF without the need for histopathologic confirmation. The radiographic pattern of UIP is not specific for IPF and can be seen in other interstitial lung diseases (ILDs). An appreciation for these other conditions, and excluding their presence, is critical to making a confident diagnosis of IPF. We will review the other major, non-IPF, causes of a UIP pattern of fibrosis on HRCT.

CHRONIC HYPERSENSITIVITY PNEUMONITIS

Hypersensitivity pneumonitis (HP) is a lung disease that results from inhalation of an antigen to which a person has been previously sensitized. It is characterized pathologically by a varying degree of inflammation and fibrosis and presents clinically in acute, and chronic forms (CHP), although there is considerable overlap among them. In the chronic form, the radiology, physiology, and clinical course can mimic IPF and distinguishing the two entities can be challenging.

Epidemiology

While HP is a rare disease, it is one of the most common causes of ILD. Using a large US administrative database with over 150 million geographically and ethnically diverse subjects, 1-year prevalence rates for HP ranged from 1.67 to 2.71 per 100,000 persons, and incidence rates ranged from 1.28 to 1.94 per 100,000 persons per year.[1] Similar to IPF, the disease increases with age and the mortality rate is higher for men than women.[1]

Diagnosis

Making a confident diagnosis of HP can be challenging. HP has an array of clinical phenotypes. There have been several, nonvalidated diagnostic criteria proposed, but there is no consensus around any one set.[2–5] In addition, in CHP (i.e., the fibrotic form), there is often a long latency between first exposure and subsequent development of lung fibrosis. Consequently, a patient's exposure to the inciting antigen (IA) may have occurred long before, or even ceased prior to, the onset of clinically apparent disease, blurring the link between antigen exposure and the disease. In many cases of CHP, the exposure goes unrecognized because a thorough and accurate environmental history is unobtainable, there is an underappreciated temporal association between a specific exposure and disease development, or there is inaccurate recollection of past or current exposures by the patient.[6]

Identifying the Inciting Antigen

Once clinical suspicion for HP is aroused, the diagnostic evaluation begins with an in-depth medical history. Using a practice-specific, geographically appropriate environmental exposure questionnaire can save time and improve the sensitivity of detecting the IA. Key elements of the exposure history are shown in Table 8.1. Although the presence of a concerning exposure does not define the disease as HP in the absence of supporting clinical-radiologic-pathologic findings, identifying exposure to a known IA is the most important predictor of the presence of HP. For instance, among subjects with CHP, the combination of a history of exposure to birds or down feathers and characteristic HRCT features has a specificity of 91% for the

diagnosis of HP (i.e., bird fancier's lung) and displays excellent performance in discriminating HP from IPF without need for an inhalation challenge test, bronchoalveolar lavage (BAL), or surgical lung biopsy.[7] In addition to its usefulness for diagnosis, identifying the IA impacts treatment decisions and prognosis. In a cohort of 142 consecutive adult patients with clinical-radiologic-pathologic CHP, even after adjusting for the presence of fibrosis, patient age, pulmonary function, and smoking history, survival was significantly longer for patients with an identified IA exposure

TABLE 8.1
Important Elements for a Detailed Environmental and Occupational History

Criteria	Comments
Understand the occupation and environmental exposure	Mnemonics can help quickly screen for a concerning exposure.
WHACS[a]: What do you do? How do you do it? Are you concerned about any of your exposures on and off the job? Coworkers or others exposed or with similar symptoms? Satisfied with your job?	
VGDF: Are you exposed to vapors, gases, dust, or fumes? or known hazard at work?	
A concerning exposure should be suspected when evaluating relationship with symptoms	
• Strength	List and type of exposure and amount (e.g., the strength of the causal relationship is higher in a person who raises and has indoor birds than a person who has one outdoor bird feeder).
• Reversibility	Reduction in exposure is followed by improvement in symptoms (e.g., antigen avoidance by moving out to a new home or significant improvement when away from work).
• Dose response	Larger exposure to cause-associated higher rates of HP in susceptible persons or lack of pharmacologic therapeutic response (e.g., degree of occupational exposure to solvent and isocyanates).
• Temporality	The exposure precedes the symptoms and HP diagnosis or symptoms aggravated during work.
• Consistency	Repeatedly observed in different places, circumstances, and times (e.g., down pillow, duvets).
• Specificity	One exposure leads to HP (e.g., several cases of HP are identified in one geographic area or family such as clustering of Japanese summer-type HP cases).
• Analogy	Cause and effect relationship already established for a similar exposure (e.g., Host HP response against *Aspergillus* species in different geographic farming regions).

HP, hypersensitivity pneumonitis.

[a] Blue AV, Chessman AW, Gilbert GE, et al. Medical students' abilities to take an occupational history: use of the WHACS mnemonic. *J Occup Environ Med.* 2000; 42:1050–1053.

than those with an unidentified IA exposure (median, 8.75 years vs. 4.88 years).[8] Identification of the IA can affect treatment decisions, including defining specific recommendations related to antigenic mitigation, guiding initial home/workplace evaluation by an industrial hygienist, establishing a legal precedent of a compensable disability due to occupational HP, and unveiling a population at risk that may benefit from preventive measures.

Once the exposure is identified, the clinician must determine the strategies for IA eradication. Although in some cases mitigation can be straightforward (e.g., indoor mold–related HP from a kitchen composter or a pipe water leak), others may require a walkthrough evaluation and visual home/workplace inspection to uncover and verify the type and extent of microbial exposure and to assess environmental health risks.[9,10] Recommended, certified, experienced technicians and inspectors can be found working in conjunction with an occupational medicine department or can be located close to the patient's home/workplace by searching the American Industrial Hygiene Association's consultants listing (www.aiha.org).

Imaging

HRCT can provide diagnostic clues (i.e., help distinguish IPF from CHP) as well as a global assessment of the extent of fibrosis in CHP. In CHP, a number of abnormal chest imaging features can be seen on HRCT: course reticular opacities, honeycomb cysts, traction bronchiectasis or bronchiolectasis, volume loss, geographic heterogeneity with expiratory air trapping, centrilobular nodules, and architectural distortion. The distribution of these abnormal features in CHP is typically peripheral in the axial plane and lower lung preponderant. This lower zone predominance, described in 11%–65% of cases, can make the distinction from IPF a challenge.[11–16] When trying to distinguish IPF from CHP by HRCT, the diagnosis is reasonably certain (up to 90% accuracy for histologic evidence of CHP) when an experienced thoracic radiologist diagnoses a pattern of CHP with a high level of confidence; however, when the diagnosis is made without a high level of confidence, the accuracy decreases to around 60%.[17] The HRCT features that best differentiate CHP from nonspecific interstitial pneumonia (NSIP) and IPF are mosaic attenuation with lobular areas of decreased attenuation and expiratory air trapping, centrilobular nodules, peribronchiolar disease distribution (i.e., features inconsistent with a definite UIP pattern). However, any or all of these findings may be absent in CHP with advanced fibrosis.

Serologic Evaluation

The diagnostic yield of circulating, antigen-specific IgG antibodies in HP varies according to the characteristics of the test and the prevalence of HP. The sensitivity and negative predictive value of the test are improved if antigens are extracted from the patient's environment, the testing utilizes antigens locally prevalent, and/or if quantitative test (e.g., enzyme-linked immunosorbent assay or ELISA) as opposed to qualitative (e.g., double immunodiffusion) are used.[10,18–21] False negatives are frequently observed when the suspected IA is not part of the routine HP panel.[20,22–24] The presence of a circulating antibody to a specific antigen is most likely a marker of exposure but not conclusive evidence of disease in the absence of the appropriate clinical-radiologic context. Moreover, the power of precipitins to discriminate patients with HP (e.g., farmer's lung) from healthy, exposed subjects is poor.[23,25,26] Therefore, the presence of precipitins in exposed, asymptomatic subjects does not predict the presence of HP or an increased risk of developing HP. The method used to identify antibodies, disease prevalence, and the type of antigen tested can influence the accuracy of precipitin testing.[18,19] Table 8.2 outlines the characteristics of the different serologic tests for HP.

Specific Inhalation Challenge

The specific inhalation challenge (SIC) is predominantly useful in the chronic forms of HP, when distinction from IPF can be challenging. In expert centers, before opting for a more invasive surgical lung biopsy, an SIC could be considered to help support the diagnosis and confirm the IA. The sensitivity and negative predictive value of SIC are highest in patients with HP caused by avian or fungal proteins.[27] Several, nonvalidated criteria for defining a positive SIC response in the diagnosis of environmental- or occupational-related HP have been reported.[27–32] Despite the reported safety of SIC in HP, the lack of standardization is a main limiting factor precluding its widespread use in clinical practice.[23,27]

Bronchoalveolar Lavage and Histopathology

The BAL cellular pattern in a healthy adult nonsmoker shows 10%–15% lymphocytes. BAL lymphocytosis is not specific for HP; however, a significant elevation in the lymphocyte percentage (e.g., >%50%) is highly suggestive of HP in the correct clinical setting.[33] BAL lymphocytosis is more prevalent in acute HP than in CHP and is more common in patients with HP who have a typical HP or NSIP-like pattern on surgical lung biopsy than those with a UIP-like pattern.[34] In

TABLE 8.2
Characteristics of Immunoassay Methods Utilized in Hypersensitivity Pneumonitis

Method	Commercial Availability	Technical Demand and Personal Training	Duration	IgG Quantification[a]	Sensitivity/ Specificity	Cost
Double immunodiffusion	Very high	Low	Hours	No	Low/low	$
Immunoelectrodiffusion	Medium-low[b]	Low	Hours	No	Medium/ low	$
ImmunoCAP[c]	Medium-low	Medium-low (automatized process)	Hours	Yes	Medium/ high	$$
ELISA	Low[c]	High	Hours	Yes	Medium-high/high	$$
Western blot	Low	High	Hours	Yes	Medium/ high	$$$
Lymphocyte proliferation test	Very low[d]	Very high	Time consuming (days—weeks)	No	Low/very high	$$$$

ELISA, enzyme-linked immunosorbent assay.
[a] The laboratory needs to determine the optimal IgG cut-off labels.
[b] Available at centers outside the United States.
[c] Commercially available for bird-specific antigen testing in the United States.
[d] A research tool. Utilized in selected centers.

patients with characteristic CHP or those with a definite UIP pattern on HRCT but with a high pretest probability of disease (i.e., a specific and clinically relevant IA has been identified), the presence of more than 30% lymphocytes in BAL fluid correlates with an increased likelihood of CHP and argues against IPF.[35] Although the lack of BAL lymphocytosis may rule out acute HP in the appropriate clinical context, it does not exclude CHP.[36,37] Early HP has been characterized by an increase in CD8+ BAL lymphocytes and inversion of the CD4+/CD8+.[38] However, T-cell subsets change during the course of the disease, and this testing is currently not recommended as a routine component of BAL cellular analysis.[33]

Transbronchial biopsy can be useful in the diagnosis of diseases with a peribronchiolar or centrilobular distribution such as HP. However, small specimen size and sampling error are significant limitations.[39,40] Video-assisted thoracoscopic biopsy is widely available and remains the surgical procedure of choice when a diagnosis cannot be obtained by less invasive tests and the clinical-radiologic assessment is inconclusive. CHP is the most challenging histopathologic pattern among HP subtypes. When present, the early

findings of lymphoplasmocytic interstitial pneumonia, bronchiolitis, air-space or interstitial nonnecrotizing granulomas, and an accentuated centrilobular/peribronchiolar distribution may help distinguish CHP from UIP/IPF.[41–44] Although nonnecrotizing poorly formed granulomas have classically been described in HP, they are not specific for HP, and there is no set threshold for how many granulomas on pathology differentiate CHP from UIP/IPF. In our experience, instead of focusing on a single feature, such as the presence or absence of granulomas, a constellation of features helps with the diagnosis, such as the predominant site of involvement and the extent and distribution of changes. Although some cases of CHP are morphologically indistinguishable from "bland" UIP, in many cases, the distinction is clear when reviewed by expert thoracic pathologists. Thus, it is highly advisable to have the slides reviewed at a specialized referral center.

Putting It all Together

When there is suspicion for HP, exclusion of alternative etiologies and multidisciplinary evaluation is needed. The importance of a thorough multidisciplinary review for diagnostic accuracy is underscored by the fact that a higher confidence for HP diagnosis relies on the meticulous evaluation of available data rather than any single test result.[45] Because antigen mitigation is critical and the HP diagnosis requires careful attention to an environmental and occupational history, it is important to have an occupational medicine specialist involved early in the multidisciplinary case review if possible.

After evaluating the HRCT pattern, consider the lower risk, less invasive test first before proceeding with a surgical lung biopsy. This approach of using serial testing maximizes specificity and positive predictive value. If some of these tests are not available (e.g., quantitative precipitins, SIC) or referral to an ILD center is not possible, performing the test with the highest specificity is most efficient (e.g., BAL rather than precipitins according to the clinical context). After the HP diagnosis is made, and if not previously done in a patient with suspected HP, IA removal and careful reevaluation for possible ongoing reexposure is vital. Fig. 8.1 outlines a diagnostic algorithm for CHP.

CONNECTIVE TISSUE DISORDER—ASSOCIATED INTERSTITIAL LUNG DISEASE

As with any interstitial lung disease (ILD), a diagnosis of IPF should be accepted only after careful evaluation for the presence of an underlying rheumatologic autoimmune disease also known as connective tissue disorder (CTD). Patients with CTD can have a radiographic and/or histopathologic pattern of UIP indistinguishable from those seen in IPF. Differences in treatment and outcomes between patients with CTD-related ILD and IPF justify an extensive evaluation to rule out CTD when IPF is suspected. This chapter reviews key features for the diagnosis and management of CTD-ILD and how to differentiate subtle forms of fibrotic CTD-ILD from IPF.

Background

CTDs are characterized by systemic organ manifestations, often affecting the musculoskeletal system, in association with autoimmune manifestations, such as the presence of autoantibodies. In all-comers with CTD-ILD, the UIP pattern on HRCT (characterized by honeycombing, reticulation, and traction bronchiectasis in a predominantly basal and/or peripheral distribution) is one of the most commonly observed interstitial lung disease patterns.[45,46]

All CTDs can present with a radiologic or pathologic UIP pattern; however, the most common CTDs associated with UIP are rheumatoid arthritis (RA) and systemic sclerosis (SSc). In fact, UIP is the most commonly observed pattern of RA-related ILD (RA-ILD).[47,48] UIP also comprises a significant percentage of the 50% —80% of patients with SSc who have ILD.[49–51]

Lung involvement, particularly UIP, can be the first manifestation of CTD, at times preceding the development of extrathoracic manifestations by several years.[52,53] In some cases, ILD and circulating autoantibodies are the only conspicuous findings pointing to the possible presence of a CTD. For instance, the presence of high titers of anticyclic citrullinated peptide antibodies is a clue to possible RA in a patient without typical RA joint symptoms who presents with UIP pattern on CT.[54] Therefore, a thorough history inquiring about CTD symptoms, a careful physical examination looking for peripheral manifestations of a CTD, and a wide autoimmune screen in all patients who present with possible IPF is warranted.

It is not uncommon for patients with ILD to present with autoantibodies or clinical, radiographic, or pathologic features suggestive of an underlying autoimmune condition while not meeting established criteria for a CTD diagnosis. Previous descriptions of such cases include undifferentiated CTD—associated ILD (UCTD-ILD),[55] lung-dominant CTD,[56] and autoimmune-featured ILD.[57] Recently, the term *interstitial pneumonia with autoimmune features (IPAF)* was created by a joint task force of the European Respiratory and American Thoracic research societies to better categorize and facilitate research in this subset of patients.[58] The criteria for IPAF are outlined in Table 8.3.

Clinical Presentation

Among patients with radiographic or histopathologic UIP, there are clues in the clinical presentation that can suggest the presence of an underlying CTD. Compared with patients with IPF, patients with CTD-UIP tend to be younger, more likely female, and nonsmokers,[59] and they may present earlier in the course of disease, with a shorter duration of symptoms, and higher total lung capacity.[60] All patients with ILD should have a thorough history and physical to identify subtle features suggestive of CTD. For example, joint pain that is worse in the morning or associated with morning stiffness or joint swelling, especially when symmetric, may suggest RA in the appropriate setting. A history of Raynaud's phenomenon, gastroesophageal reflux, skin tightening, sclerodactyly, or pericardial disease can suggest SSc. Dry mouth or dry eyes can suggest primary or secondary Sjögren's syndrome. Muscle pain or weakness, joint pain, and/or skin fissuring on the fingers (so called "mechanic's hands") can suggest the myositis spectrum of disease. Table 8.4 describes

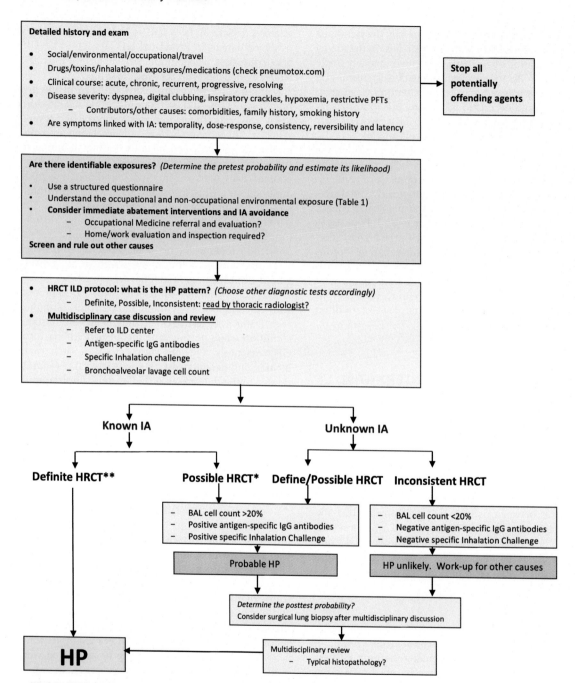

Detailed history and exam

- Social/environmental/occupational/travel
- Drugs/toxins/inhalational exposures/medications (check pneumotox.com)
- Clinical course: acute, chronic, recurrent, progressive, resolving
- Disease severity: dyspnea, digital clubbing, inspiratory crackles, hypoxemia, restrictive PFTs
    - Contributors/other causes: comorbidities, family history, smoking history
- Are symptoms linked with IA: temporality, dose-response, consistency, reversibility and latency

Stop all potentially offending agents

Are there identifiable exposures? *(Determine the pretest probability and estimate its likelihood)*

- Use a structured questionnaire
- Understand the occupational and non-occupational environmental exposure (Table 1)
- **Consider immediate abatement interventions and IA avoidance**
    - Occupational Medicine referral and evaluation?
    - Home/work evaluation and inspection required?

Screen and rule out other causes

- **HRCT ILD protocol: what is the HP pattern?** *(Choose other diagnostic tests accordingly)*
    - Definite, Possible, Inconsistent: <u>read by thoracic radiologist?</u>
- **Multidisciplinary case discussion and review**
    - Refer to ILD center
    - Antigen-specific IgG antibodies
    - Specific Inhalation challenge
    - Bronchoalveolar lavage cell count

Known IA

Unknown IA

Definite HRCT**

Possible HRCT*

Define/Possible HRCT

Inconsistent HRCT

- BAL cell count >20%
- Positive antigen-specific IgG antibodies
- Positive specific Inhalation Challenge

- BAL cell count <20%
- Negative antigen-specific IgG antibodies
- Negative specific Inhalation Challenge

Probable HP

HP unlikely. Work-up for other causes

Determine the posttest probability?
Consider surgical lung biopsy after multidisciplinary discussion

HP

Multidisciplinary review
- Typical histopathology?

**Definite HRCT fibrotic HP: Evidence of lung fibrosis (reticular abnormality and/or, traction bronchiectasis and/or, architectural distortion, and/or honeycombing) and one or more of the associated finding: a) Multilobular inspiratory mosaic attenuation, b) Multilobular air trapping on expiratory images, C) Profuse centrilobular ground glass nodular opacities
*Possible HRCT fibrotic HP: Evidence of lung fibrosis (as above) in the absence of any of above associated findings.

FIG. 8.1 Approach to suspected hypersensitivity pneumonitis. *BAL*, bronchoalveolar lavage; *HP*, hypersensitivity pneumonitis; *ILD*, interstitial lung diseases; *IA*, inciting antigen; *HRCT*, high-resolution computed tomography; *PFT*, pulmonary function testing.

TABLE 8.3
Classification Criteria for Interstitial Pneumonia With Autoimmune Features

1. Presence of interstitial pneumonia (by HRCT or surgical lung biopsy),
2. Exclusion of alternative etiologies,
3. Unmet criteria of a defined connective tissue disease, and
4. Inclusion of at least one feature from at least two of these domains:
   A. **Clinical domain**
   B. **Serologic domain**
   C. **Morphologic domain**
   A. *Clinical domain*
      1. Distal digital fissure (i.e., "mechanic hands")
      2. Distal digital tip ulceration
      3. Inflammatory arthritis or polyarticular morning joint stiffness $\geq$60 min
      4. Palmar telangiectasia
      5. Raynaud's phenomenon
      6. Unexplained digital edema
      7. Unexplained fixed rash on the digital extensor surfaces (Gottron's sign)
   B. *Serologic domain*
      1. ANA $\geq$1:320, diffuse, speckled, homogenous patterns or
         a. ANA nucleolar pattern (any titer) or
         b. ANA centromere pattern (any titer) or
      2. RF $\geq$ 2$\times$ upper limit of normal
      3. Anti-CCP
      4. Anti-dsDNA
      5. Anti-Ro (SS-A)
      6. Anti-La (SS-B)
      7. Anti-ribonucleoprotein (RNP)
      8. Anti-Smith (Sm)
      9. Anti-topoisomerase (Scl-70)
      10. Anti-tRNA synthetase (e.g., Jo-1, PL-7, PL-12, EJ, OJ, KS, Zo, tRS)
      11. Anti-PM-Scl
      12. Anti-MDA-5
   C. *Morphologic domain*
      1. Suggestive radiology patterns by HRCT:
         a. NSIP
         b. OP
         c. NSIP with OP overlap
      2. Histopathology patterns or features by surgical lung biopsy:
         a. NSIP
         b. OP
         c. NSIP with OP overlap
         d. LIP
         e. Interstitial lymphoid aggregates with germinal centers
         f. Diffuse lymphoplasmacytic infiltration (with or without lymphoid follicles)
      3. Multicompartment involvement (in addition to interstitial pneumonia):
         a. Unexplained pleural effusion or thickening
         b. Unexplained pericardial effusion or thickening
         c. Unexplained intrinsic airways disease (by PFT, imaging, or pathology)
         d. Unexplained pulmonary vasculopathy

anti-CCP, anticyclic citrullinated peptide; *ANA*, antinuclear antibody; *HRCT*, high-resolution computed tomography; *LIP*, lymphoid interstitial pneumonia; *NSIP*, nonspecific interstitial pneumonia; *OP*, organizing pneumonia; *PFT*, pulmonary function testing: includes airflow obstruction, bronchiolitis or bronchiectasis; *RF*, rheumatoid factor.
Adapted from Fischer, et al. An official European Respiratory Society/American Thoracic Society research statement: interstitial pneumonia with autoimmune features. *Eur Respir J.* 2015.

TABLE 8.4
Clinical Diagnostic Criteria for Commonly Encountered Connective Tissue Disorders

Rheumatoid Arthritis	Systemic Sclerosis	Sjögren's Syndrome	Polymyositis and Dermatomyositis
1. Morning stiffness of the joints lasting at least 1 h 2. Involvement of three or more joints (PIP, MCP, wrist, elbow, knee, ankle, MTP) 3. Arthritis of wrist, MCP, or PIP joints (Spare DIP joints) 4. Symmetrical arthritis 5. Rheumatoid nodules (subcutaneous nodules over bony prominences, extensor surfaces, or juxta-articular regions) Raised serum rheumatoid factor (RF) 6. Radiographic abnormalities of hand or wrist consistent with RA (erosions in or close to involved joints) Must meet at least four of below criteria to fulfill the classification criteria for the diagnosis RA: **Other manifestation in RA:** • Systemic: fever, weight loss, fatigue	1. **Major criterion** a. Proximal diffuse sclerosis (skin tightness, thickening, nonpitting induration of the trunk) 2. **Minor criteria** a Sclerodactyly (only fingers and/or toes) b Digital pitting scars or loss of substance of the digital finger pad (pulp loss) c Bilateral basilar pulmonary fibrosis *Must meet one major or two minor criteria to fulfill the classification criteria for SS.* **Other organ involvement in SS** • Cardiovascular Raynaud's phenomenon, cardiac conduction abnormality, pericardial effusion, congestive heart failure, diastolic dysfunction, erectile dysfunction, digital ischemic changes (nailfold capillaries abnormalities, digital pitting/ulcer, acroosteolysis)	1. Ocular symptoms Dry eyes, sensation of sand, frequent use of tear substitutes 2. Oral symptoms Dry mouth, swollen salivary glands, drinking more liquids helps with dry food 3. Ocular signs Positive Schirmer's test, high ocular dryness score 4. Histopathology Focal lymphocytic sialoadenitis in minor salivary glands 5. Salivary gland involvement Positive result for any of the following tests: unstimulated whole salivary flow, parotid sialography, salivary scintigraphy 6. Autoantibodies Detection of antibodies to Ro(SSA) or LA(SSB) *Must meet one of the following criteria:* • any four of the listed items, provided either four or six is positive; • any three of the four objective criteria items (3, 4, 5, 6) to fulfill the classification criteria for the diagnosis of SjS	1. Skin lesions Heliotrope: red-purple edematous erythema on the upper eyelid Gottron's sign: red-purple keratonic, atrophic erythema or macules on the extensor surface of finger joints Erythema on the extensor surface of extremity joints, slight raised red-purple erythema over elbows or knees 2. Proximal muscle weakness (trunk, proximal upper or lower extremities) 3. Elevated serum creatine kinase (CPK) or aldolase level 4. Muscle pain (spontaneous or on grasping) 5. "Myogenic changes on electromyography (short-duration, polyphasic motor unit potentials with spontaneous fibrillation potentials)" 6. Positive anti-Jo-1 antibody test (histidyl-tRNA synthetase) 7. Nondestructive arthritis or arthralgias

- Musculoskeletal: muscle wasting, tenosynovitis, bursitis, osteoporosis
- Hematologic: anemia, thrombocytosis, eosinophilia, Felty's syndrome, splenomegaly
- Ophtalmologic: Episcleritis, scleritis, scleromalacia.

- Skin Hyperpigmentation/depigmentation (salt and pepper skin), calcinosis, thickened skin
- Gastrointestinal GERD[1], GAVE[2] syndrome and watermelon stomach, malabsorption
- Pulmonary Pulmonary artery hypertension, interstitial lung disease, pleural disease
- Renal Renal crisis
- Musculoskeletal Puffy hands, flexion contractures, tendon friction rubs

Other systemic involvement in SjS
- Respiratory: chronic bronchitis, interstitial lung disease, pneumonia
- Gastrointestinal: GERD, dysphagia, atrophic gastritis, gastroparesis, hepatitis, primary biliary cirrhosis
- Dermatologic involvement: Xerostomy, pruritis, purpura, Raynaud's, vasculitis, vaginal dryness, vulvodynia
- Neurologic: peripheral neuropathy, cognitive impairment, dysautonomia

8. Systemic inflammatory signs (fever, elevated sedimentation rate, or C-reactive protein)
9. Pathologic findings compatible with inflammatory myositis (inflammatory infiltration or skeletal evidence of active regeneration may be seen)

In the classification criteria for DM or PM, patients presenting with at least one finding from item 1 and four findings from items 2 through 9 are said to have DM. Patients presenting with at least four findings from items 2 through 9 are said to have PM.

Other systemic involvement in PM and DM
- Pulmonary: interstitial lung disease (NSIP > UIP)
- Cardiac:
- Associated underlying cancer
- Systemic: weight loss, fatigue

DM, dermatomyositis; *PM,* polymyositis; *RA,* rheumatoid arthritis; *SjS,* Sjögren's syndrome; *SS,* systemic sclerosis.

diagnostic criteria and some of the main symptoms and physical findings to aid in the evaluation of these patients. Any signs or symptoms suggestive of CTD should prompt evaluation by a rheumatologist. Finally, among patients diagnosed with IPF, an evaluation for underlying CTD should be performed regularly during follow-up, as some patients may declare overt CTD years after their first ILD presentation.[52,53]

Role of Autoantibodies
The detection of specific autoantibodies serves a critical role in the diagnosis, prognosis, and follow-up of patients with CTD-ILD or IPAF.[54,61–63] Using an extensive autoantibody panel, specialists in ILD clinics may be able to adjust the diagnosis of patients from IPF to CTD-ILD in up to 19% of cases.[57,63,64] Antinuclear antigen (ANA) and rheumatoid factor (RF) were the most commonly occurring autoantibodies—clues for possible SSc, Sjögren's, polymyositis (PM), dermatomyositis (DM), systemic lupus erythematosus, and RA.[57,63–65]

Autoantibodies are also associated with specific CTD characteristics and prognoses.[66,67] The presence of anti-Scl-70, for example, in SSc is known to be associated with pulmonary fibrosis,[67] whereas patients with anti-centromere antibodies are usually spared from ILD but are at higher risk of developing pulmonary hypertension (PH). Table 8.5 shows some of the main clinical and prognostic characteristics associated with major autoantibodies.

In patients with ILD but no categorizable CTD, an extensive serologic screen is recommended because detection of autoantibody positivity can guide clinicians on further workup, prompt evaluation by a rheumatologist, and enhance alertness for disease manifestations that may present in the future (Table 8.3).

Pulmonary Function Testing
Pulmonary function test patterns may suggest the presence of an underlying CTD. In IPF, fibrosis of the lung parenchyma is reflected by restrictive physiology with impaired gas exchange (increased A-a O_2 gradient at rest or with exercise and decreased diffuse capacity of the lung for carbon monoxide [DLCO]). In the case of CTD-UIP, disease of another lung compartment besides the parenchyma may alert the clinician of such an association. For example, the presence of lung volumes that are reduced disproportionately to the DLCO could suggest extrapulmonary restriction, specifically respiratory muscle weakness (such as in PM or DM) and/or extrapulmonary restriction from skin changes (such as in SSc). A reduction in DLCO disproportionate to lung volumes should trigger an evaluation for PH, a condition seen more commonly in patients with SSc or mixed CTD.

Imaging Differences
The typical UIP pattern seen on chest imaging in CTD-ILD is similar to that of IPF.[68] Patients with CTD-UIP may be more likely to have atypical features on HRCT (e.g., ground glass opacities, consolidation). Additionally, in cases of CTD-ILD, soft tissue windows may show additional findings such as pleural effusions, esophageal dilation, or pericardial effusion.[69,70]

Histopathologic Features
Clinical features and imaging are usually sufficient to diagnose CTD-UIP. When doubt persists or when a diagnosis cannot be obtained by less invasive tests a video-assisted thoracoscopic surgical lung biopsy can be helpful. Histopathologic studies in patients with CTD-UIP show they have fewer fibroblastic foci and more inflammation than patients with IPF,[60,71,72] with RA-UIP demonstrating larger and more numerous lymphoid aggregates than patients with IPF.[71]

Germinal centers, thought to be where IgG autoantibodies and immune dysregulation originate,[73] are the best discriminating feature between CTD-ILD and IPF.[72] Histopathologic evidence of germinal centers, similar to those with established CTD, may be found in patients with IPF who have serologic autoimmunity (ANA or RF) but no clinical features of a CTD (patients now referred to for research purposes as having IPAF).[72] The presence of NSIP-like areas away from areas with classic UIP-pattern fibrosis is not uncommon in patients with CTD-related UIP.[71,72] As on HRCT, the additional involvement of airways, vasculature, or pleura should trigger closer investigation for an underlying CTD.[74]

Treatment Differences
With the advent of antifibrotic therapies for the treatment of IPF, the distinction between idiopathic disease and that associated with CTD becomes more important. CTD-ILD is traditionally treated with immunosuppression in contrast with IPF, for which two Food and Drug Administration (FDA)-approved antifibrotic medications are available. The data for immunosuppression in CTD-ILD are scant and limited to a few phase 3 trials in SSc-ILDs (Scleroderma Lung Studies I[75] and II[76] and the Fibrosing Alveolitis in Scleroderma Trial[77]). The availability of antifibrotic therapies in IPF has piqued interest in evaluating the effectiveness and safety of such therapy in patients with CTD-UIP. How to manage patients with UIP and features of autoimmunity who do not meet criteria for an established CTD is unclear. Historically, such patients would not have been allowed to be enrolled in trials for IPF, and yet, they would not

TABLE 8.5
Autoantibodies in Rheumatic Conditions

Autoantibody	Associated Rheumatologic Autoimmune Diseases (AID or CTD)
Antinuclear antibody (ANA; ≥1:320)	SSc, SLE, Sjogren's, PM/DM
RHEUMATOID ARTHRITIS	
Rheumatoid factor (≥60 IU/mL)	RA, Sjogren's, SLE
Anticyclic citrullinated peptide (anti-CCP)	RA
SYSTEMIC SCLEROSIS	
Antitopoisomerase (ATA/anti-Scl70)	SSc (diffuse)
Anticentromere	SSc (diffuse)
Anti-RNA polymerase (RNA-pol)	SSc
Anti-Th/To	SSc
Anti-PM/Scl-75/100	SSc-PMs overlap, SLE, Sjogren's, severe ILD
Anti-U3 ribonucleoprotein (anti-U3 RNP)	SSc
Anti-U1 ribonucleoprotein (anti-RNP or anti-U1 RNP)	SSc-overlap, MCTD, ILD
Anti-U11/U12 ribonucleoprotein (anti-U11/U12 RNP)	SSc
MYOSITIS	
Antisynthetase (Jo-1, PL-7, PL-12, EJ, OJ, KS)	PM/DM with ILD (antisynthetase syndrome)
Anti-Mi2	PM/DM, lung sparing
Anti-CADM140 (anti-MDA-5)	Amyopathic DM, ILD, poor prognosis
Anti-SRP	PM: severe necrotizing myopathy, no ILD association described
OVERLAP SYNDROMES AND SLE	
Anti-Ku	SSc, SSc-PM overlap, SLE, myositis, severe ILD
Anti-SSA/Ro, anti-SSB/La	Sjogren's, SLE, Sjogren's/SLE overlap, SSc, RA, DM, severe ILD
Systemic lupus erythematosus associated	
Anti-dsDNA	SLE
Anti-Smith	SLE

DM, dermatomyositis; *ILD*, interstitial lung diseases; *MCTD*, mixed connective tissue disease; *MDA-5*, melanoma differentiation–associated protein 5; *PM*, polymyositis; *RA*, rheumatoid arthritis; *SLE*, systemic lupus erythematosus; *SSc*, systemic sclerosis.
Adapted from Ghirardello A, et al. Myositis autoantibodies and clinical phenotypes. *Autoimmunity Highlights*. 2014;5:69–75.

have been able to be diagnosed with any CTD because they did not fulfill diagnostic criteria.

Survival Differences

In general, CTD-ILD is associated with a better prognosis than IPF.[78,79] In patients with CTD, there is no difference in survival between those with NSIP and UIP, except in the setting of RA, where UIP carries a worse prognosis.[80,81] Despite similarities in pathology, all-comers with CTD-UIP have a lower mortality rate than patients with IPF.[78,79,82] Time will tell whether these survival differences will be modified with the newly FDA-approved

antifibrotic drugs for patients with IPF.[83,84] Although some data suggest patients meeting IPAF criteria with a UIP pattern follow a course similar to those with IPF (while those with non-UIP IPAF had better survival), validation of the prognostic value of this research classification is still in its infancy, and additional research is needed. Survival studies comparing patients with IPF with and without antibodies have mixed results: Lee and colleagues found survival may indeed be longer in IPF patients with circulating autoantibodies,[85] whereas Vij and her colleagues[57] and Fischer and his colleagues[86] found no difference between the two groups.

Summary

Patients with IPF deserve an evaluation for an underlying CTD with a thorough history and physical examination, as well as a comprehensive serologic evaluation. The presence of CTD influences the workup for other involved organ systems, provides a better prognosis than IPF in most cases, and influences treatment decisions. The clinical significance of more subtle and incomplete forms of CTD, including isolated autoantibody positivity, has yet to be determined.

OTHER CAUSES OF USUAL INTERSTITIAL PNEUMONIA-PATTERN LUNG INJURY

There are other ILDs that may present with a UIP pattern on HRCT or pathology. These must be considered and excluded before placing someone in the "idiopathic" category.

Asbestosis

Asbestos, a group of fibers composed of hydrated magnesium silicates used in many different industries, is associated with a number of diseases in the thoracic cavity, including pleural disease, small airways disease, mesothelioma, lung cancer, and asbestosis.[87] Asbestosis refers to a diffuse interstitial fibrosis typically seen 15–20 years after a significant asbestos exposure. These patients may present with an HRCT or histopathologic pattern of UIP.[88] Comparisons with IPF reveal asbestosis having more pleural thickening and plaques, band-like opacities that frequently merge with the pleura, subpleural dot-like or branching opacities, subpleural curvilinear opacities and mosaic attenuation, whereas HRCTs in patients with IPF show more traction bronchiolectasis and honeycombing.[89,90] In a comparison between asbestosis and biopsy-proven UIP or NSIP, investigators found that asbestosis had coarser fibrosis and was most likely to be basilar and subpleural.[91]

Clinical presentation (with insidious onset of breathlessness) and pulmonary function abnormalities (with restriction and reduced gas transfer) resemble IPF. In early disease, histopathology differs from UIP with the fibrosing process in asbestosis centered around the bronchioles. In advanced cases, asbestosis resembles UIP but has less fibroblastic foci and concomitant mild fibrosis of the visceral pleura.[92] Arriving at a confident diagnosis of asbestosis can be hindered by the long latency between exposure and clinically apparent disease and the uncertainty of asbestos exposure in various professions.

Drug-Induced Lung Disease

A number of medications have been associated with ILD. The incidence of drug-induced lung disease (DILD) is variable depending on the medication and can occur immediately after ingestion or after many years of exposure. The severity can range from an incidental finding on chest imaging to fulminate respiratory failure. Confident diagnosis requires a temporal association between exposure to the drug and the onset of respiratory signs and/or symptoms.[93] Although HP, diffuse alveolar damage, nonspecific interstitial pneumonia, and organizing pneumonia are the most common patterns seen, UIP has been reported for a number of medications.[94]

An HRCT pattern of UIP is most commonly seen in DILD from nitrofurantoin, bleomycin, methotrexate, and amiodarone[95,96] but has also been reported less commonly in cyclophosphamide, chlorambucil, methyl-CCNU, and pindolol.[97] In nitrofurantoin toxicity, patients usually present with progressive breathlessness months to years after starting chronic nitrofurantoin therapy. Most patients will have a UIP pattern on HRCT and histopathology. Some patients with nitrofurantoin DILD have resolution of radiographic findings on HRCT with cessation of drug.[98] Early in the course of DILD from methotrexate or bleomycin, HRCT scans may show scattered or diffuse areas of ground glass opacity, whereas HRCT scans later in the course of disease may show features typical of UIP (traction bronchiectasis, honeycombing).[95] In methotrexate-induced lung disease, the progression is slower than the typical progression of UIP/IPF, and methotrexate DILD may stabilize when the drug is withdrawn.[99]

Radiation-Induced Lung Disease

The lungs are sensitive to the effects of ionizing radiation and may show acute or chronic injury patterns when exposed to significant doses. Most data are derived from the treatment of primary lung cancer. Radiation pneumonitis is typically diagnosed 3–12 weeks after completion of radiotherapy.[100] Fibrosis is a later finding, usually developing 6–12 months after completion of therapy, and radiation fibrosis may progress for up to 2 years[101] after cessation of exposure. Changes on HRCT include reticulation and traction bronchiectasis and can mimic changes seen in UIP, but sharp demarcation at the borders of injured areas in radiation fibrosis, which correspond to the treatment portal of radiation, can help distinguish the two.[101]

Hermansky-Pudlak Syndrome

Hermansky-Pudlak syndrome (HPS) is a rare, autosomal recessive disease with features of oculocutaneous albinism and bleeding diathesis. Three of the ten subtypes of HPS have highly penetrant pulmonary fibrosis as a manifestation.[102] ILD usually develops in the third decade of life, and advanced disease is characterized by a UIP pattern on HRCT and histopathology.[103]

SUMMARY

In summary, a diagnosis of IPF can only be rendered after careful consideration of other ILDs that can mimic the radiographic and/or pathologic patterns seen in IPF. Both CTD-ILD and CHP may have a UIP pattern of fibrosis on HRCT, with only subtle and elusive clinical clues pointing to the underlying diagnosis. In patients eventually diagnosed with CTD-ILD, presentation with isolated serologic autoimmunity or a constellation of clinical features that do not meet criteria for diagnosis is not uncommon. In CHP, the IA may not be apparent in up to half of the cases, and there have been recent reports of patients with IPF being rediagnosed with CHP after careful reevaluation. Finally, there are a number of other entities such as asbestosis, DILD, radiation-induced fibrosis, and HPS that can be radiographically indistinguishable from IPF and deserve consideration in any patient presenting with a fibrosing ILD. A careful history, physical examination, and serologic evaluation are critical to rule out these and other causes of a UIP pattern of fibrosis before one makes a confident diagnosis of IPF.

REFERENCES

1. Fernández Pérez ER, Kong AM, Raimundo K, Koelsch TL, Kulharni R, Cole AL. Epidemiology of hypersensitivity pneumonitis among an insured population in the United States: a claims-based cohort analysis. *Ann Am Thorac Soc.* 2018;15:460−469.
2. Richerson HB, Bernstein IL, Fink JN, et al. Guidelines for the clinical evaluation of hypersensitivity pneumonitis. Report of the Subcommittee on Hypersensitivity Pneumonitis. *J Allergy Clin Immunol.* 1989;84(5 Pt 2): 839−844.
3. Schuyler M, Cormier Y. The diagnosis of hypersensitivity pneumonitis. *Chest.* 1997;111(3):534−536.
4. Terho EO. Diagnostic criteria for farmer's lung disease. *Am J Ind Med.* 1986;10(3):329.
5. Yoshizawa Y, Ohtani Y, Hayakawa H, Sato A, Suga M, Ando M. Chronic hypersensitivity pneumonitis in Japan: a nationwide epidemiologic survey. *J Allergy Clin Immunol.* 1999;103(2 Pt 1):315−320.
6. Fernandez Perez ER, Brown KK. Fibrotic hypersensitivity pneumonitis. *Curr Respir Care Rep.* 2014;3:170−178.
7. Johannson KA, Elicker BM, Vittinghoff E, et al. A diagnostic model for chronic hypersensitivity pneumonitis. *Thorax.* 2016;71(10):951−954.
8. Fernandez Perez ER, Swigris JJ, Forssen AV, et al. Identifying an inciting antigen is associated with improved survival in patients with chronic hypersensitivity pneumonitis. *Chest.* 2013;144(5):1644−1651.
9. Kuhn DM, Ghannoum MA. Indoor mold, toxigenic fungi, and *Stachybotrys chartarum*: infectious disease perspective. *Clin Microbiol Rev.* 2003;16(1):144−172.
10. Millerick-May ML, Mulks MH, Gerlach J, et al. Hypersensitivity pneumonitis and antigen identification − an alternate approach. *Respir Med.* 2016;112:97−105.
11. Sahin H, Brown KK, Curran-Everett D, et al. Chronic hypersensitivity pneumonitis: CT features comparison with pathologic evidence of fibrosis and survival. *Radiology.* 2007;244(2):591−598.
12. Okamoto T, Miyazaki Y, Ogura T, et al. A nationwide epidemiological survey of chronic hypersensitivity pneumonitis in Japan. *Respir Investig.* 2013;51(3):191−199.
13. Morell F, Villar A, Montero MA, et al. Chronic hypersensitivity pneumonitis in patients diagnosed with idiopathic pulmonary fibrosis: a prospective case-cohort study. *Lancet Respir Med.* 2013;1(9):685−694.
14. Silva CI, Muller NL, Lynch DA, et al. Chronic hypersensitivity pneumonitis: differentiation from idiopathic pulmonary fibrosis and nonspecific interstitial pneumonia by using thin-section CT. *Radiology.* 2008;246(1): 288−297.
15. Chung JH, Zhan X, Cao M, et al. Presence of air-trapping and mosaic attenuation on chest CT predicts survival in chronic hypersensitivity pneumonitis. *Ann Am Thorac Soc.* 2017;14(10):1533−1538.
16. Chung JH, Montner SM, Adegunsoye A, et al. CT findings associated with survival in chronic hypersensitivity pneumonitis. *Eur Radiol.* 2017;27(12):5127−5135.
17. Lynch DA, Newell JD, Logan PM, King Jr TE, Muller NL. Can CT distinguish hypersensitivity pneumonitis from idiopathic pulmonary fibrosis? *AJR Am J Roentgenol.* 1995;165(4):807−811.
18. Reboux G, Piarroux R, Roussel S, Millon L, Bardonnet K, Dalphin JC. Assessment of four serological techniques in the immunological diagnosis of farmers' lung disease. *J Med Microbiol.* 2007;56(Pt 10):1317−1321.
19. Reboux G, Magy N, Dalphin J-C. *Immunological Methods.* Springer Berlin Heidelberg; 2006.
20. Fenoglio CM, Reboux G, Sudre B, et al. Diagnostic value of serum precipitins to mould antigens in active hypersensitivity pneumonitis. *Eur Respir J.* 2007;29(4): 706−712.
21. Enriquez-Matas A, Quirce S, Hernandez E, Vereda A, Carnes J, Sastre J. Hypersensitivity pneumonitis caused by domestic exposure to molds. *J Investig Allergol Clin Immunol.* 2007;17(2):126−127.
22. Cormier Y, Belanger J, Durand P. Factors influencing the development of serum precipitins to farmer's lung antigen in Quebec dairy farmers. *Thorax.* 1985;40(2): 138−142.

23. Fink JN, Ortega HG, Reynolds HY, et al. Needs and opportunities for research in hypersensitivity pneumonitis. *Am J Respir Crit Care Med.* 2005;171(7):792–798.

24. Selman M, Lacasse Y, Pardo A, Cormier Y. Hypersensitivity pneumonitis caused by fungi. *Proc Am Thorac Soc.* 2010;7(3):229–236.

25. Dalphin JC, Toson B, Monnet E, et al. Farmer's lung precipitins in Doubs (a department of France): prevalence and diagnostic value. *Allergy.* 1994;49(9):744–750.

26. Costabel U, Bonella F, Guzman J. Chronic hypersensitivity pneumonitis. *Clin Chest Med.* 2012;33(1):151–163.

27. Munoz X, Sanchez-Ortiz M, Torres F, Villar A, Morell F, Cruz MJ. Diagnostic yield of specific inhalation challenge in hypersensitivity pneumonitis. *Eur Respir J.* 2014;44(6):1658–1665.

28. Ramirez-Venegas A, Sansores RH, Perez-Padilla R, Carrillo G, Selman M. Utility of a provocation test for diagnosis of chronic pigeon Breeder's disease. *Am J Respir Crit Care Med.* 1998;158(3):862–869.

29. Ohtani Y, Kojima K, Sumi Y, et al. Inhalation provocation tests in chronic bird fancier's lung. *Chest.* 2000;118(5):1382–1389.

30. Hendrick DJ, Marshall R, Faux JA, Krall JM. Positive "alveolar" responses to antigen inhalation provocation tests: their validity and recognition. *Thorax.* 1980;35(6):415–427.

31. Morell F, Roger A, Reyes L, Cruz MJ, Murio C, Munoz X. Bird fancier's lung: a series of 86 patients. *Med (Baltim).* 2008;87(2):110–130.

32. Ishizuka M, Miyazaki Y, Tateishi T, Tsutsui T, Tsuchiya K, Inase N. Validation of inhalation provocation test in chronic bird-related hypersensitivity pneumonitis and new prediction score. *Ann Am Thorac Soc.* 2015;12(2):167–173.

33. Meyer KC, Raghu G, Baughman RP, et al. An official American Thoracic Society clinical practice guideline: the clinical utility of bronchoalveolar lavage cellular analysis in interstitial lung disease. *Am J Respir Crit Care Med.* 2012;185(9):1004–1014.

34. Gaxiola M, Buendia-Roldan I, Mejia M, et al. Morphologic diversity of chronic pigeon breeder's disease: clinical features and survival. *Respir Med.* 2011;105(4):608–614.

35. Ohshimo S, Bonella F, Cui A, et al. Significance of bronchoalveolar lavage for the diagnosis of idiopathic pulmonary fibrosis. *Am J Respir Crit Care Med.* 2009;179(11):1043–1047.

36. Munoz X, Sanchez-Ortiz M, Ojanguren I, Cruz MJ. Inhalation challenge in the differential diagnosis of usual interstitial pneumonia. *Eur Respir Rev.* 2015;24(137):542–544.

37. Ohtani Y, Saiki S, Kitaichi M, et al. Chronic bird fancier's lung: histopathological and clinical correlation. An application of the 2002 ATS/ERS consensus classification of the idiopathic interstitial pneumonias. *Thorax.* 2005;60(8):665–671.

38. Barrera L, Mendoza F, Zuniga J, et al. Functional diversity of T-cell subpopulations in subacute and chronic hypersensitivity pneumonitis. *Am J Respir Crit Care Med.* 2008;177(1):44–55.

39. Bango-Alvarez A, Ariza-Prota M, Torres-Rivas H, et al. Transbronchial cryobiopsy in interstitial lung disease: experience in 106 cases - how to do it. *ERJ Open Res.* 2017;3(1).

40. Colby TV, Tomassetti S, Cavazza A, Dubini A, Poletti V. Transbronchial cryobiopsy in diffuse lung disease: update for the pathologist. *Arch Pathol Lab Med.* 2017;141(7):891–900.

41. Churg A, Muller NL, Flint J, Wright JL. Chronic hypersensitivity pneumonitis. *Am J Surg Pathol.* 2006;30(2):201–208.

42. Akashi T, Takemura T, Ando N, et al. Histopathologic analysis of sixteen autopsy cases of chronic hypersensitivity pneumonitis and comparison with idiopathic pulmonary fibrosis/usual interstitial pneumonia. *Am J Clin Pathol.* 2009;131(3):405–415.

43. Castonguay MC, Ryu JH, Yi ES, Tazelaar HD. Granulomas and giant cells in hypersensitivity pneumonitis. *Hum Pathol.* 2015;46(4):607–613.

44. Churg A, Sin DD, Everett D, Brown K, Cool C. Pathologic patterns and survival in chronic hypersensitivity pneumonitis. *Am J Surg Pathol.* 2009;33(12):1765–1770.

45. Travis WD, Costabel U, Hansell DM, et al. An official American Thoracic Society/European Respiratory Society statement: update of the international multidisciplinary classification of the idiopathic interstitial pneumonias. *Am J Respir Crit Care Med.* 2013;188(6):733–748.

46. Tansey D, Wells AU, Colby TV, Ip S. Variations in histological patterns of interstitial pneumonia between connective tissue disorders and their relationship to prognosis. *Histopathology.* 2004;44(6):585–596.

47. Kim JS, Newell JD, Brown KK, Cool CD, Meehan R. Rheumatoid arthritis–related lung diseases: CT findings 1. *Radiology.* 2004;232(1):81–91.

48. Lee HK, Kim DS, Yoo B, Seo JB. Histopathologic pattern and clinical features of rheumatoid arthritis-associated interstitial lung disease. *Chest.* 2005;127(6):2019–2027.

49. Steen VD, Medsger TA. Changes in causes of death in systemic sclerosis, 1972-2002. *Ann Rheum Dis.* 2007;66(7):940–944.

50. Solomon JJ, Olson AL, Fischer A, Bull T, Brown KK, Raghu G. Scleroderma lung disease. *Eur Respir Rev.* 2013;22(127):6–19.

51. Desai SR, Veeraraghavan S, Hansell DM, et al. CT features of lung disease in patients with systemic sclerosis: comparison with idiopathic pulmonary fibrosis and nonspecific interstitial pneumonia. *Radiology.* 2004;232(2):560–567.

52. Homma Y, Ohtsuka Y, Tanimura K, et al. Can interstitial pneumonia as the sole presentation of collagen vascular diseases be differentiated from idiopathic interstitial pneumonia? *Respiration.* 1995;62(5):248–251.

53. Fischer A, du Bois R. Interstitial lung disease in connective tissue disorders. *Lancet.* 2012;380(9842):689–698.

54. Fischer A, Solomon JJ, du Bois RM, Deane KD. Lung disease with anti-CCP antibodies but not rheumatoid arthritis or connective tissue disease. *Respir Med.* 2012; 106(7):1040−1047.

55. Kinder BW, Collard HR, Koth L, et al. Idiopathic nonspecific interstitial pneumonia: lung manifestation of undifferentiated connective tissue disease? *Am J Respir Crit Care Med.* 2007;176(7):691−697.

56. Fischer A, West SG, Swigris JJ, Brown KK, du Bois RM. Connective tissue disease-associated interstitial lung disease: a call for clarification. *Chest.* 2010;138(2):251−256.

57. Vij R, Noth I, Strek ME. Autoimmune-featured interstitial lung disease: a distinct entity. *Chest.* 2011;140(5): 1292−1299.

58. Fischer A, Antoniou KM, Brown KK, et al. ERS/ATS Task Force on Undifferentiated Forms of CTD-ILD. An official European Respiratory Society/American Thoracic Society research statement: interstitial pneumonia with autoimmune features. *Eur Respir J.* 2015;46(4):976−987.

59. Kang EH, Lee EB, Shin KC, et al. Interstitial lung disease in patients with polymyositis, dermatomyositis and amyopathic dermatomyositis. *Rheumatology.* 2005; 44(10):1282−1286.

60. Flaherty KR, Colby TV, Travis WD. Fibroblastic foci in usual interstitial pneumonia: idiopathic versus collagen vascular disease. *Am J Respir Crit Care Med.* 2003; 167(10):1410−1415.

61. Fischer A, Meehan RT, Feghali-Bostwick CA, West SG, Brown KK. Unique characteristics of systemic sclerosis sine scleroderma-associated interstitial lung disease. *Chest.* 2006;130(4):976−981.

62. Chartrand S, Swigris JJ, Stanchev L, Lee JS, Brown KK, Fischer A. Clinical features and natural history of interstitial pneumonia with autoimmune features: a single center experience. *Respir Med.* 2016;119:150−154.

63. Jee AS, Adelstein S, Bleasel J, et al. Role of autoantibodies in the diagnosis of connective-tissue disease ILD (CTD-ILD) and interstitial pneumonia with autoimmune features (IPAF). *J Clin Med.* 2017;6(5).

64. Corte TJ, Copley SJ, Desai SR. Significance of connective tissue disease features in idiopathic interstitial pneumonia. *Eur Respir J.* 2012;39(3):661−668.

65. Kang BH, Park JK, Roh JH, Song JW. Clinical significance of serum autoantibodies in idiopathic interstitial pneumonia. *J Korean Med Sci.* 2013;28(5):731−737.

66. Kavanaugh AF, Solomon DH, American College of Rheumatology Ad Hoc Committee on Immunologic Testing Guidelines. Guidelines for immunologic laboratory testing in the rheumatic diseases: anti-DNA antibody tests. *Arthritis Rheum.* 2002;47(5):546−555.

67. Reveille JD, Solomon DH. Evidence-based guidelines for the use of immunologic tests: anticentromere, Scl-70, and nucleolar antibodies. *Arthritis Care Res.* 2003;49(3): 399−412.

68. Assayag D, Elicker BM, Urbania TH, et al. Rheumatoid arthritis-associated interstitial lung disease: radiologic identification of usual interstitial pneumonia pattern. *Radiology.* 2014;270(2):583−588.

69. Lauretis DA, Veeraraghavan S, Renzoni E. Connective tissue disease-associated interstitial lung disease: how does it differ from IPF? How should the clinical approach differ? *Chron Respir Dis.* 2011;8(1):53−82.

70. Hwang JH, Misumi S, Sahin H, Brown KK, Newell JD, Lynch DA. Computed tomographic features of idiopathic fibrosing interstitial pneumonia: comparison with pulmonary fibrosis related to collagen vascular disease. *J Comput Assist Tomogr.* 2009;33(3): 410−415.

71. Cipriani NA, Strek M, Noth I, et al. Pathologic quantification of connective tissue disease-associated versus idiopathic usual interstitial pneumonia. *Arch Pathol Lab Med.* 2012;136(10):1253−1258.

72. Song JW, Do K-HH, Kim M-YY, Jang SJ, Colby TV, Kim DS. Pathologic and radiologic differences between idiopathic and collagen vascular disease-related usual interstitial pneumonia. *Chest.* 2009;136(1):23−30.

73. Luzina IG, Atamas SP, Storrer CE. Spontaneous formation of germinal centers in autoimmune mice. *J Leukoc Biol.* 2001;70(4):578−584.

74. Fischer A, Richeldi L. Cross-disciplinary collaboration in connective tissue disease-related lung disease. *Semin Respir Crit Care Med.* 2014;35(2):159−165.

75. Tashkin DP, Elashoff R, Clements PJ, et al. Cyclophosphamide versus placebo in scleroderma lung disease. *N Engl J Med.* 2006;354(25):2655−2666.

76. Tashkin DP, Roth MD, Clements PJ, et al. Mycophenolate mofetil versus oral cyclophosphamide in scleroderma-related interstitial lung disease (SLS II): a randomised controlled, double-blind, parallel group trial. *Lancet Respir Med.* 2016;4(9):708−719.

77. Hoyles RK, Ellis RW, Wellsbury J, et al. A multicenter, prospective, randomized, double-blind, placebo-controlled trial of corticosteroids and intravenous cyclophosphamide followed by oral azathioprine for the treatment of pulmonary fibrosis in scleroderma. *Arthritis Rheum.* 2006;54(12):3962−3970.

78. Navaratnam V, Ali N, Smith CJP, McKeever T. Does the presence of connective tissue disease modify survival in patients with pulmonary fibrosis? *Respir Med.* 2011; 105(12):1925−1930.

79. Park JH, Kim DS, Park IN, Jang SJ. Prognosis of fibrotic interstitial pneumonia: idiopathic versus collagen vascular disease−related subtypes. *Am J Respir Crit Care Med.* 2007; 175(7):705−711.

80. Kim EJ, Collard HR, King TE. Rheumatoid arthritis-associated interstitial lung disease: the relevance of histopathologic and radiographic pattern. *Chest.* 2009;136(5): 1397−1405.

81. Solomon JJ, Ryu JH, Tazelaar HD, et al. Fibrosing interstitial pneumonia predicts survival in patients with rheumatoid arthritis-associated interstitial lung disease (RA-ILD). *Respir Med.* 2013;107(8):1247−1252.

82. Flaherty KR, Mumford JA, Murray S. Prognostic implications of physiologic and radiographic changes in idiopathic interstitial pneumonia. *Am J Respir Crit Care Med.* 2003; 168(5):543−548.

83. Richeldi L, du Bois RM, Raghu G. Efficacy and safety of nintedanib in idiopathic pulmonary fibrosis. *N Engl J Med*. 2014;370(22):2071−2082.

84. King Jr TE, Bradford WZ, Castro-Bernardini S. A phase 3 trial of pirfenidone in patients with idiopathic pulmonary fibrosis. *N Engl J Med*. 2014;370(22):2083−2092.

85. Lee JS, Kim EJ, Lynch KL, Elicker B, Ryerson CJ. Prevalence and clinical significance of circulating autoantibodies in idiopathic pulmonary fibrosis. *Respir Med*. 2013;107(2): 249−255.

86. Fischer A, Pfalzgraf FJ, Feghali-Bostwick CA, et al. Anti-th/ to-positivity in a cohort of patients with idiopathic pulmonary fibrosis. *J Rheumatol*. 2006;33(8):1600−1605.

87. Jamrozik E, de Klerk N, Musk AW. Asbestos-related disease. *Intern Med J*. 2011;41(5):372−380.

88. Gulati M, Redlich CA. Asbestosis and environmental causes of usual interstitial pneumonia. *Curr Opin Pulm Med*. 2015;21(2):193−200.

89. al-Jarad N, Strickland B, Pearson MC, Rubens MB, Rudd RM. High resolution computed tomographic assessment of asbestosis and cryptogenic fibrosing alveolitis: a comparative study. *Thorax*. 1992;47(8):645−650.

90. Akira M, Yamamoto S, Inoue Y, Sakatani M. High-resolution CT of asbestosis and idiopathic pulmonary fibrosis. *AJR Am J Roentgenol*. 2003;181(1):163−169.

91. Copley SJ, Wells AU, Sivakumaran P, et al. Asbestosis and idiopathic pulmonary fibrosis: comparison of thin-section CT features. *Radiology*. 2003;229(3):731−736.

92. Roggli VL, Gibbs AR, Attanoos R, et al. Pathology of asbestosis - an update of the diagnostic criteria: report of the asbestosis committee of the college of American pathologists and pulmonary pathology society. *Arch Pathol Lab Med*. 2010;134(3):462−480.

93. Matsuno O. Drug-induced interstitial lung disease: mechanisms and best diagnostic approaches. *Respir Res*. 2012; 13:39.

94. Silva CI, Muller NL. Drug-induced lung diseases: most common reaction patterns and corresponding high-resolution CT manifestations. *Semin Ultrasound CT MR*. 2006;27(2):111−116.

95. Schwaiblmair M, Behr W, Haeckel T, Markl B, Foerg W, Berghaus T. Drug induced interstitial lung disease. *Open Respir Med J*. 2012;6:63−74.

96. Papiris SA, Triantafillidou C, Kolilekas L, Markoulaki D, Manali ED. Amiodarone: review of pulmonary effects and toxicity. *Drug Saf*. 2010;33(7):539−558.

97. Myers JL, Limper AH, Swensen SJ. Drug-induced lung disease: a pragmatic classification incorporating HRCT appearances. *Semin Respir Crit Care Med*. 2003;24(4): 445−454.

98. Sheehan RE, Wells AU, Milne DG, Hansell DM. Nitrofurantoin-induced lung disease: two cases demonstrating resolution of apparently irreversible CT abnormalities. *J Comput Assist Tomogr*. 2000;24(2): 259−261.

99. Wolkove N, Baltzan M. Amiodarone pulmonary toxicity. *Can Respir J*. 2009;16(2):43−48.

100. Bledsoe TJ, Nath SK, Decker RH. Radiation pneumonitis. *Clin Chest Med*. 2017;38(2):201−208.

101. Choi YW, Munden RF, Erasmus JJ, et al. Effects of radiation therapy on the lung: radiologic appearances and differential diagnosis. *Radiographics*. 2004;24(4):985−997; discussion 998.

102. El-Chemaly S, Young LR. Hermansky-Pudlak syndrome. *Clin Chest Med*. 2016;37(3):505−511.

103. Avila NA, Brantly M, Premkumar A, Huizing M, Dwyer A, Gahl WA. Hermansky-Pudlak syndrome: radiography and CT of the chest compared with pulmonary function tests and genetic studies. *AJR Am J Roentgenol*. 2002; 179(4):887−892.

Natural History of Idiopathic Pulmonary Fibrosis and Disease Monitoring

AMEN SERGEW, MD • KEVIN K. BROWN, MD

INTRODUCTION

Idiopathic pulmonary fibrosis (IPF) is a chronic and progressive lung-limited disease with a remarkably poor prognosis. The mean survival from the time of diagnosis is 2−5 years,[1] with a 5-year survival rate of 20%−40%.[2] The significant morbidity and early mortality of IPF has prompted interest in finding easily identified clinical features indicative of disease activity and prognosis. This chapter highlights the natural, untreated history of IPF, the impact of new therapies on the disease course, and the tools available to the practitioner to predict prognosis.

THE NATURAL HISTORY OF UNTREATED IDIOPATHIC PULMONARY FIBROSIS

While recognized as inexorably progressive, the natural history of untreated IPF is surprisingly variable (Fig. 9.1). A small minority of IPF patients will remain stable for many years. Similarly, there is a relatively small subset of patients who will rapidly decline, progressing to death within a few months of diagnosis. Most IPF patients will have a gradual or intermittent but persistent decline over a few years before succumbing to respiratory failure and death. In population studies, the force vital capacity (FVC) declines about 200 mL/year (160−280 mL/year),[3] and this rate of decline appears to be independent of baseline physiologic impairment. In a recent post hoc subgroup analyses of pooled data from the two prior studies, the annual rate of decline in FVC of untreated patients with FVC >90% was −224.6 mL/year and in the patients with FVC ≤90% was −223.6 mL/year.[4]

In all IPF patients, an acute (days to a few weeks) deterioration of lung function, symptoms, and chest imaging, called an acute exacerbation (AE), is a risk.[5] AE may result from an infection, an aspiration episode, or be due to an unknown cause. IPF patients with an AE leading to hospitalization have an in-hospital mortality rate of 50% or greater.[6] Overall median survival in those who have had an AE is short, 15.5 versus 60.6 months in those without an exacerbation.[6] The 1 and 5 year survival rates following an initial AE are 56.2% and 18.4%, respectively.[6] In those that survive an AE, full recovery back to their baseline is rare. Additionally, patients who have had an AE and survive are at increased risk of a future AE.[5]

THE NATURAL HISTORY OF TREATED IDIOPATHIC PULMONARY FIBROSIS

The availability of approved medicines for IPF, pirfenidone, and nintedanib has altered the disease course. More is known about pirfenidone given its availability and use worldwide for a longer period. Both pirfenidone and nintedanib have been shown in various studies to reduce the overall rate of FVC decline in populations of IPF patients as compared with placebo.[7−11] Most of these studies were performed in patients with physiologically mild to moderate disease with the benefit seen independent of baseline FVC. For example, evaluating the effect of nintedanib therapy in physiologically early disease, pooled data from the two prior studies compared the rate of FVC decline in patients with a baseline FVC >90% with those with an FVC ≤90%.[4] The adjusted annual FVC decline in the patients with FVC >90% was −91.5 mL/year and in those with FVC ≤90% was −121.5 mL/year, suggesting a similar benefit of therapy in both cohorts. Nintedanib has also been suggested to delay the time to first AE when compared with placebo.[5,7,8]

In terms of survival, several pooled studies/meta-analyses suggest that pirfenidone treatment for 72 and 120 weeks is of benefit. In a pooled analysis of the ASCEND (Assessment of Pirfenidone to Confirm Efficacy and Safety in Idiopathic Pulmonary Fibrosis) and

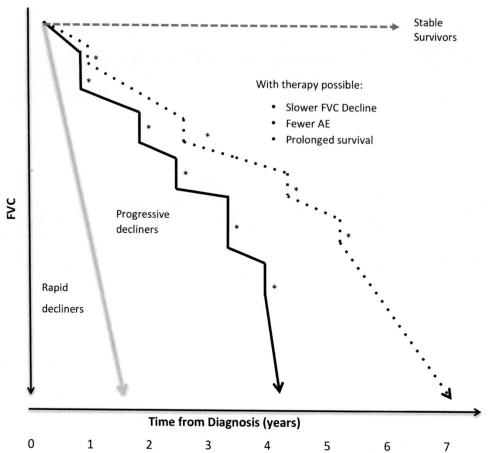

FIG. 9.1 **Disease Trajectory of Treated IPF.** The majority of patients with IPF have a slow decline in FVC over years (*black solid line*). Acute exacerbations can occur that frequently lead to death or to a faster decline (marked by the *asterisk*). A minority of patients have a stable course with a stable trajectory over years (*gray dashed line*). Additionally, a small subset of IPF patients have a rapid progression with a decline in FVC over months from the time of diagnosis (*gray solid line*). Treatment of IPF (*black dotted line*) may result in slower decline of FVC (both nintedanib and pirfenidone), delay in time to AE (nintedanib), and prolonged survival. *AE*, acute exacerbations; *FVC*, forced vital capacity; *IPF*, idiopathic pulmonary fibrosis.

CAPACITY studies (Clinical Studies Assessing Pirfenidone in Idiopathic Pulmonary Fibrosis: Research of Efficacy and Safety Outcomes), pirfenidone significantly improved progression-free survival at 1 year when compared with placebo.[10] A similar study pooled data from three multicentered randomized controlled trials and found that over 120 weeks, pirfenidone reduced the relative risk of morality compared with placebo.[12] Combined data from two prior randomized controlled studies, an open-label study, and a hospital database of patients with similar inclusion criteria suggested improved survival for patients treated with pirfenidone compared with those treated with best supportive care.[13] Overall, the mean survival was 8.72 years with pirfenidone and 6.24 years with supportive care. A metaanalysis of nine studies showed similar results.[11] Given similar primary efficacy data, nintedanib's effect on mortality appears to likely be similar.[8]

Pirfenidone may also lower the risk of respiratory hospitalization. Pooled data from three randomized control trials suggest that pirfenidone reduces the risk of respiratory hospitalization over 52 weeks compared with placebo.[14] The effect of continued pirfenidone treatment after evidence of physiologic progression was assessed in a post hoc analysis that combined subjects from two prior studies whose FVC declined $\geq$10% within the first 6 months of randomization.[15] Over the following 6 months, 5.9% of those continued on pirfenidone had a further decline of $\geq$10% in their FVC versus 27.9% in the placebo group (relative difference of 78.9%). There was also a significant difference in the number of deaths, 2.9% in the pirfenidone group (n = 1) and 20.6% (n = 14) in the placebo group (relative difference 85.7%).

While no study has directly compared pirfenidone with nintedanib, a small study of combined therapy has been performed. The INJOURNEY trial studied IPF patients with a 4–5 week run-in period of nintedanib followed by the addition of pirfenidone. Patients were followed for 12 weeks.[16] The FVC decline after 12 weeks was 13.3 mL in the nintedanib + pirfenidone group (n = 48) and 41 mL in the nintedanib + placebo group (n = 44). The safety profile suggested an increased risk of gastrointestinal adverse events in the combined treatment group. These data support the need for larger studies to get a more in-depth understanding of the impact of dual therapy.

Our current understanding of the effect of these antifibrotics on the disease course of IPF is summarized in Fig. 9.1. Given our relatively short-term experience with these medications and recognition that the current universe of patients being treated may differ from those studied in the prospective trials, the long-term effects of these antifibrotics are still unknown.

PROGNOSTIC INDICATORS

A number of clinical, physiologic, and radiologic findings have been used to predict disease progression and mortality in IPF. A number of baseline markers of disease severity have been identified (Table 9.1).

Males have been demonstrated in several reports to have a worse prognosis.[1,17,18] In IPF patients followed for a year, females had a higher survival, especially in those that did not desaturate with ambulation.[19] Males also have an increased likelihood of worse functional status, systolic pulmonary artery pressures >50 mmHg, need for supplemental oxygen, and shorter survival.[20] These survival differences, however, have not been consistent, and at least one large study showed no survival difference between the genders.[21]

Respiratory symptoms of baseline dyspnea and cough can be predictive of survival. When the level of dyspnea in 93 subjects was measured using the modified Medical Research Council (mMRC) score, the median

TABLE 9.1
Important Baseline and Longitudinal Prognostic Indicators

Baseline	Longitudinal Follow-up
Demographics: • ?Male • Age	
Symptoms: • Dyspnea score • Cough	Symptoms: • Dyspnea score
Physical Exam: • Finger clubbing • BMI <30	

Pulmonary Physiology:
• **DLCO %**
• **FVC %**
• TLC %, TGV%, FEV1%, RV%
• A-a gradient
• PaO$_2$ or oxygen saturation
• **6MW**
  • Borg scale
  • Distance (<250 m)
  • Heart rate response
  • Lowest O$_2$ saturation (<88%)
	Pulmonary Physiology:
	• **DLCO decline of $\geq$15%**
	• **FVC decline of $\geq$5–10%**
	• TLC %, TGV%, FEV1%
	• A-a gradient (change of 5 to $\geq$15 mmHg)
	• PaO$_2$ or oxygen saturation
	• **6MW**
	  • Distance (change >50 m)

Imaging: • HRCT: significant traction bronchiectasis, honeycombing, and fibrosis	Imaging: • HRCT: Increased fibrosis on HRCT
Pathology: • Number of FF	Other: • Acute exacerbation
Comorbidities: • Emphysema • GERD • Pulmonary hypertension	

6MW, six-minute walk; *A-a gradient*, alveolar–arterial oxygen gradient; *BMI*, body mass index; *DLCO*, diffusion capacity for carbon monoxide; *FEV$_1$*, forced expiratory volume in 1 second; *FF*, fibroblast foci; *FVC*, forced vital capacity; *GERD*, gastroesophageal reflux disease; *HRCT*, high-resolution computed tomography; *PaO$_2$*, partial pressure of arterial oxygen; *RV*, residual volume; *TGV*, thoracic gas volume; *TLC*, total lung capacity.

survival in those with an mMRC score of 0–1 (mild dyspnea), 2 (moderate dyspnea), and 3 (severe dyspnea) were 66.7, 30.9, and 10.2 months, respectively.[22] A number of other studies have confirmed baseline dyspnea as predictive of survival.[21,23–25] There are a variety of tools to quantify dyspnea, and there appears to be no clear advantages of a specific method. Cough has also been suggested to have prognostic significance. It appears to be more likely in those with exertional desaturation and in those with a lower FVC. Cough may also be predictive of disease progression, severity, and early or time to lung transplantation.[26]

Older age at the time of diagnosis is associated with early mortality.[1] A progressive worsening of survival with ages <50, 50–60, 60–70, and >70 has been shown.[21] On physical examination, a lower body mass index (BMI) and the presence of finger clubbing at the time of initial visit has also been shown to predict increased early mortality.[21] A single-centered study of 197 patients reviewed patients with a BMI <25, 25–30, and ≥30. The median survival was 3.6, 3.8, and 5.8 years, respectively.[27] IPF patients who survived >5 years without lung transplantation with those who died or required transplant <5 years after initial evaluation found a higher BMI to be associated with longer survival.[28]

On chest imaging, high-resolution computed tomography (HRCT) features of extensive traction bronchiectasis, honeycombing, and reticular opacities have been shown to be significant predictors of early mortality.[21,29–32] HRCT features have also been found to correspond to the level of functional impairment. Two separate studies found that those with a definite usual interstitial pneumonia (UIP) pattern on HRCT had a worse outcome than those with HRCT findings inconsistent with UIP, with a mean survival time of 30–45.7 and 77–107 months, respectively.[29,33] Patients with definite UIP pattern on HRCT are more likely to have a lower diffusion capacity for carbon monoxide (DLCO) and a higher estimated systolic pulmonary artery pressure.[33]

Commonly used pulmonary physiologic measures of disease severity include FVC, total lung capacity (TLC), and DLCO.[21–23,34] FVC has been the most commonly used marker of disease severity due to its ready availability and ease of performance, although a number of studies suggest that baseline DLCO may be a better predictor of early mortality.[34,35] In a study of 446 IPF patients, in those with mild (≥70%), moderate (55%–69%), and severe impairment in FVC % (<55%), the median survival was 55.6, 38.7, and 27.4 months, respectively.[34] In the same study, DLCO was also predictive; in those with mild (≥50%), moderate (35%–49%), or severe impairment (<35%), the median survival was 67.3, 47.8, or 31.3 months, respectively. At least one study has found DLCO and HRCT

fibrosis scores to be independent predictors of survival and together to be the strongest predictors of outcome.[36] Thoracic gas volume (TGV), residual volume and forced expiratory volume in 1 second (FEV_1), partial pressure of arterial oxygen (PaO_2), oxygen saturation, and alveolar–arterial oxygen (A-a) gradient have also been shown to be important predictors of survival.[21,23] Six-minute walk (6MW) distance, lowest pulse oximetry, and the dyspnea score associated with exercise (Borg scale) have been found useful in some studies.[22,37–39] An abnormal heart rate response 1 min after completion of a 6MW has been shown to be an independent predictor of pulmonary hypertension (PH) and of mortality.[40,41]

The presence of comorbidities impacts survival. Mild PH is common in IPF and has been demonstrated in 38.6% of the IPF patients at baseline and as high as 86.4% at the time of transplant.[42] The ARTEMIS-IPF study showed a rate of right heart catheter proven PH of 10%.[43] In this study, IPF patients with >5% honeycombing on HRCT were excluded, which may have impacted the prevalence of PH. Patients with PH and IPF have a lower DLCO and exercise capacity as well as shorter survival.[20] In IPF patients with PH, DLCO is a more important marker of prognosis than FVC.[35]

Chest imaging with evidence of emphysema has been noted in 8% of IPF patients in a study from two academic centers of 365 IPF patients.[44] A study from Mexico demonstrated it in as many as 28% patients.[45] There are mixed findings in regard to the impact of combined emphysema and IPF on prognosis when compared with those with IPF alone. Both increased and similar mortality have been reported.[44,45] In the Mexican cohort, those with IPF and emphysema had more severe desaturation with exercise, a higher mean fibrosis score on HRCT scan, and higher estimated pulmonary pressures. Other studies have also found IPF patients with emphysema have an increased risk of PH (about 50%), and these patients tend to have a higher mortality.[46,47] In patients with combined IPF and emphysema, DLCO and change in FEV_1 are the best predictors of early mortality.[35,48]

The prevalence of gastroesophageal reflux disease (GERD) in IPF patients has been reported to occur in up to 90% of patients with IPF.[49,50] Treatment of GERD has been associated with mixed outcomes. A retrospective study of 204 patients demonstrated IPF patients who had been treated with antacid therapy had a slower decline in FVC and DLCO and improved prognosis.[51] A similar retrospective study of data collected during three prior randomized controlled trials showed that IPF subjects who reported taking antacid therapy had a smaller decline in FVC after 30 weeks when compared with those not taking antacid therapy.[52] In contrast, a more recent post hoc analysis of three prior studies compared the outcome of patients who reported taking antacid therapy with those who reported not taking therapy for 52 weeks in 624 IPF patients and found no significant difference between groups for disease progression, survival, or decline in FVC. There was a trend toward increased hospitalizations in the antacid-treated group. In patients with an FVC <70%, the antacid-treated group had higher overall infections and lung infections.[53] The role of antacid therapy in patients with IPF remains uncertain.

RECOMMENDATIONS FOR DISEASE MONITORING

Various measures have been demonstrated to be useful in the monitoring of the longitudinal disease activity and are summarized in Table 9.1. Worsening dyspnea scores over 6 and 12 months are significant predictors of early mortality.[23,25] Both a relative and absolute decline of FVC over 6 or 12 months have negative prognostic implications.[23,54−57] Longitudinal change is a better predictor of mortality than baseline values.[34,58] The risk of 1-year mortality if the FVC has declined 5%−10% may be increased >twofold when compared with those with stable FVC, and in those with an FVC decline >10% the increased risk is as high as fivefold.[58] Even small declines in FVC of 2%−6% may represent a clinically significant change; however, because the intratest variability of spirometry approaches or exceeds 5%, interpretation of small changes in individual patients must be made with significant caution. One single study of patients performing daily home FVC monitoring with a portable spirometer suggested changes can be predictive of mortality within 3 months.[59]

A longitudinal decline in DLCO is suggestive of disease activity. A >15% decline in the DLCO has been associated with shortened survival.[56] Additionally, changes at 6 and 12 months in TLC, PaO_2, oxygen saturation, and A-a gradient, as well as the 6-month change in TGV and FEV_1 have been shown to be predictive of survival time.[22,23,28] A large study of 822 IPF patients found that a decline of >50 m in 6MW distance over 6 months was associated with a >fourfold increase in 1 year mortality.[60] Other studies support the usefulness of change in 6MW distance in evaluating prognosis.[38,39] The minimum clinically significant change in distance walked is suggested to be approximately 30 m with a range of 21.7−37 m.[61,62] Separately, desaturation

during 6MW has been associated with increased mortality even if the saturation was >88%.[63]

Longitudinal changes in chest imaging evaluated with semiquantitative CT have been shown to have prognostic significance. An increase in traction bronchiectasis, honeycombing, and/or fibrosis predicts a worse outcome.[31,64] Progressive fibrosis over 6 months predicts poor prognosis, even in the setting of unchanged FVC.[65] Analysis with automated software to quantify the amount of global parenchymal lung abnormalities on HRCT has been shown to be predictive of worsened survival in those with interval changes.[66]

There have been a number of composite measures of prognosis published that use a variety of clinical variables to increase the accuracy and sensitivity of prognostication. These are summarized in Table 9.2. The initial clinical−radiographic−physiologic (CRP) score was published in 1986 and incorporated seven variables: dyspnea, chest imaging with the extent of fibrosis/changes suggestive of PH, spirometry, lung volume, diffusion capacity, resting A-a gradient, and exercise O_2.[67] The CRP score correlates with disease severity and prognosis. The modified CRP scoring system was developed in 2001 and was demonstrated to be a better predictor.[21] It incorporated age, smoking history, presence of clubbing, TLC, PaO_2 at maximal exercise, and changes on chest imaging associated with fibrosis and PH. The abbreviated CRP excluding maximal exercise PaO_2 also predicted survival, although inferior to the modified CRP.

The composite physiologic index (CPI) uses the DLCO, FVC, and FEV_1 and is more accurate in predicting early mortality than any of the individual measures.[68] The Risk stratificatiOn ScorE (ROSE) index incorporates the CPI score with the mMRC dyspnea score and 6MW distance and can be used to predict 3-year mortality in those with newly diagnosed IPF.[69] Another simplified scoring system was developed using data collected during prospective treatment trials. Using age, history of respiratory hospitalization, FVC, and 6-month change in FVC, the score was predictive of 1-year mortality.[70] In a follow-up study, this was modified with the addition of 6MW distance and change in 6MW distance after 6 months, which improved its accuracy.[39]

The GAP index is an easily derived metric for evaluating prognosis that has seen increasing use. The index involves gender (G), age (A), and physiology (P).[71] Patients can be staged based on their score. Stage I, a score of 0−3 points, correlates with a 1-year mortality of 6%, Stage II, a score of 4−5 points, correlates with a 1-year mortality of 16%, and Stage III, a score of 6−8 points,

TABLE 9.2 Composite Measures of Prognosis	
Index	**Variables**
Clinical–radiographic–physiologic[67]	• Dyspnea • Chest imaging with the extent of fibrosis/changes suggestive of pulmonary hypertension • FEV_1, FVC, TGV • DLCO • Resting A-a gradient • Exercise PaO_2
Modified CRP[21]	• Age • Smoking history • Clubbing • Dyspnea • Chest imaging with the extent of fibrosis/changes suggestive of pulmonary hypertension • TLC • Exercise PaO_2
Abbreviated CRP[21]	• Age • Smoking history • Clubbing • Dyspnea • Chest imaging with the extent of fibrosis/changes suggestive of pulmonary hypertension • TLC
Composite physiologic index[68]	• DLCO • FVC • FEV_1
Risk stratificatiOn ScorE[69]	• mMRC Dyspnea score • 6MW distance • CPI
du Bois[70]	• Age • History of respiratory hospitalization over 6 months • FVC • 6-month change in FVC
Modified du Bois[39]	• Age • History of respiratory hospitalization over 6 months • FVC • 6-month change in FVC • 6MW distance • 6-month change in 6MW distance
GAP index[71,73]	• Gender (G) • Age (A) • Physiology (P): DLCO and FVC
Longitudinal GAP index[72]	• Gender (G) • Age (A)

TABLE 9.2 Composite Measures of Prognosis—cont'd	
Index	**Variables**
	• Physiology (P): DLCO and FVC • 6-month change in FVC • 6-month history of hospitalization
CT-GAP[73]	• Gender (G) • Age (A) • Physiology (P): FVC • Semiquantitative CT fibrosis score

6MW, six-minute walk; *A-a gradient*, alveolar–arterial oxygen gradient; *CPI*, composite physiologic index; *CRP*, clinical–radiographic–physiologic; *CT*, computed tomography; *DLCO*, diffusion capacity for carbon monoxide; *FEV₁*, forced expiratory volume in 1 second; *FVC*, forced vital capacity; *PaO₂*, partial pressure of arterial oxygen; *TGV*, thoracic gas volume, *TLC*, total lung capacity.

correlates with a 1-year mortality of 39%. Additional variations of the GAP index have been created. The longitudinal GAP index added a 24-week relative change in FVC and history of hospitalization and adjusts for changes over a 6-month period.[72] CT-GAP adds semiquantitative CT fibrosis score to take the place of DLCO measures from the original GAP index. This measure can be used when the DLCO is unobtainable, unavailable, or felt to be unreliable.[73]

CONCLUSION

IPF has a poor prognosis. The natural history of IPF is variable. While both acute declines and prolonged stability are possible, a slow progression over years resulting in death from respiratory failure is common. Markers of prognosis include both baseline and follow-up symptom scores, pulmonary physiology, and chest imaging. In the past few years, with the advent of two new medications for IPF, the natural history appears to be altered with a slower decline in FVC and potentially prolonged survival.

REFERENCES

1. Ley B, Collard HR, King Jr TE. Clinical course and prediction of survival in idiopathic pulmonary fibrosis. *Am J Respir Crit Care Med*. 2011;183:431−440.
2. Kim DS, Collard HR, King Jr TE. Classification and natural history of the idiopathic interstitial pneumonias. *Proc Am Thorac Soc*. 2006;3:285−292.
3. Kim HJ, Perlman D, Tomic R. Natural history of idiopathic pulmonary fibrosis. *Respir Med*. 2015;109:661−670.

4. Kolb M, Richeldi L, Behr J, et al. Nintedanib in patients with idiopathic pulmonary fibrosis and preserved lung volume. *Thorax.* 2017;72:340−346.

5. Collard HR, Ryerson CJ, Corte TJ, et al. Acute exacerbation of idiopathic pulmonary fibrosis. An International Working Group Report. *Am J Respir Crit Care Med.* 2016;194: 265−275.

6. Song JW, Hong SB, Lim CM, Koh Y, Kim DS. Acute exacerbation of idiopathic pulmonary fibrosis: incidence, risk factors and outcome. *Eur Respir J.* 2011;37:356−363.

7. Richeldi L, Costabel U, Selman M, et al. Efficacy of a tyrosine kinase inhibitor in idiopathic pulmonary fibrosis. *N Engl J Med.* 2011;365:1079−1087.

8. Richeldi L, du Bois RM, Raghu G, et al. Efficacy and safety of nintedanib in idiopathic pulmonary fibrosis. *N Engl J Med.* 2014;370:2071−2082.

9. Noble PW, Albera C, Bradford WZ, et al. Pirfenidone in patients with idiopathic pulmonary fibrosis (CAPACITY): two randomised trials. *Lancet.* 2011;377:1760−1769.

10. King Jr TE, Bradford WZ, Castro-Bernardini S, et al. A phase 3 trial of pirfenidone in patients with idiopathic pulmonary fibrosis. *N Engl J Med.* 2014;370:2083−2092.

11. Fleetwood K, McCool R, Glanville J, et al. Systematic review and network meta-analysis of idiopathic pulmonary fibrosis treatments. *J Manag Care Spec Pharm.* 2017;23: S5−S16.

12. Nathan SD, Albera C, Bradford WZ, et al. Effect of pirfenidone on mortality: pooled analyses and meta-analyses of clinical trials in idiopathic pulmonary fibrosis. *Lancet Respir Med.* 2017;5:33−41.

13. Fisher M, Nathan SD, Hill C, et al. Predicting life expectancy for pirfenidone in idiopathic pulmonary fibrosis. *J Manag Care Spec Pharm.* 2017;23:S17−S24.

14. Ley B, Swigris J, Day BM, et al. Pirfenidone reduces respiratory-related hospitalizations in idiopathic pulmonary fibrosis. *Am J Respir Crit Care Med.* 2017;196: 756−761.

15. Nathan SD, Albera C, Bradford WZ, et al. Effect of continued treatment with pirfenidone following clinically meaningful declines in forced vital capacity: analysis of data from three phase 3 trials in patients with idiopathic pulmonary fibrosis. *Thorax.* 2016;71:429−435.

16. Vancheri C, Kreuter M, Richeldi L, et al. Nintedanib with add-on pirfenidone in idiopathic pulmonary fibrosis. Results of the INJOURNEY trial. *Am J Respir Crit Care Med.* 2018;197:356−363.

17. Raghu G, Collard HR, Egan JJ, et al. An official ATS/ ERS/JRS/ALAT statement: idiopathic pulmonary fibrosis: evidence-based guidelines for diagnosis and management. *Am J Respir Crit Care Med.* 2011;183: 788−824.

18. Flaherty KR, Toews GB, Travis WD, et al. Clinical significance of histological classification of idiopathic interstitial pneumonia. *Eur Respir J.* 2002;19:275−283.

19. Han MK, Murray S, Fell CD, et al. Sex differences in physiological progression of idiopathic pulmonary fibrosis. *Eur Respir J.* 2008;31:1183−1188.

20. Nadrous HF, Pellikka PA, Krowka MJ, et al. Pulmonary hypertension in patients with idiopathic pulmonary fibrosis. *Chest.* 2005;128:2393−2399.

21. King Jr TE, Tooze JA, Schwarz MI, Brown KR, Cherniack RM. Predicting survival in idiopathic pulmonary fibrosis: scoring system and survival model. *Am J Respir Crit Care Med.* 2001;164:1171−1181.

22. Nishiyama O, Taniguchi H, Kondoh Y, et al. A simple assessment of dyspnoea as a prognostic indicator in idiopathic pulmonary fibrosis. *Eur Respir J.* 2010;36:1067−1072.

23. Collard HR, King Jr TE, Bartelson BB, Vourlekis JS, Schwarz MI, Brown KK. Changes in clinical and physiologic variables predict survival in idiopathic pulmonary fibrosis. *Am J Respir Crit Care Med.* 2003;168:538−542.

24. King Jr TE, Schwarz MI, Brown K, et al. Idiopathic pulmonary fibrosis: relationship between histopathologic features and mortality. *Am J Respir Crit Care Med.* 2001;164: 1025−1032.

25. Khadawardi H, Mura M. A simple dyspnoea scale as part of the assessment to predict outcome across chronic interstitial lung disease. *Respirology.* 2017;22:501−507.

26. Ryerson CJ, Abbritti M, Ley B, Elicker BM, Jones KD, Collard HR. Cough predicts prognosis in idiopathic pulmonary fibrosis. *Respirology.* 2011;16:969−975.

27. Alakhras M, Decker PA, Nadrous HF, Collazo-Clavell M, Ryu JH. Body mass index and mortality in patients with idiopathic pulmonary fibrosis. *Chest.* 2007;131:1448−1453.

28. Brown AW, Shlobin OA, Weir N, et al. Dynamic patient counseling: a novel concept in idiopathic pulmonary fibrosis. *Chest.* 2012;142:1005−1010.

29. Sumikawa H, Johkoh T, Colby TV, et al. Computed tomography findings in pathological usual interstitial pneumonia: relationship to survival. *Am J Respir Crit Care Med.* 2008;177:433−439.

30. Lynch DA, Godwin JD, Safrin S, et al. High-resolution computed tomography in idiopathic pulmonary fibrosis: diagnosis and prognosis. *Am J Respir Crit Care Med.* 2005;172:488−493.

31. Lee HY, Lee KS, Jeong YJ, et al. High-resolution CT findings in fibrotic idiopathic interstitial pneumonias with little honeycombing: serial changes and prognostic implications. *Am J Roentgenol.* 2012;199:982−989.

32. Edey AJ, Devaraj AA, Barker RP, Nicholson AG, Wells AU, Hansell DM. Fibrotic idiopathic interstitial pneumonias: HRCT findings that predict mortality. *Eur Radiol.* 2011; 21:1586−1593.

33. Le Rouzic O, Bendaoud S, Chenivesse C, Remy J, Wallaert B. Prognostic value of the initial chest high-resolution CT pattern in idiopathic pulmonary fibrosis. *Sarcoidosis Vasc Diffuse Lung Dis.* 2016;32:353−359.

34. Nathan SD, Shlobin OA, Weir N, et al. Long-term course and prognosis of idiopathic pulmonary fibrosis in the new millennium. *Chest.* 2011;140:221−229.

35. Gonzalez AT, Maher T. Predicting mortality in idiopathic pulmonary fibrosis. Which parameters should be used to determine eligibility for treatment? Analysis of a UK prospective cohort. *Eur Respir J.* 2016;48:OA282.

36. Mogulkoc N, Brutsche MH, Bishop PW, et al. Pulmonary function in idiopathic pulmonary fibrosis and referral for lung transplantation. *Am J Respir Crit Care Med.* 2001; 164:103–108.

37. Lama VN, Flaherty KR, Toews GB, et al. Prognostic value of desaturation during a 6-minute walk test in idiopathic interstitial pneumonia. *Am J Respir Crit Care Med.* 2003; 168:1084–1090.

38. du Bois RM, Albera C, Bradford WZ, et al. 6-Minute walk distance is an independent predictor of mortality in patients with idiopathic pulmonary fibrosis. *Eur Respir J.* 2014;43:1421–1429.

39. du Bois RM, Albera C, Bradford WZ, Costabel U, Noble PW, Sahn SA. A novel clinical prediction model for near-term mortality in patients with idiopathic pulmonary fibrosis (IPF). *Am J Respir Crit Care Med.* 2013;187: A2357.

40. Swigris JJ, Swick J, Wamboldt FS, et al. Heart rate recovery after 6-min walk test predicts survival in patients with idiopathic pulmonary fibrosis. *Chest.* 2009;136:841–848.

41. Swigris JJ, Olson AL, Shlobin OA, Ahmad S, Brown KK, Nathan SD. Heart rate recovery after six-minute walk test predicts pulmonary hypertension in patients with idiopathic pulmonary fibrosis. *Respirology.* 2011;16:439–445.

42. Nathan SD, Shlobin OA, Ahmad S, et al. Serial development of pulmonary hypertension in patients with idiopathic pulmonary fibrosis. *Respiration.* 2008;76:288–294.

43. Raghu G, Behr J, Brown KK, et al. Treatment of idiopathic pulmonary fibrosis with ambrisentan: a parallel, randomized trial. *Ann Intern Med.* 2013;158:641–649.

44. Ryerson CJ, Hartman T, Elicker BM, et al. Clinical features and outcomes in combined pulmonary fibrosis and emphysema in idiopathic pulmonary fibrosis. *Chest.* 2013;144:234–240.

45. Mejia M, Carrillo G, Rojas-Serrano J, et al. Idiopathic pulmonary fibrosis and emphysema: decreased survival associated with severe pulmonary arterial hypertension. *Chest.* 2009;136:10–15.

46. Cottin V. The impact of emphysema in pulmonary fibrosis. *Eur Respir Rev.* 2013;22:153–157.

47. Cottin V, Nunes H, Brillet PY, et al. Combined pulmonary fibrosis and emphysema: a distinct underrecognised entity. *Eur Respir J.* 2005;26:586–593.

48. Schmidt SL, Nambiar AM, Tayob N, et al. Pulmonary function measures predict mortality differently in IPF versus combined pulmonary fibrosis and emphysema. *Eur Respir J.* 2011;38:176–183.

49. Raghu G, Freudenberger TD, Yang S, et al. High prevalence of abnormal acid gastro-oesophageal reflux in idiopathic pulmonary fibrosis. *Eur Respir J.* 2006;27:136–142.

50. Tobin RW, Pope 2nd CE, Pellegrini CA, Emond MJ, Sillery J, Raghu G. Increased prevalence of gastroesophageal reflux in patients with idiopathic pulmonary fibrosis. *Am J Respir Crit Care Med.* 1998;158:1804–1808.

51. Lee JS, Ryu JH, Elicker BM, et al. Gastroesophageal reflux therapy is associated with longer survival in patients with idiopathic pulmonary fibrosis. *Am J Respir Crit Care Med.* 2011;184:1390–1394.

52. Lee JS, Collard HR, Anstrom KJ, et al. Anti-acid treatment and disease progression in idiopathic pulmonary fibrosis: an analysis of data from three randomised controlled trials. *Lancet Respir Med.* 2013;1:369–376.

53. Kreuter M, Wuyts W, Renzoni E, et al. Antacid therapy and disease outcomes in idiopathic pulmonary fibrosis: a pooled analysis. *Lancet Respir Med.* 2016;4:381–389.

54. Jegal Y, Kim DS, Shim TS, et al. Physiology is a stronger predictor of survival than pathology in fibrotic interstitial pneumonia. *Am J Respir Crit Care Med.* 2005;171:639–644.

55. King Jr TE, Safrin S, Starko KM, et al. Analyses of efficacy end points in a controlled trial of interferon-gamma1b for idiopathic pulmonary fibrosis. *Chest.* 2005;127:171–177.

56. Zappala CJ, Latsi PI, Nicholson AG, et al. Marginal decline in forced vital capacity is associated with a poor outcome in idiopathic pulmonary fibrosis. *Eur Respir J.* 2010;35: 830–836.

57. Richeldi L, Ryerson CJ, Lee JS, et al. Relative versus absolute change in forced vital capacity in idiopathic pulmonary fibrosis. *Thorax.* 2012;67:407–411.

58. du Bois RM, Weycker D, Albera C, et al. Forced vital capacity in patients with idiopathic pulmonary fibrosis: test properties and minimal clinically important difference. *Am J Respir Crit Care Med.* 2011;184:1382–1389.

59. Russell AM, Adamali H, Molyneaux PL, et al. Daily home spirometry: an effective tool for detecting progression in idiopathic pulmonary fibrosis. *Am J Respir Crit Care Med.* 2016;194:989–997.

60. du Bois RM, Weycker D, Albera C, et al. Six-minute-walk test in idiopathic pulmonary fibrosis: test validation and minimal clinically important difference. *Am J Respir Crit Care Med.* 2011;183:1231–1237.

61. Nathan SD, du Bois RM, Albera C, et al. Validation of test performance characteristics and minimal clinically important difference of the 6-minute walk test in patients with idiopathic pulmonary fibrosis. *Respir Med.* 2015;109: 914–922.

62. Swigris JJ, Wamboldt FS, Behr J, et al. The 6 minute walk in idiopathic pulmonary fibrosis: longitudinal changes and minimum important difference. *Thorax.* 2010;65: 173–177.

63. Flaherty KR, Andrei AC, Murray S, et al. Idiopathic pulmonary fibrosis: prognostic value of changes in physiology and six-minute-walk test. *Am J Respir Crit Care Med.* 2006;174:803–809.

64. Hwang JH, Misumi S, Curran-Everett D, Brown KK, Sahin H, Lynch DA. Longitudinal follow-up of fibrosing interstitial pneumonia: relationship between physiologic testing, computed tomography changes, and survival rate. *J Thorac Imaging.* 2011;26:209–217.

65. Oda K, Ishimoto H, Yatera K, et al. High-resolution CT scoring system-based grading scale predicts the clinical outcomes in patients with idiopathic pulmonary fibrosis. *Respir Res.* 2014;15:10.

66. Maldonado F, Moua T, Rajagopalan S, et al. Automated quantification of radiological patterns predicts survival in idiopathic pulmonary fibrosis. *Eur Respir J.* 2014;43: 204–212.

67. Watters LC, King TE, Schwarz MI, Waldron JA, Stanford RE, Cherniack RM. A clinical, radiographic, and physiologic scoring system for the longitudinal assessment of patients with idiopathic pulmonary fibrosis. *Am Rev Respir Dis.* 1986;133:97–103.
68. Wells AU, Desai SR, Rubens MB, et al. Idiopathic pulmonary fibrosis: a composite physiologic index derived from disease extent observed by computed tomography. *Am J Respir Crit Care Med.* 2003;167:962–969.
69. Mura M, Porretta MA, Bargagli E, et al. Predicting survival in newly diagnosed idiopathic pulmonary fibrosis: a 3-year prospective study. *Eur Respir J.* 2012;40:101–109.
70. du Bois RM, Weycker D, Albera C, et al. Ascertainment of individual risk of mortality for patients with idiopathic pulmonary fibrosis. *Am J Respir Crit Care Med.* 2011;184:459–466.
71. Ley B, Ryerson CJ, Vittinghoff E, et al. A multidimensional index and staging system for idiopathic pulmonary fibrosis. *Ann Intern Med.* 2012;156:684–691.
72. Ley B, Bradford WZ, Weycker D, Vittinghoff E, du Bois RM, Collard HR. Unified baseline and longitudinal mortality prediction in idiopathic pulmonary fibrosis. *Eur Respir J.* 2015;45:1374–1381.
73. Ley B, Elicker BM, Hartman TE, et al. Idiopathic pulmonary fibrosis: CT and risk of death. *Radiology.* 2014;273:570–579.

CHAPTER 10

Biomarkers in IPF

ZULMA X. YUNT, MD • YAEL ASCHNER, MD • KEVIN K. BROWN, MD

INTRODUCTION

Idiopathic pulmonary fibrosis (IPF) is a progressive fibrotic lung disorder of unknown etiology with an incidence of 4–17 per 100,000.[1] Its incidence increases with advancing age. Clinically, IPF presents with insidious onset of shortness of breath, cough, and fatigue and is frequently misdiagnosed for other more common lung conditions, including chronic obstructive pulmonary disease (COPD) and asthma. Its nonspecific presentation, alongside a lack of overt systemic symptoms, makes early diagnosis challenging.

IPF disease pathogenesis remains elusive; however, currently the disease is thought to result from repetitive microinjury to lung airway epithelium followed by aberrant wound healing responses. This almost assuredly occurs in the setting of an injurious environmental exposure on a background of genetic predisposition. Aberrant repair responses in airway epithelium begin with normal activation of proinflammatory and procoagulant cascades but lead to abnormal epithelial cell signaling with the development and activation of profibrotic myofibroblasts. These cells produce collagen and extracellular matrix that ultimately leads to irreversible fibrosis.

The prognosis in IPF remains poor with a mean survival of 3–5 years.[1] However, prognosis in any one individual is difficult to predict. Disease course is highly variable, with some patients experiencing rapid, unrelenting progression of disease from the onset and others experiencing a slowly progressive course with or without episodic worsening.[2] All patients with IPF are at risk for acute exacerbations (AEs) which carry a poor prognosis. However, annually, only 5%–10% of patients with IPF will experience an exacerbation, and currently we are unable to predict who will be affected.[3–5]

A biomarker is an objectively measured indicator of a normal biological or pathologic process or an indicator of pharmacologic response to a therapeutic agent. Molecular biomarkers are molecules that can be measured within biologic specimens and are often used to gain information regarding clinical disease including risk, diagnosis, prognosis, or activity. The ideal biomarker is one that is easily obtained (low risk), affordable, widely available, and accurate. Currently, no commercially available biomarkers have been confirmed as useful adjuncts to standard diagnosis and clinical assessments in IPF. However, several molecular biomarkers, both individual and in combination, are being investigated for IPF, and it is possible that in the future these will have a place in clinical practice. The currently proposed biomarkers in IPF serve primarily as indicators of disease risk and prognosis. While a small number of potential diagnostic biomarkers have been identified, these have not been validated across broad populations and are not included in current practice guidelines for the diagnosis of IPF.

IDIOPATHIC PULMONARY FIBROSIS: BIOMARKERS OF DISEASE SUSCEPTIBILITY

Disease risk in IPF is believed to be multifactorial and linked to both environment and genetics. The last 10 years have seen considerable progress in our knowledge of genetic risk in IPF, and this is outlined in the following section. To the contrary, biomarkers reflective of environmental risk have not been identified. The greatest currently recognized environmental risk factor for the development of IPF is smoking, and until recently, there has been no way to assess cumulative long-term smoke exposure in an individual person. However promising epigenome-wide association studies have now identified several blood DNA methylation markers with strong correlation to smoking history and cumulative smoke exposure. A systematic review of 17 studies examining methylation changes and active smoke exposure identified multiple genetic loci of interest, most notably genes *AHRR*, *F2RL3*, *GPR15*, and gene regions *2q37.1* and *6p21.33*.[6,7] Furthermore, demethylation at three gene sites—*AHRR, 6p21.33, and F2RL3*—has recently been shown to correlate with lung cancer incidence.[8] There is interest in investigating this finding in relation to other smoking-related conditions, but at present, the relationship between blood DNA demethylation, smoking history, and disease incidence in IPF has not been examined.

Currently, the biomarkers for disease risk in IPF with the most data are genetic markers. Genetics contribute to disease risk in IPF, and some specific gene polymorphisms associated with heightened risk of disease development are known. While an initial recognition of genetic risk in IPF came from familial cases of lung fibrosis, today it is evident that genetics play a role in sporadic cases as well. Known gene variants that increase the risk of developing IPF are outlined in Table 10.1.

Genetic Risk in Familial Fibrosis

Genetic predisposition in IPF was first recognized through identification of familial clusters of pulmonary fibrosis and nonpulmonary genetic conditions characterized by fibrosis. Familial pulmonary fibrosis (FPF) is defined as the occurrence of pulmonary fibrosis in

TABLE 10.1
Genetic Variants Associated With Idiopathic Pulmonary Fibrosis

Gene	Gene Product
MUC5B	Encodes a gel-forming mucin important in mucociliary transport and lung airway defense
TOLLIP	Encodes a protein that interacts with components of the toll-like receptor (TLR) signaling cascade, TGF-β signaling, and IL-1 receptor functions
TERT	Telomerase reverse transcriptase—a catalytic subunit of the telomerase enzyme
TERC	RNA component of telomerase enzyme
DKC1	Dyskerin pseudouridine synthase 1 involved in telomerase stabilization
SFTPC	Surfactant protein C
SFTPA2	Surfactant protein A
ABCA3	ATP-binding cassette transporter protein involved in lipid transport
TINF2	Encodes a protein of the shelterin complex
RTELI	DNA helicase involved in telomere maintenance
PARN	Poly-A-specific ribonuclease involved in mRNA maintenance
AKAP13	Rho guanine nucleotide exchange factor that regulates RhoA
TLR3	TLR family protein important for pathogen recognition and innate immunity
HLA-DRB1	Major histocompatibility complex protein
DSP	Desmoplakin protein important for desmosome structure and adhesion
IL1RN	Interleukin-1 receptor antagonist
FAM13A	Family with sequence similarity 13, member A—function related to GTPase activation
IL8	Interleukin-8 inflammatory cytokine
OBFC1	Protein involved in DNA polymerase-α-primase activity
MUC2	Mucin component protein
ATP11A	Membrane ATPase
TGFB1	TGF-β-associated ligand involved in various cell functions
SPPL2C	Signal peptide peptidase-like 2C
DPP9	Serine protease with aminopeptidase activity
MAPT	Microtubule-associated protein tau—functions to promote microtubule structure and stability
MDGA2	MAM Domain Containing Glycosylphosphatidylinositol Anchor 2

at least two first-degree relatives. FPF accounts for only a fraction of total IPF cases (0.5%—10%).[9-11] As such, the incidence of recognized genetic variants linked with familial fibrosis is low overall. However, within families with FPF, the prevalence of these genetic variants can be quite high. Many of these genetic variants occur in genes associated with telomerase activity (TERT, TERC, DKC1, TINF2, RTEL1, and PARN). Others are related to alveolar maintenance, including SFTPC, SFTPA1, SFTPA2, ABCA3, and NAF1.

Telomerase abnormalities

Telomeres are repetitive nucleotide sequences found at the ends of DNA strands that shorten with advancing age until eventually triggering cell death by apoptosis. Mutations in genes responsible for telomere maintenance are responsible for a rare heritable, clinically recognized condition commonly associated with lung fibrosis called dyskeratosis congenita. In 2007, two studies examining the telomerase genes TERT and TERC in FPF found abnormalities in 8%—14% of these families.[12,13] TERT encodes "telomerase reverse transcriptase," which is a catalytic subunit of the telomerase enzyme, and TERC encodes the RNA component of this enzyme. Abnormalities in these genes lead to shortened telomere length. Other studies have revealed that even in sporadic cases of IPF, telomere length is significantly shorter than in control populations, in the absence of a genetic mutation.[14] A study published in 2008 found that 24% of individuals with sporadic IPF had leukocyte telomere length in the <10th percentile of normal even in the absence of a mutation in TERT or TERC.[14]

Surfactant protein mutations

Surfactant proteins are collagen-containing lectins critical for pulmonary alveolar immunity and homeostasis. Genetic mutations in two of these surfactant proteins—surfactant A (A1 and A2) and surfactant C—have been reported in small familial studies of pulmonary fibrosis. The first report, published in 2001, identified a mutation in surfactant protein C (SP—C) occurring in a child and her mother, both of whom were diagnosed with interstitial pneumonia during infancy.[15] Subsequent studies identified mutations in surfactant proteins A1 and A2 (SP-A1 and SP-A2) within small familial cohorts of pulmonary fibrosis.[16,17] Notably, these mutations occurred in families with both FPF and lung cancer, suggesting a pathogenic link between lung fibrosis and lung cancer. The incidence of surfactant protein mutations in sporadic IPF is very low. However, surfactant protein *levels* as measured in blood and lung lavage fluid (independent of genetics) have been studied as potential molecular biomarkers in IPF (see the following section).

Genetic Risk in Sporadic Idiopathic Pulmonary Fibrosis

Genetic polymorphisms linked to sporadic forms of IPF were identified following the advent of large genome-wide association and linkage studies. These have now identified several genetic risk variants for familial and sporadic IPF[18-22] (Table 10.1). The most replicated finding is a specific variant (rs35705950)—a single nucleotide polymorphism (SNP) within the promoter region of *MUC5B*. Most of the currently identified polymorphisms associated with IPF affect genes linked with epithelial cell function and host defense, suggesting that these biologic processes are important for IPF disease pathogenesis. The link between genetic variants and biologic function is an area of active investigation.

MUC5B promoter variant as a molecular biomarker

In 2011, a hallmark study using combined genetic linkage and association analysis reported a common variant (rs35705950) within the promoter region of *MUC5B* that occurred in 34% of FPF cases, 38% of sporadic IPF cases, and 9% of healthy controls.[23] This study provided the first major insight into genetic risk in sporadic IPF. Several studies have since confirmed this risk variant in large, diverse cohorts of IPF, although the variant seems to occur in lower frequency within Asian populations.[18-22,24] Notably the *MUC5B* polymorphism shows no association with a population of interstitial lung disease (ILD) related to systemic sclerosis, suggesting a disease specificity.[25]

Mucin 5B is a gel-forming mucin in airway epithelial cells. The (rs35705950) variant within the *MUC5B* promoter leads to increased mucin production in airway epithelial cells, which may increase endoplasmic reticulum stress and lead to fibrosis.[2] Precise mechanisms are unknown. Despite being associated with an increased risk of disease development, the *MUC5B* polymorphism is associated with improved survival. *MUC5B* may therefore serve as a marker of both disease risk and prognosis. Studies from two separate IPF cohorts—one a US cohort and the other a multinational cohort—showed that the presence of *MUC5B* was independently associated with decreased mortality when compared with the wild-type SNP.[26] Additionally, when included in a clinical prediction model, the presence of *MUC5B* significantly improved the model's ability to predict mortality.[26]

From these studies, it is evident that MUC5B may have a role in risk assessment and prognostication in IPF. However, at present, the feasibility and clinical utility of testing for genetic polymorphisms in an at-risk population is unclear, and no genetic testing has yet been adopted into standard clinical practice guidelines.

TOLLIP

Two large genome-wide association studies of IPF and control patients have identified SNPs in the TOLLIP gene (Toll-interacting protein) to be associated with an increased risk of developing IPF relative to controls.[18,19] One of these studies specifically examined patients with Euro-American ancestry and identified three separate susceptibility SNPs in the TOLLIP gene.[19] This study was of interest because it also identified increased mortality risk associated with one SNP, rs3750920, within TOLLIP exon 3. TOLLIP is an intracellular protein that acts downstream of Toll-like receptor (TLR) 3 and participates in TGF-β signaling.[27] The precise link between this protein and IPF disease pathogenesis is unknown.

IDIOPATHIC PULMONARY FIBROSIS: DIAGNOSTIC BIOMARKERS

Under current guidelines, diagnosis of IPF is made clinically through simultaneous exclusion of nonidiopathic cause of ILD and identification of a usual interstitial pneumonia (UIP) pattern on high resolution computed tomography (HRCT) or surgical lung biopsy. Most often, diagnostic evaluation for IPF commences once patients have become symptomatic and presented to medical attention. An accurate clinical diagnosis of IPF is challenging even among experts, particularly in cases of discordance between imaging and pathology.[28] Multidisciplinary review confers better diagnostic accuracy, but these conferences are not widely available and may lack accuracy outside of academic centers.[29,30]

An IPF-specific biomarker that can distinguish it from other ILDs would be a tremendous advance in current diagnostic practice. However, the available diagnostic biomarkers in IPF have not demonstrated superiority to standard clinical methods thus far. Here we will summarize the data for currently recognized diagnostic biomarkers in IPF. Many of these have also been shown to correlate with parameters of disease activity.

KL-6

Krebs von den Lungen-6 (KL-6)/mucin 1 (MUC1) is a cell surface–associated glycoprotein member of the mucin family. In the lung, it is present on type II alveolar epithelial cells (AECs) and on bronchial epithelial cells. AECs are considered central to disease pathogenesis in IPF, and as such, there is growing interest in examining KL-6 as a biomarker in IPF. Cell surface

expression of KL-6 increases dramatically within damaged regions of lung in interstitial pneumonia, particularly within regenerating AECs.[31] In vitro, KL-6 is chemotactic for human fibroblasts.[32] Furthermore, KL-6 demonstrates profibroproliferative and antiapoptotic effects on lung fibroblasts, and this activity is inhibited by anti-KL-6 antibodies.[33] Limited data have demonstrated an effect of anti-KL-6 treatment on fibrosis in animal models.[34]

KL-6 has been extensively investigated as a biomarker for various forms of ILD. However, its validity in non-Asian populations has not been established.

In Asian populations, serum levels KL-6 are elevated in various forms of ILD relative to healthy controls. A study of 32 patients with ILD and 82 controls showed that serum KL-6 had higher diagnostic accuracy than surfactant protein A (SP-A), surfactant protein D (SP-D), and monocyte chemoattractant protein-1 (MCP-1) for the presence of ILD.[35] Similarly, a study of KL-6, MMP-7, CCL18, SP-A, and SP-D in IPF found that serum levels of all five markers were elevated in IPF relative to controls, but KL-6 had the highest diagnostic accuracy at 98% on receiver operating characteristic (ROC) curve analysis.[36] To date, KL-6 has not been shown to effectively discriminate IPF from other ILDs such as CTD-ILD or chronic hypersensitivity pneumonitis.

Several studies have examined KL-6 as a prognostic marker in ILD. These have demonstrated that high levels of KL-6 at the time of diagnosis are associated with poor outcome. Two studies—one examining 219 patients with various ILDs and another examining 27 patients with IPF—demonstrated that a KL-6 value of >1000 U/mL was significantly associated with worse survival.[37,38] However, other larger studies in IPF patients have not replicated these findings.[39] There is also interest in exploring KL-6 as a marker of AEs of IPF (AE-IPF). In one study of 47 patients with AE-IPF, KL-6 was able to discriminate between AE-IPF, stable IPF, and acute lung injury not due to AE-IPF.[40] Studies are currently under way to examine KL-6 and its utility as an IPF biomarker in cohorts outside of Asia.

Surfactant Proteins

Surfactant proteins are critical to alveolar homeostasis and are produced by type II AECs. Type II AEC hyperplasia is a pathologic feature of IPF. These cells are considered to play a role in disease pathogenesis, so abnormalities in surfactant proteins may be reflective of disease processes. Genetic abnormalities in genes encoding surfactant proteins A1, A2, and C have been identified in small familial cohorts of IPF.

However, independent of genetic makeup, serum, and bronchoalveolar lavage (BAL) fluid, levels of surfactant proteins may provide diagnostic and prognostic information.

Several studies have determined that serum levels of SP-A and SP-D are elevated in patients with ILD, although their ability to distinguish IPF from other ILDs is less clear.[35,41] However, a recent metaanalysis incorporating data from 21 studies found that serum SP-A and SP-D could distinguish IPF from other ILDs, particularly in Caucasian populations.[42] A study examining 57 patients with various forms of ILD found that serum SP-A was significantly higher in patients with UIP than those with nonspecific interstitial pneumonia (NSIP), whereas BAL fluid levels of SP-D were significantly lower in UIP than in NSIP.[43] Several studies have shown that BAL fluid levels SP-A and SP-D are decreased in patients with IPF relative to healthy controls.[44,45] Furthermore, the biophysical properties of surfactant proteins are altered in IPF patients relative to other ILDs, and this seems to correlate with the level of physiologic restriction.[46] However, obtaining BAL fluid involves performing a semiinvasive procedure, making these measurements considerably less useful in routine practice.

Serum SP-A and SP-D have been shown to independently predict survival time in IPF, and they appear to independently strengthen some (although not all) clinical prediction models.[39,41,45,47,48] BAL fluid SP-A may likewise be predictive of survival: lower levels predict worse survival.[49]

The relationship between SP-A and SP-D levels and disease activity has also been examined. Small studies have identified a link between SP-A and SP-D levels and disease activity, including AE-IPF.[50,51] However, there was no difference in serial measures of SP-A and SP-D in patients receiving pirfenidone versus placebo in larger prospective trials.[4,52] A retrospective trial of 60 patients in Japan did show that baseline SP-D level predicted ≥10% decline in force vital capacity (FVC) over 12 months in patients starting pirfenidone.[53]

Matrix Metalloproteinases

Matrix metalloproteinases (MMPs) are a family of structurally related zinc-containing endopeptidases. A total of 23 MMPs have been identified. MMPs are produced by diverse cell types, including immune cells, epithelial cells, and fibroblasts. MMP functions include degradation of components of the extracellular matrix (ECM) and cleavage of nonmatrix molecules, resulting in altered cell-matrix and cell-cell interactions and activation or inactivation of cytokines, growth factors, and

cell surface receptors. As such, MMPs play critical roles in many physiologic processes including immune responses, tissue remodeling, and wound repair.[54-56] MMPs are highly expressed in IPF, and several MMPs have been implicated in its pathogenesis.[57]

MMP1

MMP1, or collagenase-1, is the prototypical MMP, functioning primarily to degrade collagen types 1 and 3.[56] It is localized to the alveolar and bronchial epithelial cells that line honeycomb cysts in IPF, while absent in the interstitium and fibroblast foci.[58] While expression is low in normal lung, it is highly upregulated both transcriptionally and immunohistochemically in IPF.[57,59,60] A precise rodent ortholog does not exist; thus, no knockout murine studies are available.[56]

MMP7

MMP7 (also called matrilysin) is also expressed in AECs and is capable of degrading multiple ECM components. MMP7 knockout mice are protected from bleomycin-induced pulmonary fibrosis, suggesting a plausible role in the process of fibrogenesis.[57] MMP7 and osteopontin may participate in bidirectional regulation in the pathogenesis of IPF.[61] In humans, MMP7 expression is observed in IPF lung tissue but not healthy control samples.[62] MMP7 is also detectable in BAL fluid where levels are increased in patients with IPF and inversely correlated with FVC.[62,63] A similar relationship is noted in plasma, with a negative correlation between MMP7 levels and both FVC and diffusing capacity of the lungs for carbon monoxide (DLCO).[59] In a separate study, elevated plasma MMP7 levels were independently associated with increased mortality.[64] MMP7 may not be specific for IPF, as expression is also increased in other ILDs.[62,63,65] However, in combination, threshold serum levels of MMP1 and MMP7 are able to distinguish IPF patients from healthy controls and IPF from HP patients, while each marker alone was inadequate.[59]

MMP3

MMP3 is upregulated in the lungs of IPF patients as well as in the lungs of mice treated with bleomycin.[66] Elevated BAL MMP3 levels have also been documented in rapid IPF progressors compared with slow progressors.[67] MMP3 knockout mice were protected from bleomycin-induced fibrosis, whereas expression of recombinant MMP3 in rat lung resulted in fibrosis. In vitro, cultured lung epithelial cells exposed to purified MMP3 upregulated β-catenin signaling pathways, with resultant epithelial-to-mesenchymal transition.[66] MMP3 also cleaves and activates osteopontin.[61]

Several other MMPs have been implicated in the pathogenesis of IPF. Among these are MMP2, MMP8, and MMP9, which play roles in fibrocyte migration into lung tissue.[68]

Osteopontin

Osteopontin (also called secreted phosphoprotein 1) is a phosphorylated glycoprotein that binds integrins and functions as a mediator of cell adhesion, migration, immune responses, and tissue repair.[55,69] In mice, osteopontin expression is increased in bleomycin-induced pulmonary fibrosis.[69] Osteopontin knockout mice are protected from the development of fibrosis and have reduced levels of active TGF-β1 and MMP2 expression.[69,70] In vitro, osteopontin promotes fibroblast and AEC proliferation and migration and increased fibroblast deposition of ECM,[70,71] suggesting a plausible link to the pathogenesis of IPF.

In humans, osteopontin expression is increased in UIP lung tissue compared with normal controls and localizes to areas of epithelium and immune cells (macrophages and lymphocytes) while showing no staining within the fibrotic matrix or fibroblast foci.[69,71] Gene expression levels are similarly elevated in IPF lungs.[71,72] Osteopontin can also be detected in BAL fluid[71] and in plasma, where levels are higher in patients with IPF as well as those with other interstitial lung diseases compared with healthy control patients. Levels of 300–380 ng/mL are 100% sensitive and specific for distinguishing patients with ILD and healthy controls. While plasma levels correlate with worse oxygenation, there appears to be no correlation with FVC or DLCO measurements.[73]

IDIOPATHIC PULMONARY FIBROSIS: PROGNOSTIC BIOMARKERS

Prognostic biomarkers hold promise as novel tools in the management of IPF. Currently, practitioners rely largely on clinical markers, particularly the change in these markers over time, as predictors of disease outcome in IPF. However, clinicians recognize that there is considerable variability in disease course from patient to patient, and, at least in theory, biologic specimens could provide unique information regarding disease activity or prognosis for individual patients.

Several prognostic biomarkers have been identified in IPF, but none have been adopted into routine clinical practice, in part due to lack of validation in large, prospective cohorts. Many of these including KL-6, SP-A, SP-D, and MMP-7 were previously introduced in this chapter as diagnostic markers, but they may demonstrate superior utility as prognostic indicators. Please refer to the previous section for information regarding prognostic utility of these biomarkers. Given that validated diagnostic tools and algorithms already exist in IPF, there is active interest in developing tools for prognosis and disease activity, and it is likely that these may become more routinely incorporated into clinical assessments in the future.

Matrix Metalloproteinase Degradation Products

MMPs are critical to ECM deposition and remodeling in IPF. These processes are central to IPF disease pathogenesis. Biomarkers of matrix turnover have therefore been targeted as indicators of disease activity and prognosis. Recently, a prospective study of 189 patients with IPF examined the predictive capacity of a panel of 11 novel MMP-degraded ECM protein fragments (neoepitopes) with respect to disease progression.[74] The study included a 55-patient discovery cohort and a 134-patient validation cohort. Serum samples from patients were examined at baseline, 1, 3, and 6 months and compared with a decline in FVC (>10%) at 12 months or death. The study identified six neoepitopes whose levels were significantly higher in subjects with progressive versus stable IPF as well as two epitopes whose baseline levels predicted mortality. The 3-month rate of change from baseline in six epitopes was a strong predictor of survival in a dose-dependent fashion such that a greater magnitude of increase correlated with worse outcome.[74]

Gene Profiling

As previously reviewed in this chapter, genomic studies have identified gene variants with prognostic implications in IPF. Specifically, polymorphisms in *MUC5B* and *TOLLIP* have demonstrated prognostic utility as predictors of mortality in IPF.[19,26] More recently, analysis of a 52-gene signature profile in six separate UK and US cohorts was found to predict outcome in IPF.[75] The 52-gene signature identified two subgroups of IPF patients with disparate transplant-free survival defined as "low-risk" and "high-risk" validated in all cohorts (hazard ratio between 2.03 and 4.37 in each of the six cohorts). The addition of this gene signature to a preexisting clinical prediction model—the gender, age, and physiology index—significantly strengthened the tool's ability to predict mortality in patients with IPF.[75] The efficacy of this gene signature as an indicator of response to therapy merits further investigation.

Toll-Like Receptors

TLRs are a central component of the innate immune response, host defense, and tissue homeostasis. TLRs participate in the activation of key inflammatory mediators and pathways, including the transcription factor nuclear-factor-κβ, interferons, and interferon regulatory factors 3 (IRF3), among others.[76] It has been postulated that abnormal TLR function could drive aberrant repair mechanisms in IPF. To this end, a polymorphism within the TLR3 gene L412F was examined in two independent IPF cohorts—one, a UK cohort (170 subjects) and the other the INSPIRE IPF trial cohort (138 subjects). This study found that among IPF patients, a variant allele in L412F was associated with increased risk of mortality and more rapid decline in FVC relative to wild type.[77] Of a total of 308 subjects, 25 died during the 12 months of recruitment for this study, and of these, 18 (72%) carried a variant L412F allele. Pending further validation, polymorphisms in this gene could serve as important biomarkers for early transplant referral and prognostic counseling.

CCL18

CC Chemokine ligand 18 (CCL18) is a profibrotic chemokine produced by alveolar macrophages. CCL18 is increased in lung macrophages of patients with ILD, and longitudinal serum levels correlate inversely with lung function in these patients.[78] CCL18 appears to stimulate collagen production in lung fibroblasts with a positive feedback loop mechanism.[79] In a prospective study of 72 IPF patients, baseline serum levels of CCL18 predicted 6-month decline in FVC and TLC, and baseline CCL18 greater than 150 ng/mL correlated with significantly higher mortality.[80]

YKL40

YKL40 is a chitinase-like protein with roles in inflammation, tissue remodeling, fibrosis, and wound healing. In the lung, YKL40 is linked to asthma disease severity and COPD.[81–83] Serum levels of YKL40 are elevated in IPF and other fibrotic conditions including liver fibrosis.[84,85] A study of 85 IPF patients from the Netherlands found that IPF patients with high serum or BAL levels of YKL40 had significantly worse survival relative to those with low levels.[86] YKL40 from both serum and BAL was significantly higher in IPF patients than in healthy controls.

T Cells

T cells are central to adaptive immunity and have long been implicated in aberrant inflammatory mechanisms in IPF. Early studies identified increased numbers of CD4+ T lymphocytes and T cell–derived mediators in both IPF lung tissue and peripheral blood.[87–90] IPF patients demonstrate clonal expansion of circulating CD4+ T cells, increased IgG autoantibodies, and differential phenotypic and functional CD4+ T cells in peripheral blood relative to controls.[91] A study of 89 patients with IPF examined the relationship between CD4+CD28null T lymphocytes and clinical outcome in this disease. The study identified an increased frequency of CD4+CD28null cells in IPF patients relative to controls.[92] CD4+CD28null cells (in contrast to the normal CD4+CD28+ T lymphocyte phenotype) reflect repetitive adaptive immune stimulation, and in IPF patients, %CD28+ correlated with reduced DLCO and increased mortality.[92] Furthermore, change in CD4+CD28null percentage over time correlated with the decline in FVC.[92] A microarray analysis of peripheral blood mononuclear cells in IPF patients identified four genes (CD28, ICOS, LCK, and ITK) within a T cell activation pathway that were predictive of transplant-free survival when used alongside clinical markers of age, gender, and FVC% predicted.[93] CD4+28+ T lymphocyte levels correlated with expression of these four genes, suggesting that these cells were a likely source of this increased gene expression.

Regulatory T cells (Tregs) modulate T cell immune responses and are reduced in BAL fluid and the peripheral blood of patients with IPF.[94] Semaphorin 7a (Sema 7a) is a glycophosphatidylinositol-anchored membrane protein expressed on both macrophages and CD4+ T cells in IPF lungs.[95] In peripheral blood, circulating CD4+CD25+FoxP3+ Tregs expressing Sema 7a were found to be increased in IPF patients relative to controls and identified patients with rapidly progressive disease.[95]

CXCL13

C-X-C motif chemokine 13 (CXCL13) is a small circulating cytokine that is chemotactic for B cells. The role of B cells in IPF disease pathogenesis is little known; however, a single study examining the relationship between CXCL13 and IPF found significantly increased lung mRNA and blood plasma concentrations of CXCL13 in subjects with IPF relative to COPD and controls.[96] CXCL13 levels were highest in IPF patients who had pulmonary hypertension or AE. On immunostaining, CXCL13 localized to lymphoid aggregates within IPF lung tissue. Notably, high levels of this molecule correlated with increased 6-month mortality, suggesting CXCL13 may have value as a prognostic biomarker if this finding is validated in other cohorts.[96]

IDIOPATHIC PULMONARY FIBROSIS: BIOMARKERS OF DISEASE ACTIVITY AND ACUTE EXACERBATION

Few biomarkers of disease activity or progression have been identified in IPF. Given the heterogeneity of disease behavior in IPF, accurate markers of disease activity would prove useful in its management, particularly if these could serve as markers of response to therapy or likelihood of a future AE. Recent studies examining multimarker panels and gene profiles in IPF may provide information pertinent to disease activity and progression and merit further investigation.[74,75] These (MMP degradation products and 52-gene profile) were reviewed in the previous section. Limited data regarding KL-6 and surfactant proteins (SP-A and SP-D) as markers of AE were also previously reviewed.

Defensins

The defensins are antimicrobial peptides secreted primarily by neutrophils but also by epithelial cells in the lung. In addition to having well-known antimicrobial functions, these molecules participate in innate and adaptive immune responses in lung and other tissues.[97] One subclass—the α-defensins—is elevated in peripheral blood from patients with IPF and shows promise as markers of AE-IPF.[98] In a gene expression profiling study of 23 stable IPF lungs and 8 AE-IPF lungs, there was significant upregulation of α-defensin genes and α-defensin protein levels in AE-IPF lungs compared with stable IPF lungs.[99] In addition, α-defensin protein levels were increased in the peripheral blood of these patients, making this a feasible AE-IPF biomarker pending further investigation. Another study of 130 IPF patients examined gene signatures in peripheral blood RNA from patients with mild versus severe IPF compared with controls. This study found that α-defensins A3 and A4 were differentially expressed in mild versus severe IPF determined by DLCO (but not FVC).[100]

Fibrocytes

Fibrocytes are bone marrow–derived, circulating mesenchymal progenitor cells that express both hematopoietic markers (CD45, CD34) and mesenchymal markers (Col-1, fibronectin).[101,102] In the healthy state, fibrocytes make up <1% of the pool of circulating leukocytes.[103] Fibrocytes migrate to sites of tissue injury in response to the chemokine CXCR12 and may differentiate into fibroblast-like cells and produce ECM components.[102,103] In murine models, circulating fibrocytes are recruited to the lungs of bleomycin-treated mice. Fibrocyte recruitment and extent of fibrosis can be reduced with CXCL12-neutralizing antibodies.[103]

In human studies, levels of circulating fibrocytes ($CD45^+Col-1^+$ cells) are increased threefold in the blood of stable IPF patients as compared with health controls. In the setting of AE-IPF, levels are further increased to approximately 15% of total peripheral blood leukocytes, recovering to preexacerbations levels in those patients who resolved their exacerbations.[102] Fibrocyte numbers are not correlated with measurements of lung function, 6MWT, or radiographic severity of fibrosis. However, a circulating level of >5% total blood leukocytes is associated with increased mortality.[102] Other studies have not confirmed high levels of fibrocytes in the peripheral blood of IPF patients, but they have demonstrated a reduction in the percentage of circulating fibrocytes in patients after treatment with nintedanib or pirfenidone.[104] Thus, levels of circulating fibrocytes may provide a promising surrogate for disease severity or progression, as well as response to treatment. Usefulness may be limited, however, by the overall rarity of these circulating cells.

Periostin

Periostin is matricellular protein that plays essential roles in wound healing, ECM deposition, mesenchymal cell proliferation, and tissue fibrosis.[55,105,106] Periostin is strongly expressed in fibroblasts in human UIP lung tissue, particularly in areas of active fibrosis and fibroblast foci. In addition, serum levels of periostin are significantly elevated in IPF patients.[106,107] Levels correlate with worse lung function (FVC, DLCO, and HRCT honeycombing score)[106,108,109] but do not correlate with AE-IPF.[106] In murine models of bleomycin-induced fibrosis, periostin expression is increased, and periostin accumulates within the ECM of treated mice. $Periostin^{-/-}$ mice (genetically lacking periostin) are protected from bleomycin-induced fibrosis. Similarly, blockade of periostin with a monoclonal antibody to block its interaction with cellular integrins also results in improved survival and reduced fibrosis after treatment with bleomycin.[107]

In patients with asthma, periostin levels have been used as a marker of IL-13 expression and correlate with favorable responses to treatment with an IL-13 monoclonal antibody.[110] IL-13 has also been implicated in the pathogenesis of IPF.[111] Periostin may therefore serve as a marker of disease progression, a possible therapeutic target, and a marker of treatment response, although further studies will be required.

CONCLUSION

The field of biomarkers in IPF remains in its infancy. Biomarkers do not play a role in current clinical guidelines or routine practice for the diagnosis or management of IPF. However, several markers show promise, particularly as indicators of disease risk and prognosis. In recent years, genetic biomarkers have advanced the field significantly, and as genetic testing becomes more accessible, these will likely influence clinical trial design and eventually clinical practice. Furthermore, as understanding of IPF disease pathogenesis grows, new biomarker targets will be identified. Biomarkers are poised to add tremendous value to the management of this otherwise clinically heterogeneous and devastating disease.

REFERENCES

1. Raghu G, Collard HR, Egan JJ, et al. An official ATS/ERS/JRS/ALAT statement: idiopathic pulmonary fibrosis: evidence-based guidelines for diagnosis and management. *Am J Respir Crit Care Med.* 2011;183(6):788–824. https://doi.org/10.1164/rccm.2009-040GL. PMID: 21471066.
2. Ley B, Collard HR, King Jr TE. Clinical course and prediction of survival in idiopathic pulmonary fibrosis. *Am J Respir Crit Care Med.* 2011;183(4):431–440. https://doi.org/10.1164/rccm.201006-0894CI. PMID: 20935110.
3. Kim DS, Park JH, Park BK, Lee JS, Nicholson AG, Colby T. Acute exacerbation of idiopathic pulmonary fibrosis: frequency and clinical features. *Eur Respir J.* 2006;27(1):143–150. https://doi.org/10.1183/09031936.06.00114004. PMID: 16387947.
4. Azuma A, Nukiwa T, Tsuboi E, et al. Double-blind, placebo-controlled trial of pirfenidone in patients with idiopathic pulmonary fibrosis. *Am J Respir Crit Care Med.* 2005;171(9):1040–1047. https://doi.org/10.1164/rccm.200404-571OC. PMID: 15665326.
5. Collard HR, Ryerson CJ, Corte TJ, et al. Acute exacerbation of idiopathic pulmonary fibrosis. An International Working Group report. *Am J Respir Crit Care Med.* 2016;194(3):265–275. https://doi.org/10.1164/rccm.201604-0801CI. PMID: 27299520.
6. Gao X, Jia M, Zhang Y, Breitling LP, Brenner H. DNA methylation changes of whole blood cells in response to active smoking exposure in adults: a systematic review of DNA methylation studies. *Clin Epigenet.* 2015;7:113. https://doi.org/10.1186/s13148-015-0148-3. PMID: 26478754; PMCID: PMC4609112.
7. Zhang Y, Yang R, Burwinkel B, Breitling LP, Brenner H. F2RL3 methylation as a biomarker of current and lifetime smoking exposures. *Environ Health Perspect.* 2014;122(2):131–137. https://doi.org/10.1289/ehp.1306937. PMID: 24273234; PMCID: PMC3915264.
8. Zhang Y, Elgizouli M, Schottker B, Holleczek B, Nieters A, Brenner H. Smoking-associated DNA methylation markers predict lung cancer incidence. *Clin Epigenet.* 2016;8:127. https://doi.org/10.1186/s13148-016-0292-4. PMID: 27924164; PMCID: PMC5123284.
9. Marshall RP, Puddicombe A, Cookson WO, Laurent GJ. Adult familial cryptogenic fibrosing alveolitis in the United Kingdom. *Thorax.* 2000;55(2):143–146. PMID: 10639533; PMCID: PMC1745672.
10. Hodgson U, Laitinen T, Tukiainen P. Nationwide prevalence of sporadic and familial idiopathic pulmonary fibrosis: evidence of founder effect among multiplex families in Finland. *Thorax.* 2002;57(4):338–342. PMID: 11923553; PMCID: PMC1746288.
11. van Moorsel CH, van Oosterhout MF, Barlo NP, et al. Surfactant protein C mutations are the basis of a significant portion of adult familial pulmonary fibrosis in a Dutch cohort. *Am J Respir Crit Care Med.* 2010;182(11):1419–1425. https://doi.org/10.1164/rccm.200906-0953OC. PMID: 20656946.
12. Armanios MY, Chen JJ, Cogan JD, et al. Telomerase mutations in families with idiopathic pulmonary fibrosis. *N Engl J Med.* 2007;356(13):1317–1326. https://doi.org/10.1056/NEJMoa066157. PMID: 17392301.
13. Tsakiri KD, Cronkhite JT, Kuan PJ, et al. Adult-onset pulmonary fibrosis caused by mutations in telomerase. *Proc Natl Acad Sci USA.* 2007;104(18):7552–7557. https://doi.org/10.1073/pnas.0701009104. PMID: 17460043; PMCID: PMC1855917.
14. Cronkhite JT, Xing C, Raghu G, et al. Telomere shortening in familial and sporadic pulmonary fibrosis. *Am J Respir Crit Care Med.* 2008;178(7):729–737. https://doi.org/10.1164/rccm.200804-550OC. PMID: 18635888; PMCID: PMC2556455.
15. Nogee LM, Dunbar 3rd AE, Wert SE, Askin F, Hamvas A, Whitsett JA. A mutation in the surfactant protein C gene associated with familial interstitial lung disease. *N Engl J Med.* 2001;344(8):573–579. https://doi.org/10.1056/NEJM200102223440805. PMID: 11207353.
16. Wang Y, Kuan PJ, Xing C, et al. Genetic defects in surfactant protein A2 are associated with pulmonary fibrosis and lung cancer. *Am J Hum Genet.* 2009;84(1):52–59. https://doi.org/10.1016/j.ajhg.2008.11.010. PMID: 19100526; PMCID: PMC2668050.
17. Nathan N, Giraud V, Picard C, et al. Germline SFTPA1 mutation in familial idiopathic interstitial pneumonia and lung cancer. *Hum Mol Genet.* 2016;25(8):1457–1467. https://doi.org/10.1093/hmg/ddw014. PMID: 26792177.
18. Fingerlin TE, Murphy E, Zhang W, et al. Genome-wide association study identifies multiple susceptibility loci for pulmonary fibrosis. *Nat Genet.* 2013;45(6):613–620. https://doi.org/10.1038/ng.2609. PMID: 23583980; PMCID: PMC3677861.

19. Noth I, Zhang Y, Ma SF, et al. Genetic variants associated with idiopathic pulmonary fibrosis susceptibility and mortality: a genome-wide association study. *Lancet Respir Med.* 2013;1(4):309–317. https://doi.org/10.1016/S2213-2600(13)70045-6. PMID: 24429156; PMCID: PMC3894577.

20. Mushiroda T, Wattanapokayakit S, Takahashi A, et al. A genome-wide association study identifies an association of a common variant in TERT with susceptibility to idiopathic pulmonary fibrosis. *J Med Genet.* 2008;45(10):654–656. https://doi.org/10.1136/jmg.2008.057356. PMID: 18835860.

21. Fingerlin TE, Zhang W, Yang IV, et al. Genome-wide imputation study identifies novel HLA locus for pulmonary fibrosis and potential role for auto-immunity in fibrotic idiopathic interstitial pneumonia. *BMC Genet.* 2016;17(1):74. https://doi.org/10.1186/s12863-016-0377-2. PMID: 27266705; PMCID: PMC4895966.

22. Allen RJ, Porte J, Braybrooke R, et al. Genetic variants associated with susceptibility to idiopathic pulmonary fibrosis in people of European ancestry: a genome-wide association study. *Lancet Respir Med.* 2017;5(11):869–880. https://doi.org/10.1016/S2213-2600(17)30387-9. PMID: 29066090; PMCID: PMC5666208.

23. Seibold MA, Wise AL, Speer MC, et al. A common MUC5B promoter polymorphism and pulmonary fibrosis. *N Engl J Med.* 2011;364(16):1503–1512. https://doi.org/10.1056/NEJMoa1013660. PMID: 21506741; PMCID: PMC3379886.

24. Horimasu Y, Ohshimo S, Bonella F, et al. MUC5B promoter polymorphism in Japanese patients with idiopathic pulmonary fibrosis. *Respirology.* 2015;20(3):439–444. https://doi.org/10.1111/resp.12466. PMID: 25581455.

25. Borie R, Crestani B, Dieude P, et al. The MUC5B variant is associated with idiopathic pulmonary fibrosis but not with systemic sclerosis interstitial lung disease in the European Caucasian population. *PLoS One.* 2013;8(8):e70621. https://doi.org/10.1371/journal.pone.0070621. PMID: 23940607; PMCID: PMC3734256.

26. Peljto AL, Zhang Y, Fingerlin TE, et al. Association between the MUC5B promoter polymorphism and survival in patients with idiopathic pulmonary fibrosis. *JAMA.* 2013;309(21):2232–2239. https://doi.org/10.1001/jama.2013.5827. PMID: 23695349; PMCID: PMC4545271.

27. Selman M, Pardo A. Revealing the pathogenic and aging-related mechanisms of the enigmatic idiopathic pulmonary fibrosis. An integral model. *Am J Respir Crit Care Med.* 2014;189(10):1161–1172. https://doi.org/10.1164/rccm.201312-2221PP. PMID: 24641682.

28. Salisbury ML, Xia M, Zhou Y, et al. Idiopathic pulmonary fibrosis: gender-age-physiology index stage for predicting future lung function decline. *Chest.* 2016;149(2):491–498. https://doi.org/10.1378/chest.15-0530. PMID: 26425858; PMCID: PMC4944785.

29. Flaherty KR, King Jr TE, Raghu G, et al. Idiopathic interstitial pneumonia: what is the effect of a multidisciplinary approach to diagnosis? *Am J Respir Crit Care Med.* 2004;170(8):904–910. https://doi.org/10.1164/rccm.200402-147OC. PMID: 15256390.

30. Flaherty KR, Andrei AC, King Jr TE, et al. Idiopathic interstitial pneumonia: do community and academic physicians agree on diagnosis? *Am J Respir Crit Care Med.* 2007;175(10):1054–1060. https://doi.org/10.1164/rccm.200606-833OC. PMID: 17255566; PMCID: PMC1899268.

31. Ohtsuki Y, Fujita J, Hachisuka Y, et al. Immunohisto-chemical and immunoelectron microscopic studies of the localization of KL-6 and epithelial membrane antigen (EMA) in presumably normal pulmonary tissue and in interstitial pneumonia. *Med Mol Morphol.* 2007;40(4):198–202. https://doi.org/10.1007/s00795-007-0382-7. PMID: 18085378.

32. Hirasawa Y, Kohno N, Yokoyama A, Inoue Y, Abe M, Hiwada K. KL-6, a human MUC1 mucin, is chemotactic for human fibroblasts. *Am J Respir Cell Mol Biol.* 1997;17(4):501–507. https://doi.org/10.1165/ajrcmb.17.4.2253. PMID: 9376125.

33. Ohshimo S, Yokoyama A, Hattori N, Ishikawa N, Hirasawa Y, Kohno N. KL-6, a human MUC1 mucin, promotes proliferation and survival of lung fibroblasts. *Biochem Biophys Res Commun.* 2005;338(4):1845–1852. https://doi.org/10.1016/j.bbrc.2005.10.144. PMID: 16289035.

34. Xu L, Yang D, Zhu S, et al. Bleomycin-induced pulmonary fibrosis is attenuated by an antibody against KL-6. *Exp Lung Res.* 2013;39(6):241–248. https://doi.org/10.3109/01902148.2013.798056. PMID: 23672275.

35. Ohnishi H, Yokoyama A, Kondo K, et al. Comparative study of KL-6, surfactant protein-A, surfactant protein-D, and monocyte chemoattractant protein-1 as serum markers for interstitial lung diseases. *Am J Respir Crit Care Med.* 2002;165(3):378–381. https://doi.org/10.1164/ajrccm.165.3.2107134. PMID: 11818324.

36. Hamai K, Iwamoto H, Ishikawa N, et al. Comparative study of circulating MMP-7, CCL18, KL-6, SP-A, and SP-D as disease markers of idiopathic pulmonary fibrosis. *Dis Markers.* 2016;2016:4759040. https://doi.org/10.1155/2016/4759040. PMID: 27293304; PMCID: PMC4886062.

37. Yokoyama A, Kondo K, Nakajima M, et al. Prognostic value of circulating KL-6 in idiopathic pulmonary fibrosis. *Respirology.* 2006;11(2):164–168. https://doi.org/10.1111/j.1440-1843.2006.00834.x. PMID: 16548901.

38. Satoh H, Kurishima K, Ishikawa H, Ohtsuka M. Increased levels of KL-6 and subsequent mortality in patients with interstitial lung diseases. *J Intern Med.* 2006;260(5):429–434. https://doi.org/10.1111/j.1365-2796.2006.01704.x. PMID: 17040248.

39. Song JW, Do KH, Jang SJ, Colby TV, Han S, Kim DS. Blood biomarkers MMP-7 and SP-A: predictors of outcome in idiopathic pulmonary fibrosis. *Chest*. 2013; 143(5):1422−1429. https://doi.org/10.1378/chest.11-2735. PMID: 23715088.

40. Collard HR, Calfee CS, Wolters PJ, et al. Plasma biomarker profiles in acute exacerbation of idiopathic pulmonary fibrosis. *Am J Physiol Lung Cell Mol Physiol*. 2010;299(1):L3−L7. https://doi.org/10.1152/ajplung.90637.2008. PMID: 20418386; PMCID: PMC2904092.

41. Greene KE, King Jr TE, Kuroki Y, et al. Serum surfactant proteins-A and -D as biomarkers in idiopathic pulmonary fibrosis. *Eur Respir J*. 2002;19(3):439−446. PMID: 11936520.

42. Wang K, Ju Q, Cao J, Tang W, Zhang J. Impact of serum SP-A and SP-D levels on comparison and prognosis of idiopathic pulmonary fibrosis: a systematic review and meta-analysis. *Medicine (Baltimore)*. 2017;96(23):e7083. https://doi.org/10.1097/MD.0000000000007083. PMID: 28591049; PMCID: PMC5466227.

43. Ishii H, Mukae H, Kadota J, et al. High serum concentrations of surfactant protein A in usual interstitial pneumonia compared with non-specific interstitial pneumonia. *Thorax*. 2003;58(1):52−57. PMID: 12511721; PMCID: PMC1746446.

44. McCormack FX, King Jr TE, Voelker DR, Robinson PC, Mason RJ. Idiopathic pulmonary fibrosis. Abnormalities in the bronchoalveolar lavage content of surfactant protein A. *Am Rev Respir Dis*. 1991;144(1):160−166. https://doi.org/10.1164/ajrccm/144.1.160. PMID: 2064123.

45. Barlo NP, van Moorsel CH, Ruven HJ, Zanen P, van den Bosch JM, Grutters JC. Surfactant protein-D predicts survival in patients with idiopathic pulmonary fibrosis. *Sarcoidosis Vasc Diffuse Lung Dis*. 2009;26(2):155−161. PMID: 20560296.

46. Gunther A, Schmidt R, Nix F, et al. Surfactant abnormalities in idiopathic pulmonary fibrosis, hypersensitivity pneumonitis and sarcoidosis. *Eur Respir J*. 1999;14(3):565−573. PMID: 10543276.

47. Kinder BW, Brown KK, McCormack FX, et al. Serum surfactant protein-A is a strong predictor of early mortality in idiopathic pulmonary fibrosis. *Chest*. 2009; 135(6):1557−1563. https://doi.org/10.1378/chest.08-2209. PMID: 19255294; PMCID: PMC2716710.

48. Takahashi H, Fujishima T, Koba H, et al. Serum surfactant proteins A and D as prognostic factors in idiopathic pulmonary fibrosis and their relationship to disease extent. *Am J Respir Crit Care Med*. 2000;162(3 Pt 1):1109−1114. https://doi.org/10.1164/ajrccm.162.3.9910080. PMID: 10988138.

49. McCormack FX, King Jr TE, Bucher BL, Nielsen L, Mason RJ. Surfactant protein A predicts survival in idiopathic pulmonary fibrosis. *Am J Respir Crit Care Med*. 1995;152(2):751−759. https://doi.org/10.1164/ajrccm.152.2.7633738. PMID: 7633738.

50. Honda Y, Kuroki Y, Matsuura E, et al. Pulmonary surfactant protein D in sera and bronchoalveolar lavage fluids. *Am J Respir Crit Care Med*. 1995;152(6 Pt 1):1860−1866. https://doi.org/10.1164/ajrccm.152.6.8520747. PMID: 8520747.

51. Honda Y, Kuroki Y, Shijubo N, et al. Aberrant appearance of lung surfactant protein A in sera of patients with idiopathic pulmonary fibrosis and its clinical significance. *Respiration*. 1995;62(2):64−69. PMID: 7784711.

52. Taniguchi H, Ebina M, Kondoh Y, et al. Pirfenidone in idiopathic pulmonary fibrosis. *Eur Respir J*. 2010;35(4):821−829. https://doi.org/10.1183/09031936.00005209. PMID: 19996196.

53. Ikeda K, Shiratori M, Chiba H, et al. Serum surfactant protein D predicts the outcome of patients with idiopathic pulmonary fibrosis treated with pirfenidone. *Respir Med*. 2017;131:184−191. https://doi.org/10.1016/j.rmed.2017.08.021. PMID: 28947028.

54. Aschner Y, Zemans RL, Yamashita CM, Downey GP. Matrix metalloproteinases and protein tyrosine kinases: potential novel targets in acute lung injury and ARDS. *Chest*. 2014;146(4):1081−1091. https://doi.org/10.1378/chest.14-0397. PMID: 25287998; PMCID: 4188143.

55. Ley B, Brown KK, Collard HR. Molecular biomarkers in idiopathic pulmonary fibrosis. *Am J Physiol Lung Cell Mol Physiol*. 2014;307(9):L681−L691. https://doi.org/10.1152/ajplung.00014.2014. PMID: 25260757; PMCID: 4280147.

56. Pardo A, Selman M. Matrix metalloproteases in aberrant fibrotic tissue remodeling. *Proc Am Thorac Soc*. 2006;3(4):383−388. https://doi.org/10.1513/pats.200601-012TK. PMID: 16738205.

57. Zuo F, Kaminski N, Eugui E, et al. Gene expression analysis reveals matrilysin as a key regulator of pulmonary fibrosis in mice and humans. *Proc Natl Acad Sci USA*. 2002;99(9):6292−6297. https://doi.org/10.1073/pnas.092134099. PMID: 11983918; PMCID: 122942.

58. Fukuda Y, Ishizaki M, Kudoh S, Kitaichi M, Yamanaka N. Localization of matrix metalloproteinases-1, -2, and -9 and tissue inhibitor of metalloproteinase-2 in interstitial lung diseases. *Lab Investig*. 1998;78(6):687−698. PMID: 9645759.

59. Rosas IO, Richards TJ, Konishi K, et al. MMP1 and MMP7 as potential peripheral blood biomarkers in idiopathic pulmonary fibrosis. *PLoS Med*. 2008;5(4):e93. https://doi.org/10.1371/journal.pmed.0050093. PMID: 18447576; PMCID: 2346504.

60. Pardo A, Cabrera S, Maldonado M, Selman M. Role of matrix metalloproteinases in the pathogenesis of idiopathic pulmonary fibrosis. *Respir Res*. 2016;17:23. https://doi.org/10.1186/s12931-016-0343-6. PMID: 26944412; PMCID: 4779202.

61. Agnihotri R, Crawford HC, Haro H, Matrisian LM, Havrda MC, Liaw L. Osteopontin, a novel substrate for matrix metalloproteinase-3 (stromelysin-1) and matrix metalloproteinase-7 (matrilysin). *J Biol Chem.* 2001;276(30):28261–28267. https://doi.org/10.1074/jbc.M103608200. PMID: 11375993.

62. Fujishima S, Shiomi T, Yamashita S, et al. Production and activation of matrix metalloproteinase 7 (matrilysin 1) in the lungs of patients with idiopathic pulmonary fibrosis. *Arch Pathol Lab Med.* 2010;134(8):1136–1142. https://doi.org/10.1043/2009-0144-OA.1. PMID: 20670133.

63. Vuorinen K, Myllarniemi M, Lammi L, et al. Elevated matrilysin levels in bronchoalveolar lavage fluid do not distinguish idiopathic pulmonary fibrosis from other interstitial lung diseases. *Acta Pathol Microbiol Immunol Scand.* 2007;115(8):969–975. https://doi.org/10.1111/j.1600-0463.2007.apm_697.x. PMID: 17696954.

64. Richards TJ, Kaminski N, Baribaud F, et al. Peripheral blood proteins predict mortality in idiopathic pulmonary fibrosis. *Am J Respir Crit Care Med.* 2012;185(1):67–76. https://doi.org/10.1164/rccm.201101-0058OC. PMID: 22016448; PMCID: 3262037.

65. Huh JW, Kim DS, Oh YM, et al. Is metalloproteinase-7 specific for idiopathic pulmonary fibrosis? *Chest.* 2008;133(5):1101–1106. https://doi.org/10.1378/chest.07-2116. PMID: 18071010.

66. Yamashita CM, Radisky DC, Aschner Y, Downey GP. The importance of matrix metalloproteinase-3 in respiratory disorders. *Expert Rev Respir Med.* 2014;8(4):411–421. https://doi.org/10.1586/17476348.2014.909288. PMID: 24869454.

67. McKeown S, Richter AG, O'Kane C, McAuley DF, Thickett DR. MMP expression and abnormal lung permeability are important determinants of outcome in IPF. *Eur Respir J.* 2009;33(1):77–84. https://doi.org/10.1183/09031936.00060708. PMID: 18829682.

68. Garcia-de-Alba C, Becerril C, Ruiz V, et al. Expression of matrix metalloproteases by fibrocytes: possible role in migration and homing. *Am J Respir Crit Care Med.* 2010;182(9):1144–1152. https://doi.org/10.1164/rccm.201001-0028OC. PMID: 20622038.

69. Berman JS, Serlin D, Li X, et al. Altered bleomycin-induced lung fibrosis in osteopontin-deficient mice. *Am J Physiol Lung Cell Mol Physiol.* 2004;286(6):L1311–L1318. https://doi.org/10.1152/ajplung.00394.2003. PMID: 14977630.

70. Takahashi F, Takahashi K, Okazaki T, et al. Role of osteopontin in the pathogenesis of bleomycin-induced pulmonary fibrosis. *Am J Respir Cell Mol Biol.* 2001;24(3):264–271. https://doi.org/10.1165/ajrcmb.24.3.4293. PMID: 11245625.

71. Pardo A, Gibson K, Cisneros J, et al. Up-regulation and profibrotic role of osteopontin in human idiopathic pulmonary fibrosis. *PLoS Med.* 2005;2(9):e251. https://doi.org/10.1371/journal.pmed.0020251. PMID: 16128620; PMCID: 1198037.

72. Yang IV, Coldren CD, Leach SM, et al. Expression of cilium-associated genes defines novel molecular subtypes of idiopathic pulmonary fibrosis. *Thorax.* 2013;68(12):1114–1121. https://doi.org/10.1136/thoraxjnl-2012-202943. PMID: 23783374.

73. Kadota J, Mizunoe S, Mito K, et al. High plasma concentrations of osteopontin in patients with interstitial pneumonia. *Respir Med.* 2005;99(1):111–117. PMID: 15672859.

74. Jenkins RG, Simpson JK, Saini G, et al. Longitudinal change in collagen degradation biomarkers in idiopathic pulmonary fibrosis: an analysis from the prospective, multicentre PROFILE study. *Lancet Respir Med.* 2015;3(6):462–472. https://doi.org/10.1016/S2213-2600(15)00048-X. PMID: 25770676.

75. Herazo-Maya JD, Sun J, Molyneux PL, et al. Validation of a 52-gene risk profile for outcome prediction in patients with idiopathic pulmonary fibrosis: an international, multicentre, cohort study. *Lancet Respir Med.* 2017;5(11):857–868. https://doi.org/10.1016/S2213-2600(17)30349-1. PMID: 28942086; PMCID: PMC5677538.

76. Ranjith-Kumar CT, Miller W, Sun J, et al. Effects of single nucleotide polymorphisms on Toll-like receptor 3 activity and expression in cultured cells. *J Biol Chem.* 2007;282(24):17696–17705. https://doi.org/10.1074/jbc.M700209200. PMID: 17434873.

77. O'Dwyer DN, Armstrong ME, Trujillo G, et al. The Toll-like receptor 3 L412F polymorphism and disease progression in idiopathic pulmonary fibrosis. *Am J Respir Crit Care Med.* 2013;188(12):1442–1450. https://doi.org/10.1164/rccm.201304-0760OC. PMID: 24070541.

78. Prasse A, Pechkovsky DV, Toews GB, et al. CCL18 as an indicator of pulmonary fibrotic activity in idiopathic interstitial pneumonias and systemic sclerosis. *Arthritis Rheum.* 2007;56(5):1685–1693. https://doi.org/10.1002/art.22559. PMID: 17469163.

79. Prasse A, Pechkovsky DV, Toews GB, et al. A vicious circle of alveolar macrophages and fibroblasts perpetuates pulmonary fibrosis via CCL18. *Am J Respir Crit Care Med.* 2006;173(7):781–792. https://doi.org/10.1164/rccm.200509-1518OC. PMID: 16415274.

80. Prasse A, Probst C, Bargagli E, et al. Serum CC-chemokine ligand 18 concentration predicts outcome in idiopathic pulmonary fibrosis. *Am J Respir Crit Care Med.* 2009;179(8):717–723. https://doi.org/10.1164/rccm.200808-1201OC. PMID: 19179488.

81. James AJ, Reinius LE, Verhoek M, et al. Increased YKL-40 and chitotriosidase in asthma and chronic obstructive pulmonary disease. *Am J Respir Crit Care Med.* 2016;193(2):131–142. https://doi.org/10.1164/rccm.201504-0760OC. PMID: 26372680.

82. Konradsen JR, James A, Nordlund B, et al. The chitinase-like protein YKL-40: a possible biomarker of inflammation and airway remodeling in severe pediatric asthma. *J Allergy Clin Immunol.* 2013;132(2):328–335.e5. https://doi.org/10.1016/j.jaci.2013.03.003. PMID: 23628340.

83. Chupp GL, Lee CG, Jarjour N, et al. A chitinase-like protein in the lung and circulation of patients with severe asthma. *N Engl J Med.* 2007;357(20):2016–2027. https://doi.org/10.1056/NEJMoa073600. PMID: 18003958.

84. Furuhashi K, Suda T, Nakamura Y, et al. Increased expression of YKL-40, a chitinase-like protein, in serum and lung of patients with idiopathic pulmonary fibrosis. *Respir Med.* 2010;104(8):1204−1210. https://doi.org/10.1016/j.rmed.2010.02.026. PMID: 20347285.

85. Johansen JS, Christoffersen P, Moller S, et al. Serum YKL-40 is increased in patients with hepatic fibrosis. *J Hepatol.* 2000;32(6):911−920. PMID: 10898311.

86. Korthagen NM, van Moorsel CH, Barlo NP, et al. Serum and BALF YKL-40 levels are predictors of survival in idiopathic pulmonary fibrosis. *Respir Med.* 2011;105(1):106−113. https://doi.org/10.1016/j.rmed.2010.09.012. PMID: 20888745.

87. Homolka J, Ziegenhagen MW, Gaede KI, Entzian P, Zissel G, Muller-Quernheim J. Systemic immune cell activation in a subgroup of patients with idiopathic pulmonary fibrosis. *Respiration.* 2003;70(3):262−269. https://doi.org/10.1159/000072007. PMID: 12915745.

88. Daniil Z, Kitsanta P, Kapotsis G, et al. CD8$^+$ T lymphocytes in lung tissue from patients with idiopathic pulmonary fibrosis. *Respir Res.* 2005;6:81. https://doi.org/10.1186/1465-9921-6-81. PMID: 16042790; PMCID: PMC1199622.

89. Groen H, Hamstra M, Aalbers R, van der Mark TW, Koeter GH, Postma DS. Clinical evaluation of lymphocyte sub-populations and oxygen radical production in sarcoidosis and idiopathic pulmonary fibrosis. *Respir Med.* 1994;88(1):55−64. PMID: 8029515.

90. Costabel U, Guzman J. Bronchoalveolar lavage in interstitial lung disease. *Curr Opin Pulm Med.* 2001;7(5):255−261. PMID: 11584173.

91. Feghali-Bostwick CA, Tsai CG, Valentine VG, et al. Cellular and humoral autoreactivity in idiopathic pulmonary fibrosis. *J Immunol.* 2007;179(4):2592−2599. PMID: 17675522.

92. Gilani SR, Vuga LJ, Lindell KO, et al. CD28 down-regulation on circulating CD4 T-cells is associated with poor prognoses of patients with idiopathic pulmonary fibrosis. *PLoS One.* 2010;5(1):e8959. https://doi.org/10.1371/journal.pone.0008959. PMID: 20126467; PMCID: PMC2813297.

93. Herazo-Maya JD, Noth I, Duncan SR, et al. Peripheral blood mononuclear cell gene expression profiles predict poor outcome in idiopathic pulmonary fibrosis. *Sci Transl Med.* 2013;5(205):205ra136. https://doi.org/10.1126/scitranslmed.3005964. PMID: 24089408; PMCID: PMC4175518.

94. Kotsianidis I, Nakou E, Bouchliou I, et al. Global impairment of CD4$^+$CD25$^+$FOXP3$^+$ regulatory T cells in idiopathic pulmonary fibrosis. *Am J Respir Crit Care Med.* 2009;179(12):1121−1130. https://doi.org/10.1164/rccm.200812-1936OC. PMID: 19342412.

95. Reilkoff RA, Peng H, Murray LA, et al. Semaphorin 7a$^+$ regulatory T cells are associated with progressive idiopathic pulmonary fibrosis and are implicated in transforming growth factor-beta1-induced pulmonary fibrosis. *Am J Respir Crit Care Med.* 2013;187(2):180−188. https://doi.org/10.1164/rccm.201206-1109OC. PMID: 23220917; PMCID: PMC3570653.

96. Vuga LJ, Tedrow JR, Pandit KV, et al. C-X-C motif chemokine 13 (CXCL13) is a prognostic biomarker of idiopathic pulmonary fibrosis. *Am J Respir Crit Care Med.* 2014;189(8):966−974. https://doi.org/10.1164/rccm.201309-1592OC. PMID: 24628285; PMCID: PMC4098096.

97. Tecle T, Tripathi S, Hartshorn KL. Review: defensins and cathelicidins in lung immunity. *Innate Immun.* 2010;16(3):151−159. https://doi.org/10.1177/1753425910365734. PMID: 20418263.

98. Mukae H, Iiboshi H, Nakazato M, et al. Raised plasma concentrations of alpha-defensins in patients with idiopathic pulmonary fibrosis. *Thorax.* 2002;57(7):623−628. PMID: 12096207; PMCID: PMC1746385.

99. Konishi K, Gibson KF, Lindell KO, et al. Gene expression profiles of acute exacerbations of idiopathic pulmonary fibrosis. *Am J Respir Crit Care Med.* 2009;180(2):167−175. https://doi.org/10.1164/rccm.200810-1596OC. PMID: 19363140; PMCID: PMC2714820.

100. Yang IV, Luna LG, Cotter J, et al. The peripheral blood transcriptome identifies the presence and extent of disease in idiopathic pulmonary fibrosis. *PLoS One.* 2012;7(6):e37708. https://doi.org/10.1371/journal.pone.0037708. PMID: 22761659; PMCID: PMC3382229.

101. Guiot J, Moermans C, Henket M, Corhay JL, Louis R. Blood biomarkers in idiopathic pulmonary fibrosis. *Lung.* 2017;195(3):273−280. https://doi.org/10.1007/s00408-017-9993-5. PMID: 28353114; PMCID: 5437192.

102. Moeller A, Gilpin SE, Ask K, et al. Circulating fibrocytes are an indicator of poor prognosis in idiopathic pulmonary fibrosis. *Am J Respir Crit Care Med.* 2009;179(7):588−594. https://doi.org/10.1164/rccm.200810-1534OC. PMID: 19151190.

103. Phillips RJ, Burdick MD, Hong K, et al. Circulating fibrocytes traffic to the lungs in response to CXCL12 and mediate fibrosis. *J Clin Investig.* 2004;114(3):438−446. https://doi.org/10.1172/JCI20997. PMID: 15286810; PMCID: 484979.

104. De Biasi S, Cerri S, Bianchini E, et al. Levels of circulating endothelial cells are low in idiopathic pulmonary fibrosis and are further reduced by anti-fibrotic treatments. *BMC Med.* 2015;13:277. https://doi.org/10.1186/s12916-015-0515-0. PMID: 26552487; PMCID: 4640202.

105. Kudo A. Periostin in fibrillogenesis for tissue regeneration: periostin actions inside and outside the cell. *Cell Mol Life Sci.* 2011;68(19):3201−3207. https://doi.org/10.1007/s00018-011-0784-5. PMID: 21833583; PMCID: 3173633.

106. Okamoto M, Hoshino T, Kitasato Y, et al. Periostin, a matrix protein, is a novel biomarker for idiopathic interstitial pneumonias. *Eur Respir J.* 2011;37(5):1119−1127. https://doi.org/10.1183/09031936.00059810. PMID: 21177844.

107. Naik PK, Bozyk PD, Bentley JK, et al. Periostin promotes fibrosis and predicts progression in patients with idiopathic pulmonary fibrosis. *Am J Physiol Lung Cell Mol Physiol.* 2012;303(12):L1046−L1056. https://doi.org/10.1152/ajplung.00139.2012. PMID: 23043074; PMCID: 3532583.

108. Ohta S, Okamoto M, Fujimoto K, et al. The usefulness of monomeric periostin as a biomarker for idiopathic pulmonary fibrosis. *PLoS One*. 2017;12(3):e0174547. https://doi.org/10.1371/journal.pone.0174547. PMID: 28355256; PMCID: 5371347.

109. Tajiri M, Okamoto M, Fujimoto K, et al. Serum level of periostin can predict long-term outcome of idiopathic pulmonary fibrosis. *Respir Investig*. 2015;53(2):73–81. https://doi.org/10.1016/j.resinv.2014.12.003. PMID: 25745852.

110. Corren J, Lemanske RF, Hanania NA, et al. Lebrikizumab treatment in adults with asthma. *N Engl J Med*. 2011;365(12):1088–1098. https://doi.org/10.1056/NEJMoa1106469. PMID: 21812663.

111. Vij R, Noth I. Peripheral blood biomarkers in idiopathic pulmonary fibrosis. *Transl Res*. 2012;159(4): 218–227. https://doi.org/10.1016/j.trsl.2012.01.012. PMID: 22424426; PMCID: 3308120.

FURTHER READING

1. Orens JB, Kazerooni EA, Martinez FJ, et al. The sensitivity of high-resolution CT in detecting idiopathic pulmonary fibrosis proved by open lung biopsy. A prospective study. *Chest*. 1995;108(1):109–115. PMID: 7606943.

CHAPTER 11

Therapeutic Options for Patients With Idiopathic Pulmonary Fibrosis

DEEPA RAMADURAI, MD • YOSAFE WAKWAYA, MD • BRIDGET A. GRANEY, MD •
MARJORIE PATRICIA GEORGE, MD • AMY L. OLSON, MD, MSPH •
JEFFREY J. SWIGRIS, DO, MS

INTRODUCTION

Long gone are the days when idiopathic pulmonary fibrosis (IPF) was accepted as a condition for which "there is nothing to do." Although there is still no cure for IPF, several therapeutic options—both non-pharmacologic and pharmacologic—are now available to patients with IPF. As with any condition, for IPF, the overarching goals of therapy are to improve how patients feel, function, and survive. Clearly, there is work to be done, but mounting evidence suggests substantial headway is being made toward attaining these goals. Over the last two decades, rigorously conducted studies have yielded data to support various therapeutic interventions for patients with IPF. For the first time ever, there are medications, approved by regulatory agencies around the world, to treat patients with IPF. These medications and a host of research efforts have renewed hope in all factions of the IPF field—from patients to practitioners to researchers.

Each therapy for IPF (exercise programs, supplemental oxygen, antifibrotic medications, lung transplantation) has potential merits and shortcomings. Thus, detailed discussions about available options should be undertaken with each patient whose goals, values, and judgments about therapy must be considered. And shared decision-making should be employed to determine the most appropriate treatment regimen for any individual with IPF.

In this chapter, we review data for pulmonary rehabilitation, supplemental oxygen, and the two Food and Drug Administration (FDA)-approved antifibrotic medications. We also discuss two comorbid conditions that affect many patients with IPF: gastroesophageal reflux (GERD), which some studies suggest occurs in the vast majority of patients with IPF and could play a role in its pathogenesis; and pulmonary hypertension (PH), which occurs in up to a third or more patients with IPF, worsens symptoms, impairs quality of life, and creates significant challenges in the therapeutic approach. The chapter concludes with a brief summary of lung transplantation and its role as a therapy for some patients with IPF.

EXERCISE AND PULMONARY REHABILITATION

The impetus to recommend physical exercise and pulmonary rehabilitation as a therapeutic modality in IPF stems from the abundance of data supporting their use in patients with chronic obstructive pulmonary disease (COPD) and a growing literature on its beneficial effects in patients with IPF. Pulmonary rehabilitation programs consist of exercise training, as their backbone, and other components of disease education and psychosocial support. The goal of these programs is to augment day-to-day physical functioning to achieve optimal participation in life's compulsory and leisure activities and therefore to enhance physical and emotional well-being.[1] Studies of patients with COPD have demonstrated that by reducing respiratory rate, increasing tidal volumes, increasing fat-free body mass, and promoting skeletal muscle fatigue resistance, the physical exercise component of pulmonary rehabilitation induces physiologic changes that lead to significant improvements in a number of clinically relevant, patient-centered outcomes.[1–4] Although the pathophysiologic mechanisms of COPD differ from IPF, patients with IPF appear to receive the same clinical benefits of pulmonary rehabilitation as patients with COPD.

The core of any pulmonary rehabilitation program is physical exercise, consisting of endurance (aerobic) training and resistance (strength) training. Lower extremity aerobic training is accomplished via ground or treadmill walking, stationary cycle ergometry, or step-type trainers. Upper extremity aerobic training may be incorporated with the lower extremity work (e.g., via a NuStep or similar machine) or done separately via repetitive arm raises or arm ergometry. The resistance component of the program employs free weights, elastic bands, or machines used to target upper- or lower-body muscle groups in alternating fashion.

Most pulmonary rehabilitation programs are run by physical therapists who use a goal-directed approach to the exercise component. Once a patient is enrolled, some form of exercise testing (either a 6-min walk [6MWT] or cardiopulmonary exercise test [CPET]) is performed to establish baseline functional capacity and to derive physiologic targets. Commonly used targets for aerobic training include beginning exercise at 70%–80% of the average walk speed from the 6MWT,[5–7] 60% of the peak workload from the CPET, or 60%–80% of the patient's age-based, maximal predicted heart rate.[8–10] The resistance training component is not nearly as precise: typically, weight or resistance is set low to begin and increased when a patient completes a prespecified number of repetitions (e.g., 10–20).

The educational component of pulmonary rehabilitation varies from program to program but typically includes information on medications (including supplemental oxygen), breathing techniques, nutrition, mechanisms of energy conservation, and psychologic well-being, which encompasses coping with the physical and emotional stresses of the disease and end-of-life planning. Some programs include stretching and a nutritional component (which involves assessment by a nutritionist/dietician and recommendations for dietary modifications).

Since 2008, results from numerous studies of patients with IPF have demonstrated clear benefits of pulmonary rehabilitation on maximal or submaximal exercise,[6,7,11,12] health status or quality of life,[6–8,11,12] fatigue and dyspnea.[7,12] The data are nicely summarized in a Cochrane review.[13] Evidence in support of pulmonary rehabilitation for patients with IPF is generally of low quality but most robust for postprogram improvements in distance covered in a 6MWT (6MWD). In 4 studies that included 111 subjects with IPF, pulmonary rehabilitation was associated with a mean 35.6 m improvement in 6MWD. One of the challenges facing the field is how to ensure the improvements from pulmonary rehabilitation are durable, as benefits wane after program completion. On average,

improvements in every outcome decline back to baseline by 6 months postpulmonary rehabilitation. Whether longer programs (most are 6–12 weeks), protocolized home-based maintenance programs with close supervision and frequent follow-up visits, online programs with remote monitoring of data captured via wearable technology, or other modalities confer durability is unclear. Likewise, it is unknown whether interval training (e.g., short bursts of exercise separated by rest periods) might be more beneficial than the universally employed endurance training approach. Several studies aimed at answering this question are underway. Furthermore, whether or how the resistance training component should be modified to best suit patients with IPF is uncertain. In two studies, patients with IPF were found to have significantly reduced quadriceps force[14] or global lower extremity strength compared with age-matched controls.[15] Whether implementing a more targeted approach to strengthening large muscle groups of the lower extremities would bolster beneficial effects of pulmonary rehabilitation is uncertain, but we believe this merits investigation.

Based on available data and our experience caring for patients with IPF, we offer the following general recommendations:

1. All patients with IPF, regardless of disease severity, should be encouraged to complete a formal pulmonary rehabilitation program. Although some studies suggest that patients with the greatest impairments in submaximal exercise benefit most, no study has convincingly identified a baseline 6MWD above which pulmonary rehabilitation is ineffective.[5,7,16] Thus, even patients with early or very mild disease should be given the opportunity to participate in pulmonary rehabilitation and encouraged to exercise daily. Given the high prevalence of coronary artery disease in patients with IPF, there should be a low threshold to perform cardiac stress testing before program initiation.

2. Pulmonary rehabilitation programs should—at a minimum—include educational and training components; stretching and nutritional components are optional (but considered beneficial).

3. Sessions should occur at least twice weekly for at least 6 weeks, but we believe programs lasting at least 12 weeks are better. Regardless of the length of the program, patients should be strongly encouraged to exercise between sessions and to continue daily exercise after the program concludes.

4. During exercise sessions, supplemental oxygen should be provided to maintain a peripheral oxygen saturation (SpO_2) > 89% during exercise. Once

SpO_2 is measured at various levels of exertion (and supplemental oxygen flow is adjusted as needed), continuous monitoring is not required.

5. An educational component specific to IPF should be offered. Suggested topics include disease education, symptom management, clinical tests, autonomy (i.e., how to become or remain self-sufficient and "take charge of their disease"[17]), appropriate oxygen use, medications, and end-of-life counseling.

6. Patients' goals, exercise capacity, and various patient-reported outcomes should be assessed before and after completion of the program. Doing so will help determine a patient-centered care plan that best prioritizes individual goals.

Standard pulmonary rehabilitation programs provide tangible benefits in outcomes meaningful to patients with IPF, including physical functional capacity, dyspnea, health status, and quality of life. In a disease with effective treatment options in short but growing supply, the volume of evidence suggests pulmonary rehabilitation should be incorporated into every IPF patient's therapeutic regimen. Several questions about pulmonary rehabilitation in IPF remain to be answered, including when it should be prescribed, how long the program should last, what exercise prescription leads to the greatest benefits (e.g., endurance vs. interval training, whether there should be more focus on resistance training of large muscle groups of the lower extremities), and what the educational component should include and how best to deliver it.

SUPPLEMENTAL OXYGEN

Most patients with IPF will need supplemental oxygen at some point in their disease course. The cache of data supporting the use of supplemental oxygen in hypoxemic patients with IPF is surprisingly sparse. Even for COPD, a condition with far greater prevalence than IPF, studies assessing the effects of supplemental oxygen on clinical outcomes are few and dated.[18,19] There is little doubt that supplemental oxygen prolongs life in patients with COPD who are hypoxemic at rest or who have signs of right heart failure.[18,19] It is far less clear whether supplemental oxygen is beneficial for patients who are normoxic at rest but become hypoxemic with activity. In a landmark trial that included patients with COPD who desaturate to a moderate degree with exertion, supplemental oxygen did not improve mortality, time to hospitalization, health-related quality of life, anxiety, depression, or 6MWD.[20]

However, scientific rationale, clinical experience, and a small handful of published studies suggest supplemental oxygen has beneficial effects among patients with IPF who desaturate to a significant degree during sleep or with activity. Thus, despite a lack of robust data, experts recommend that, for patients with IPF, oxygen needs should be assessed at each clinic visit.[21] Our practice is to follow these recommendations; we assess patients' needs and prescribe supplemental oxygen in flows that will maintain $SpO_2 > 89\%$ regardless of the level of physical activity. Interestingly, it appears as though, for any level of disease severity, patients with IPF desaturate more (and thus require greater oxygen flow rates) than patients with COPD,[22] and patients with IPF are more likely than patients with other forms of fibrotic interstitial lung disease (ILD)[23] to be prescribed supplemental oxygen.

In a randomized, placebo-controlled, crossover trial of 20 Japanese patients with IPF who desaturated to less than 88% during a 6MWT, compared with ambient air, supplemental oxygen had no beneficial effects on dyspnea, 6MWD, or leg fatigue. However, a major criticism of this study is that oxygen was not titrated to achieve a peripheral oxygen saturation >89% (mean saturation after 6MWD was 84% despite using oxygen at a flow of 4 L/min).[24] In two small, single-center studies that included a total of 34 patients with IPF or fibrotic nonspecific interstitial pneumonia (fNSIP), supplemental oxygen (appropriately titrated to achieve saturations of >88% or 90%[25,26]) was associated with significantly increased 6MWD[25,26] and/or improved dyspnea.[26] In another trial published only in abstract form,[27] Visca and colleagues used a randomized, crossover design to compare effects of supplemental oxygen (vs. no oxygen) on numerous, patient-centered outcomes in 83 subjects with fibrotic ILD (half with IPF) who desaturated with activity. Oxygen improved health status, dyspnea, and physical activity.

It is important to remind patients that supplemental oxygen will not completely alleviate dyspnea, and for many patients, the effects on dyspnea and physical functioning are modest.[28] Whether those modest benefits are worth the hassles and hardships for patients is a question that has never been directly assessed. We would argue that for the sick lungs of patients with IPF, doing anything possible to try to prevent additional problems (e.g., the development of PH) seems like a reasonable goal.

Although nasal cannula is the predominant mode of supplemental oxygen delivery, we believe transtracheal oxygen (TTO) is a viable but underutilized option that may be advantageous in certain IPF patients. To deliver oxygen directly into the trachea, a 10–13 cm long catheter is surgically inserted through the skin of the neck and rests in the distal trachea, providing a conduit for supplemental oxygen delivery. Besides alleviating skin irritation, nasal irritation, mucosal drying, or bleeding that occurs in many patients who use a nasal cannula, TTO delivery allows oxygen flows to be reduced by an average of 50% at rest and 30% with exertion. In contrast with many patients whose chronic lung disease causes copious amounts of sputum production, patients with IPF would seem to be an ideal group for this modality of oxygen delivery.[29] And we typically discuss TTO with any IPF patient who requires oxygen at rest.

Supplemental oxygen definitely has its challenges and potential drawbacks. Patients describe feeling tethered to their oxygen delivery device and may feel stigmatized by having to lug their delivery devices around or wear a nasal cannula in public. Delivery devices are heavy and can be unwieldy, thus limiting activity. Patients whose oxygen needs are not met by portable oxygen concentrators are particularly constrained, unable to travel via airplane. Given the challenges, we believe supplemental oxygen should be prescribed to patients with IPF who need it but only after a detailed discussion of oxygen and how to use it appropriately. Because supplemental oxygen will affect everyone in the home, we believe patients' caregivers should be involved in this discussion. Qualitative studies have documented the challenges supplemental oxygen imposes on caregivers of patients with IPF who describe it as a physical "barrier" to living a normal life.[30]

Available data, scientific rationale, and expert opinion suggest that assessing oxygen needs in patients with IPF—and prescribing supplemental oxygen to meet those needs—is a reasonable endeavor. Many, but not all, patients will derive benefit from using it, and for some, the challenges supplemental oxygen poses are profound. Research is currently underway to better define benefits and drawbacks of using supplemental oxygen in the IPF population and to identify more efficient ways to deliver it.

ANTIFIBROTIC THERAPIES

In 2018, there is still no cure for IPF. Over the last few decades, research has launched the field to a heightened level of understanding of the pathophysiologic mechanisms involved in fibrosis formation and progression. That improved understanding of the profibrotic cascade has exposed a number of potential therapeutic targets in IPF. The ultimate effect of drugs that target pathways or components of the cascade—generally referred to as antifibrotic agents—is to reduce fibroblast proliferation

and/or activity. The intended result of such medications, then, is to halt or at least decrease the formation of scar/fibrosis.

In 2014, the US FDA approved two medications for the treatment of IPF, nintedanib and pirfenidone. In large, multinational confirmatory trials, each drug was shown to slow the progression of IPF to similar degrees. Among 1066 subjects enrolled in either of two, replicate, 52-week trials, nintedanib 150 mg twice daily reduced the modeled decline in forced vital capacity (FVC) by 50% compared with placebo. For subjects in the placebo groups, modeled FVC declined by an average 240 mL compared with subjects in the nintedanib groups whose modeled FVC declined by an average 115 mL, for a mean between-group difference of 125 mL ($P < .001$). Startlingly similarly, among 555 subjects enrolled in a 52-week trial, pirfenidone 2403 mg divided into three daily doses reduced the decline in FVC by 48% compared with placebo. For subjects in the placebo group, modeled FVC declined by an average 280 mL compared with subjects in the pirfenidone group whose modeled FVC declined by an average 164 mL, for a mean between-group difference of 116 mL ($P < .001$).

The aggregate of the published data—many stemming from post hoc analyses—suggest nintedanib and pirfenidone have other beneficial effects, including prolonging survival[31–33] and reducing hospitalizations.[33,34] As in other chronic illnesses (e.g., diabetes or infection with human immunodeficiency virus), experts theorize that using antifibrotic drugs in combination to inhibit multiple pathways in the profibrotic cascade may be more beneficial than monotherapy.[35] Research around this issue is ongoing.

Both nintedanib and pirfenidone have potential adverse effects that must be discussed in detail with patients to whom they are prescribed. By not using shared decision-making, managing patient expectations (e.g., making patients fully aware that the average effect of the drugs is to slow—not even halt—progression), or outlining detailed plans for monitoring and addressing side effects, the chance for poor adherence is very high. Both nintedanib and pirfenidone are long-term medications that we regard as similar to antihypertensives: they are taken not to necessarily make patients feel better (unfortunately) but in hopes of preventing or delaying onset of poor outcomes down the road.

The most frequent adverse effect of nintedanib is diarrhea, which occurred in greater than 60% of subjects in the confirmatory trials. However, less than 5% of subjects who developed diarrhea discontinued the drug.[36] Adequate counseling about dietary modifications, hydration, and initiation of antidiarrheals (e.g., loperamide) at the first clinical sign of diarrhea typically alleviates symptoms and allows nintedanib to be continued. Nintedanib is contraindicated in patients with Child Pugh B or C liver disease, and screening liver enzymes (including AST, ALT, ALP, and bilirubin) should be obtained before starting nintedanib and serially thereafter. The most frequent adverse effects of pirfenidone are nausea and anorexia. In addition, sun protective clothing and sunscreen should be used to avoid the photosensitivity rash that can occur in a significant minority of patients. The three daily doses of pirfenidone must be taken with food (on a full stomach). Liver enzymes should be checked at baseline and monitored serially throughout the course of therapy. Both nintedanib and pirfenidone affect a CYP enzyme (3A4 in nintedanib and 1A2 in pirfenidone), thus, drug-drug interactions should be assessed before initiating either antifibrotic and if any new drug is started afterward.

Available longitudinal, observational data suggest the effects of nintedanib and pirfenidone on slowing disease progression are durable. Whether benefits wane over even longer periods of time is unknown.[36–38] In our opinion, the drugs are equally effective, and either could be offered to any given patient with IPF after a detailed discussion of expected benefits, potential adverse effects, and required monitoring. In the majority of patients, side effects of nintedanib and pirfenidone are manageable; however, we strongly encourage very close clinical follow-up and frequent monitoring of patients prescribed either of these drugs.[39]

GASTROESOPHAGEAL REFLUX

A growing body of evidence suggests a link between GERD, microaspiration, and lung disease. In observational studies, GERD has been identified in greater than 90% of patients with IPF.[40,41] In retrospective case series, there appeared to be an association between halting IPF progression and aggressive treatment of GERD. Gavini and colleagues showed that reflux and prolonged reflux bolus clearance time (detected via esophageal impedance monitoring) was associated with the severity of pulmonary physiologic dysfunction in pretransplant patients with IPF.[42] Although not strongly supporting causation, the evidence suggesting a relationship between GERD and IPF is quite intriguing, and the issue remains an area of interest for physician-scientists and one of the key areas of research encouraged by IPF experts around the world.[40]

Obviously, reflux itself (i.e., retrograde flow of gastric contents into the esophagus) cannot cause lung injury; the link—if there truly is one—between GERD and the development or progression of lung fibrosis must be aspiration (i.e., inhalation, advancement, leakage, drip, or drainage of oropharyngeal, esophageal or gastric contents, through the glottis (vocal cords), and into the lower respiratory tract). In a study of patients with IPF, Hoppo and colleagues identified proximal reflux events in greater than half their sample, and 85% had a defective lower esophageal sphincter (LES).[41] Diminished tone of the LES can be spontaneous or be due to a hiatal hernia; traction from the diaphragm; or induced by foods, beverages, or medications.[43] However, diminished LES tone, or even proximal reflux, is not equivalent to aspiration; and to date, the presence of overt or occult aspiration has not been studied in IPF.

Many experts theorize that episodic, recurrent microaspiration of gastric contents (that reach the glottis via reflux up the esophagus) could be a cause of epithelial injury in IPF. The basilar predominance (where aspirate collects in the upright or semirecumbent lung) and the temporal heterogeneity of the UIP pattern suggest plausibility for recurrent microaspiration as an instigator of injury in IPF.

More data implicating GERD/aspiration as a potential source of lung injury in IPF come from animal models, in which repetitive tracheal injections of gastric contents can lead to the development of pulmonary fibrosis.[45,46] Also, higher concentrations of bile acids and pepsin have been found in the lungs of IPF patients compared with controls with (ILD) other than IPF or healthy people.[46] In laboratory studies, Chen and colleagues demonstrated that bile acids promote molecular mechanisms that drive pulmonary fibrosis, including activation of lung fibroblasts and differentiation to the myofibroblast phenotype.[44] Some of the effects of bile acids were mediated via farnesoid X receptor, a bile acid–activated nuclear receptor found in alveolar epithelial cells.[44] Bile acids have also been shown to induce alveolar epithelial cells to generate transforming growth factor beta, the downstream effects of which include fibroblast proliferation.[47]

Clinically, IPF patients with GERD are likely to lack typical symptoms of reflux, including heartburn, regurgitation, or dysphagia.[43] Thus, clinical symptoms are not a reliable screening tool for pathologic reflux in IPF patients. Using questionnaires to screen for GERD in patients with IPF has a sensitivity of 65% and specificity of 71% when compared with gold standard 24-h pH monitoring.[43] In a prospective study with a broad range of outcomes, Savarino and colleagues examined associations between impedance-pH monitors, tests of esophageal motility, salivary and bronchoalveolar lavage (BAL) fluid bile acid, and pepsin levels with clinical markers of IPF severity among 40 patients with IPF, 40 patients with non-IPF ILD, and 50 healthy controls. Patients with IPF had more acid and weakly acidic reflux episodes (76%) than patients with non-IPF ILD (47%) and healthy controls (32%).[46] Patients with IPF also had more episodes of proximal reflux and higher levels of both pepsin and bile acids in saliva and BAL fluid than the comparator groups. There was strong correlation between the extent of fibrosis (on high-resolution computed tomography [HRCT]) and BAL pepsin and bile acids and the number of distal and proximal reflux episodes.[46]

Thus, patients with IPF have more distal and proximal reflux and higher quantities of moieties from the gastrointestinal tract in their lungs than other patients. Experts have pondered whether patients with IPF have these abnormalities because lung fibrosis alters the mechanics of the LES; that is, they have reflux because they have fibrosis, not the other way around. In two retrospective analyses, investigators observed improved clinical outcomes among patients with IPF treated with antireflux/antacid therapy. In a study of 204 patients with IPF,[48] the use of acid-suppressing medications was an independent predictor of longer survival.[48] There was no association between GERD symptoms and IPF severity. There was no objective measurement of reflux; investigators were forced to rely on patient-reported use of medications, and there was no assessment of adequacy of acid suppression. In an analysis of all subjects randomized to the placebo arms in one of three NIH-sponsored drug trials conducted by sites in the IPF Network (IPFnet), antacid (i.e., proton pump inhibitor or PPI) therapy was associated with less decline in FVC (-0.06 L compared with -0.12 L in subjects not on antacid therapy [$P = .05$]) and fewer acute exacerbations.[43] Interestingly, some experts have theorized that PPIs could exert beneficial effects in IPF via antiinflammatory and/or antifibrotic activities by directly suppressing proinflammatory cytokines, profibrotic proteins, and the proliferation of lung fibroblasts, rather than simply suppressing acid.[49]

Acid suppression has no effect on nonacid reflux, which appears to be common in patients with IPF. Maybe in IPF, any reflux (and presumably the microaspiration that follows) can promote fibrosis. In patients with end-stage lung disease awaiting transplant, antireflux surgery was safe, led to stabilization of lung function decline, and prevented increasing oxygen requirements observed in patients who did not undergo antireflux surgery.[50] In another retrospective study, investigators observed an association between fundoplication surgery and prolonged survival in patients with IPF.[51] These compelling data raise the question of whether preventing acidic, weakly acidic, and nonacidic reflux is required to interrupt the pathogenetic mechanisms of IPF. Results from a prospective, multicenter, randomized controlled trial (Weighing Risks and Benefits of Laparoscopic Anti-Reflux Surgery in Patients with IPF—NCT01982968[52]) are eagerly awaited.

Currently accepted guidelines recommend antacid therapy for all patients with IPF.[40] However, additional research is needed to answer a multitude of questions around the role of GERD and aspiration in the pathogenesis of IPF.

PULMONARY HYPERTENSION

Pulmonary vascular disease is a significant comorbidity in IPF. In patients with IPF, the prevalence of PH, defined as a mean pulmonary arterial pressure ≥ 25 mmHg on right heart catheterization, is relatively low, ranging between 8.1% and 14.9%.[53,54] However PH is found in 31.6%—46.1% of patients with severe IPF who have been referred for lung transplantation.[55—57]

In IPF, the presence of PH is associated with a disproportionately low diffusion capacity of carbon monoxide (DLCO), higher than expected oxygen requirements, and increased risk of death.[55,58] Patients with IPF and PH (PH-IPF) have also reduced exercise tolerance and increased ventilatory inefficiency on CPET.[59,60]

There are several challenges in addressing PH in the setting of IPF. Predicting which IPF patients will develop PH is difficult because PH is not necessarily associated with disease severity as determined by pulmonary function testing or chest imaging.[57,61] Echocardiography is highly inaccurate in the setting of parenchymal lung disease and can overestimate or underestimate pulmonary artery pressures.[62—64] Chest computed tomography (CT)-derived measurements of the pulmonary artery are of limited utility in identifying PH in IPF.[64,65]

Once a diagnosis of PH is made in a patient with IPF, the approach to treating it is extremely challenging. As a first step, accepted guidelines recommend optimizing treatment of patients' underlying lung disease, including providing adequate supplemental oxygen therapy.[66] As detailed earlier, supplemental oxygen therapy is believed to be a critical component of therapy in patients who are hypoxemic or desaturated, but most evidence is extrapolated from studies performed in COPD patients.[67,68] To date, there is no clinical evidence supporting routine use of vasodilator therapy in patients with PH-IPF. However, little research has been done to assess the effectiveness of therapy for PH-IPF. Research into the pathophysiology of IPF suggests that endothelin-1 could play a role in the development and progression of fibrosis. In response, major trials of endothelin receptor antagonists (ERAs) (Table 11.1) were designed to target fibrosis without regard to PH. As in other trials of therapies for IPF, patients with more severe fibrosis were excluded.[69–71] While the nonselective ERAs bosentan and macitentan were well-tolerated but were not associated with benefit, ambrisentan, a selective endothelin-A (ET-A) receptor antagonist, was associated with progression of fibrosis.[72]

In the Sildenafil Trial of Exercise Performance in IPF, sildenafil was associated with improvement in secondary endpoints, including dyspnea and quality of life. In a substudy of subjects with available echocardiographic data, compared with subjects without right ventricular (RV) systolic dysfunction, in those with RV systolic dysfunction, sildenafil was associated with less decline over time in 6MWD and improved dyspnea.[73,74] A trial of the soluble guanylate cyclase stimulator, riociguat, in patients with PH associated with idiopathic interstitial pneumonia (including IPF) was terminated early because of adverse outcomes.[75] Trials examining inhaled use of prostacyclin and inhaled nitric oxide in PH associated with IPF are underway.

Given there seems to be a percentage of patients with IPF who suffer from precapillary disease that appears to behave similarly to that seen in patients with a pulmonary arterial hypertension (PAH) phenotype, recommendations were made at the 2013 World Symposium on PH for ways to think about PH in ILD. Seeger and colleagues suggest that there are likely different phenotypes of disease in the spectrum of PH associated with parenchymal lung disease (i.e., World Health Organization [WHO] Group 3 PH) and that categorizing patients at the time of considering therapy is important in the management of this disease.[76] In their recommendations for management (Table 11.2), they suggested considering IPF patients on the basis of the severity of the parenchymal disease and pulmonary vascular abnormalities. Thus, in patients with IPF and a mean pulmonary artery pressure (mPAP) < 25 mmHg at rest, they recommended no vasodilator therapy. In IPF patients with mPAP between 25 and

35 mmHg, they recognized that currently there are no data supporting treatment with vasodilator therapy. In patients with IPF and with FVC ≥ 70% predicted, minimal changes on HRCT scan and mPAP ≥ 35 mmHg at rest, it is important to try to discriminate between WHO Group 1 (a PAH phenotype) and WHO Group 3 phenotype; in these cases, referral to a center with expertise in PH and lung disease is recommended. In patients with more advanced IPF (FVC < 70% predicted, more extensive fibrosis on HRCT scan), and mPAP between 25 and 35 mmHg, referral to a center for individualized care (for both PH and IPF) is recommended. And, in this group of patients, clinical trials are needed. These recommendations were acknowledged in the 2015 European Respiratory Society Guidelines, which state "patients with suspected PAH in addition to their lung diseases characterized by (1) mild parenchymal lung abnormalities, (2) symptoms insufficiently explained by mechanical disturbances, and (3) a hemodynamic "PAH phenotype," (i.e., severe PAH with high PVR and low CO) may be treated according to recommendations for PAH, keeping in mind the potential implications of coexisting lung disease on symptoms and response to therapy."[66]

Since the World Symposium on PH in 2013, researchers have begun exploring the use of vasodilator therapy in patients with a PAH phenotype in the setting of chronic lung disease. Brewis and colleagues studied patients with lung disease and severe PH (defined as mPAP ≥ 35 mmHg with a pulmonary artery wedge pressure ≤ 15 mmHg and normal or reduced cardiac output)[77] and analyzed data after stratifying on criteria proposed by Seeger and colleagues (i.e., on FVC ≥ 70% or <70%). Interestingly, they observed no difference in survival between subgroups, but patients with the most severe lung disease had overall increased mortality. All patients were treated with PH-specific therapy for a minimum of 3 months, with treating physicians choosing the agent(s). The authors observed no benefits of vasodilator therapy on 6MWD or New York Heart Association functional class. They postulated that this may be due to the fact that their subjects had ventilatory limitations due to their underlying lung disease. They did note a reduction in N-terminal prohormone of brain natriuretic peptide (NT-proBNP) in some subjects who had improved survival compared with subjects whose NT-proBNP remained elevated (>1449 pg/mL).[77]

In a systemic review and metaanalysis of PAH-specific therapy in WHO Group 3 PH, single-arm trials suggested beneficial effects, but in two randomized, controlled trials, PAH therapy had no effect on

TABLE 11.1
Clinical Trials of Vasodilator Therapy in ILD

Trial	Type	Agent	Design	Primary Outcome	Results
ARTEMIS-IPF Raghu et al.[72]	Randomized, double-blind placebo-controlled trial	Ambrisentan selective ET-A antagonist	Ambrisentan given to all patients with mild IPF (minimal to no honeycombing on HRCT)	Time to disease progression, event-driven trial	Terminated early because of increased disease progression and hospitalization in ambrisentan-treated patients
BUILD-1 King et al.[69]	Randomized, double-blind placebo-controlled trial	Bosentan	Bosentan given to patients with IPF for 12 months	Improvement in 6MWD	No difference from placebo, but trend toward improved time to death/disease progression and improved HRQOL
BUILD-3 King et al.[70]	Randomized, double-blind placebo-controlled trial	Bosentan	Bosentan given to patients with biopsy-confirmed IPF and minimal HRCT changes, event-driven study	Time to IPF worsening or death	No difference from placebo. No effects on HRQOL or dyspnea
MUSIC Raghu et al.[71]	Randomized, double-blind, placebo-controlled trial	Macitentan	Macitentan given to patients with surgical lung biopsy—confirmed UIP and mild disease (minimal HRCT changes)	Change in FVC from baseline	No difference from placebo in pulmonary function testing, or time to disease worsening or death
STEP-IPF IPF Clinical Research Network Zisman et al.[74]	Randomized, double-blind, placebo-controlled trial	Sildenafil	Sildenafil 20 mg TID given to advanced stage IPF patients (DLCO ≤ 35%)	20% improvement in 6MWD over 12 weeks	No significant difference in primary outcome but improvement in dyspnea and HRQOL. Stabilization of DLCO.
STEP-IPF substudy Han et al.[73]	Subgroup analysis of subjects in STEP-IPF with echocardiograms	Sildenafil	Compare those with RVH or RVSD with those without	6MWD, SGRQ, SF-36	Subjects with RVSD had significantly less decline in 6MWD and greater improvement in SGRQ. Subjects with RVH had greater improvement in SGRQ.
RISE-IIP Nathan et al.[75]	Randomized, double-blind, placebo-controlled trial	Riociguat	Change from baseline to 26-week 6MWD	6MWD	Terminated early because of an increase in SAEs and mortality in riociguat arm

6MWD, 6-min walk distance; *DLCO*, diffusion capacity of carbon monoxide; *FVC*, forced vital capacity; *HRCT*, high-resolution computed tomography; *HRQOL*, health-related quality of life; *ILD*, interstitial lung disease; *IPF*, idiopathic pulmonary fibrosis; *RVH*, right ventricular hypertrophy; *RVSD*, right ventricular systolic dysfunction; *SAEs*, severe adverse events; *STEP-IPF*, Sildenafil Trial of Exercise Performance in IPF; *UIP*, usual interstitial pneumonia.

TABLE 11.2
Management of PH in the Context of IPF

Severity of IPF	mPAP ≤25 mmHg at Rest	mPAP >25 mmHg, ≤35 mmHg at Rest	mPAP ≥35 mmHg at Rest
FVC ≥ 70% predicted Mild or no CT evidence of parenchymal abnormalities	No PH No PH treatment	PH classification uncertain No data support treatment with PAH-specific vasodilators	PH classification uncertain Discrimination between WHO Group 1 and WHO Group 3 phenotypes Refer to a center with expertise in both PH and lung disease
FVC < 70% predicted CT findings of CPFE	No PH No PH treatment	PH-IPF, PH-CPFE No data support treatment with PAH-specific vasodilators	Severe PH-IPF, Severe PH-CPFE Refer to a center with expertise in both PH and lung for personalized treatment disease because of poor prognosis Clinical trials needed

CPFE, combined pulmonary fibrosis emphysema syndrome; CT, computed tomography; FVC, forced vital capacity; IPF, idiopathic pulmonary fibrosis; PAH, pulmonary arterial hypertension; PH, pulmonary hypertension; WSPH, World Symposium on pulmonary hypertension.
From WSPH 2013, Seeger W, Adir Y, Barbera JA, et al. Pulmonary hypertension in chronic lung diseases. J Am Coll Cardiol. 2013;62(25 Suppl.): D109–D116.

6MWD.[78] In an open-label, single-arm study by Saggar and colleagues, 15 patients with PH-IPF referred for lung transplantation were placed on IV treprostinil as a bridge to transplant. This therapy was associated with significant improvements in hemodynamics and RV function (as seen on echocardiogram) without significant changes in systemic blood pressure, heart rate, or oxygenation.[79]

By identifying patients with mild ILD and exercise-associated PH, invasive cardiopulmonary exercise testing (iCPET) could provide a way to more precisely phenotype patients with pulmonary vascular disease and underlying lung disease. Degani-Costa and colleagues used iCPET[80] to categorize patients with ILD and pulmonary vascular disease; those with a mPAP-Q'T slope ≥ 3 mmHg min/L had low peak oxygen consumption, increased dead space, and inefficient ventilation.[80] Such markers might help us identify patients earlier in the course of PH and find those who may be candidates for PH-specific therapy.

In summary, among patients with IPF, when concomitant PAH is suspected (e.g., very low DLCO, symptoms out of proportion to what is expected based on pulmonary physiology or HRCT, elevation in

NT-BNP), noninvasive testing and/or right heart catheterization should be considered. Currently accepted guidelines suggest referral to specialty PH centers for evaluation and consideration of PH-directed therapy in addition to optimizing treatment of the patient's underlying lung disease. In the future, adjunctive studies such as CPET and iCPET may help us to more precisely phenotype and monitor patients and to assess their responses to PH-specific therapy. It is our practice to refer potential candidates with PH-IPF for lung transplant evaluation.

LUNG TRANSPLANTATION

Although there have been advances in therapy for IPF, it remains a chronic and progressive disease, and in 2018, the only cure for IPF is lung transplantation. IPF has the poorest prognosis among common lung diseases for which patients are referred to lung transplantation.[81] Because of this, criteria for referral for lung transplant evaluation have expanded.[82] Because of the poor survival in IPF, it is recommended that patients with IPF be referred for lung transplant evaluation at the time of diagnosis.[81] Other indications for referral of patients with IPF to lung transplant include an FVC < 80% predicted; DLCO < 40% predicted; any dyspnea or functional limitation attributed to lung disease; and the need for supplemental oxygen, even if only with exertion.[81] To these recommendations, we would also suggest referral of patients with PH-IPF.

Earlier referral permits a more comprehensive evaluation of patients and their comorbid conditions. Early referral may allow physicians and patients to optimize management of comorbidities, shore up the patient's social support network, and give patients time to consider and discuss the pros and cons of lung transplantation. It is important for referring providers and patients to realize that early referral does not necessarily mean immediate listing for transplant but allows both the center to get to know the patient and the patient to prepare for the transplant. Criteria for listing for transplant include an FVC decline of 5%–10% or more over 6 months; DLCO decline by 15% or more in 6 months of follow-up; desaturation to <88% or distance covered <250 m on 6MWT over a 6-month period; PH on echocardiogram or right heart catheterization; or hospitalization due to exacerbation, respiratory decline, or pneumothorax.[81]

Although survival after lung transplant has improved over time, median survival in patients with IPF (or fNSIP) is 4.9 years, the lowest of the major diagnostic categories for lung transplant (COPD, cystic fibrosis [CF], and PAH).[83] However, transplant still confers a survival benefit (given the median survival of 2–3 years post IPF diagnosis) and improved quality of life.[21] In the United States, IPF is the second most common referring diagnosis for lung transplantation and has the highest waiting list mortality compared with the other three common diagnostic categories.[84]

Factors contributing to posttransplant mortality in IPF include age (this patient population tends to be older), concomitant morbidities (increased risk of heart disease or occult malignancies that could flourish in the posttransplant, immunosuppressed patient), and type of procedure performed (single vs. double lung transplantation).[85] Although increased age is a risk factor for posttransplant mortality, outcomes in septuagenarians have improved recently. Compared with outcomes before use of the lung allocation score (LAS), after implementation of the LAS, survival in patients aged 70 years and older has improved and is not significantly different from patients aged 60–69 years.[86]

Development and implementation of the LAS has been one of the most significant recent advancements in lung transplantation. Before 2005, lungs were allocated to patients based on time accrued on the waiting list. The LAS is a score that reflects disease severity and balances the risk of dying on the waiting list with potential posttransplant survival. Every year since institution of the LAS, the number of patients with IPF who have received transplants in the United States has increased—this is not true for the other diagnostic groups. The LAS has reduced both waiting list time and mortality.[85] Additionally, the LAS has allowed for transplantation of sicker patients who are at greatest risk for death.[87] In general, patients with IPF have a higher LAS than patients in other diagnostic categories; as such, although they appear to have the greatest risk for posttransplant mortality, outcomes have improved among transplant recipients in the upper LAS quartile.[88]

Posttransplant survival is better in double lung transplant recipients than in single lung transplant recipients. Because single lung transplantation is more common in IPF than in other disease categories, and posttransplant survival is worse in patients with lung fibrosis that in patients with other lung diseases, experts have debated whether all patients with IPF should receive a double lung transplant.[83] In the 2015 update of the 2011 clinical practice guidelines for the treatment of IPF, the authors performed a pooled survival analysis of three studies and found no survival difference between patients with IPF who received single versus double lung transplant (HR 0.47; 95% confidence interval 0.19–1.17).[40] Although the current trend is to perform more double lung transplants, the choice is far from simple. Brown and colleagues state that performing a single lung transplantation may be preferable to double lung transplantation because wait times are shorter, patients spend less time under general anesthesia or on cardiopulmonary bypass, they receive fewer transfusions, and there is less surgeon fatigue. They discuss how long-term outcomes need to be balanced against risk of death on the waiting list and perioperative comorbidities, especially in older patients. Thus, in certain settings, single lung transplantation may be preferred in older patients, but double lung transplantation may be more beneficial in younger patients or in patients with PH-IPF.[85]

In summary, it is important to consider lung transplantation as a therapeutic option in patients with IPF. Early referral, soon after diagnosis, allows for adequate patient education and time to address and optimize the patient's comorbidities in preparation for surgery. The LAS has made IPF one of the most common conditions for which patients are transplanted. For patients with IPF, transplant leads to improved survival and quality of life; however, average survival after transplant remains frustratingly low—around 5 years or so. There is debate around whether all patients with IPF should receive double lung transplantation, which appears to confer a survival advantage over single lung transplantation.

REFERENCES

1. Rochester CL, Vogiatzis I, Holland AE, et al. An Official American Thoracic Society/European Respiratory Society Policy Statement: enhancing implementation, use, and delivery of pulmonary rehabilitation. *Am J Respir Crit Care Med.* 2015;192(11):1373–1386.
2. Bianchi R, Gigliotti F, Romagnoli I, et al. Impact of a rehabilitation program on dyspnea intensity and quality in patients with chronic obstructive pulmonary disease. *Respir Int Rev Thorac Dis.* 2011;81(3):186–195.
3. Bernard S, Whittom F, Leblanc P, et al. Aerobic and strength training in patients with chronic obstructive pulmonary disease. *Am J Respir Crit Care Med.* 1999;159(3):896–901.
4. Mador MJ, Kufel TJ, Pineda LA, et al. Effect of pulmonary rehabilitation on quadriceps fatiguability during exercise. *Am J Respir Crit Care Med.* 2001;163(4):930–935.
5. Ryerson CJ, Cayou C, Topp F, et al. Pulmonary rehabilitation improves long-term outcomes in interstitial lung disease: a prospective cohort study. *Respir Med.* 2014;108(1):203–210.
6. Dowman LM, McDonald CF, Hill CJ, et al. The evidence of benefits of exercise training in interstitial lung disease: a randomised controlled trial. *Thorax.* 2017;72(7):610–619.
7. Holland AE, Hill CJ, Conron M, Munro P, McDonald CF. Short term improvement in exercise capacity and symptoms following exercise training in interstitial lung disease. *Thorax.* 2008;63(6):549–554.
8. Gaunaurd IA, Gomez-Marin OW, Ramos CF, et al. Physical activity and quality of life improvements of patients with idiopathic pulmonary fibrosis completing a pulmonary rehabilitation program. *Respir Care.* 2014;59(12):1872–1879.
9. Jackson RM, Gomez-Marin OW, Ramos CF, et al. Exercise limitation in IPF patients: a randomized trial of pulmonary rehabilitation. *Lung.* 2014;192(3):367–376.
10. Vainshelboim B, Oliveira J, Fox BD, Soreck Y, Fruchter O, Kramer MR. Long-term effects of a 12-week exercise training program on clinical outcomes in idiopathic pulmonary fibrosis. *Lung.* 2015;193(3):345–354.
11. Nishiyama O, Kondoh Y, Kimura T, et al. Effects of pulmonary rehabilitation in patients with idiopathic pulmonary fibrosis. *Respirology.* 2008;13(3):394–399.
12. Vainshelboim B, Oliveira J, Yehoshua L, et al. Exercise training-based pulmonary rehabilitation program is clinically beneficial for idiopathic pulmonary fibrosis. *Respir Int Rev Thorac Dis.* 2014;88(5):378–388.
13. Dowman L, Hill CJ, Holland AE. Pulmonary rehabilitation for interstitial lung disease. *Cochrane Database Syst Rev.* 2014;(10):CD006322.
14. Nishiyama O, Taniguchi H, Kondoh Y, et al. Quadriceps weakness is related to exercise capacity in idiopathic pulmonary fibrosis. *Chest.* 2005;127(6):2028–2033.
15. Olson AL, Swigris JJ, Belkin A, et al. Physical functional capacity in idiopathic pulmonary fibrosis: performance characteristics of the continuous-scale physical function performance test. *Expert Rev Respir Med.* 2015;9(3):361–367.
16. Ferreira A, Garvey C, Connors GL, et al. Pulmonary rehabilitation in interstitial lung disease: benefits and predictors of response. *Chest.* 2009;135(2):442–447.
17. Morisset J, Dube BP, Garvey C, et al. The unmet educational needs of patients with interstitial lung disease. Setting the stage for tailored pulmonary rehabilitation. *Ann Am Thorac Soc.* 2016;13(7):1026–1033.
18. Heebink DM. The NOTT study. *Respir Care.* 1981;26(1):63–65.
19. Continuous or nocturnal oxygen therapy in hypoxemic chronic obstructive lung disease: a clinical trial. Nocturnal Oxygen Therapy Trial Group. *Ann Intern Med.* 1980;93(3):391–398.
20. Long-Term Oxygen Treatment Trial Research Group, Albert RK, Au DH, et al. A randomized trial of long-term oxygen for COPD with moderate desaturation. *N Engl J Med.* 2016;375(17):1617–1627.
21. Raghu G, Collard HR, Egan JJ, et al. An official ATS/ERS/JRS/ALAT statement: idiopathic pulmonary fibrosis: evidence-based guidelines for diagnosis and management. *Am J Respir Crit Care Med.* 2011;183(6):788–824.
22. Du Plessis JP, Fernandes S, Jamal R, et al. Exertional hypoxemia is more severe in fibrotic interstitial lung disease than in COPD. *Respirology.* 2018;23(4):392–398. https://doi.org/10.1111/resp.13226. Epub 2017 Nov 28.
23. Olson AL, Graney B, Baird S, et al. Tracking dyspnea up to supplemental oxygen prescription among patients with pulmonary fibrosis. *BMC Pulm Med.* 2017;17(1):152.
24. Nishiyama O, Miyajima H, Fukai Y, et al. Effect of ambulatory oxygen on exertional dyspnea in IPF patients without resting hypoxemia. *Respir Med.* 2013;107(8):1241–1246.
25. Visca D, Montgomery A, de Lauretis A, et al. Ambulatory oxygen in interstitial lung disease. *Eur Respir J.* 2011;38(4):987–990.
26. Frank RC, Hicks S, Duck AM, Spencer L, Leonard CT, Barnett E. Ambulatory oxygen in idiopathic pulmonary fibrosis: of what benefit? *Eur Respir J.* 2012;40(1):269–270.
27. Visca D, Tsipouri V, Mori L, et al. Ambulatory oxygen in fibrotic lung disease (AmbOx): study protocol for a randomised controlled trial. *Trials.* 2017;18(1):201.

28. Khor YH, Goh NSL, McDonald CF, Holland AE. Oxygen therapy for interstitial lung disease. A mismatch between patient expectations and experiences. *Ann Am Thorac Soc.* 2017;14(6):888–895.

29. Christopher KL, Spofford BT, Petrun MD, McCarty DC, Goodman JR, Petty TL. A program for transtracheal oxygen delivery. Assessment of safety and efficacy. *Ann Intern Med.* 1987;107(6):802–808.

30. Belkin A, Albright K, Swigris JJ. A qualitative study of informal caregivers' perspectives on the effects of idiopathic pulmonary fibrosis. *BMJ Open Respir Res.* 2014;1(1):e000007.

31. Rochwerg B, Neupane B, Zhang Y, et al. Treatment of idiopathic pulmonary fibrosis: a network meta-analysis. *BMC Med.* 2016;14:18.

32. Fisher M, Nathan SD, Hill C, et al. Predicting life expectancy for pirfenidone in idiopathic pulmonary fibrosis. *J Manag Care Spec Pharm.* 2017;23(3-b suppl):S17–S24.

33. Richeldi L, Cottin V, du Bois RM, et al. Nintedanib in patients with idiopathic pulmonary fibrosis: combined evidence from the TOMORROW and INPULSIS(®) trials. *Respir Med.* 2016;113:74–79.

34. Ley B, Swigris J, Day BM, et al. Pirfenidone reduces respiratory-related hospitalizations in idiopathic pulmonary fibrosis. *Am J Respir Crit Care Med.* 2017;196(6):756–761.

35. Vancheri C, Kreuter M, Richeldi L, et al. Nintedanib with add-on pirfenidone in idiopathic pulmonary fibrosis. Results of the INJOURNEY trial. *Am J Respir Crit Care Med.* 2018;197(3):356–363.

36. Hughes G, Toellner H, Morris H, Leonard C, Chaudhuri N. Real world experiences: pirfenidone and nintedanib are effective and well tolerated treatments for idiopathic pulmonary fibrosis. *J Clin Med.* 2016;5(9).

37. Nathan SD, Albera C, Bradford WZ, et al. Effect of continued treatment with pirfenidone following clinically meaningful declines in forced vital capacity: analysis of data from three phase 3 trials in patients with idiopathic pulmonary fibrosis. *Thorax.* 2016;71(5):429–435.

38. Valeyre D, Albera C, Bradford WZ, et al. Comprehensive assessment of the long-term safety of pirfenidone in patients with idiopathic pulmonary fibrosis. *Respirology.* 2014;19(5):740–747.

39. Loveman E, Copley VR, Scott DA, Colquitt JL, Clegg AJ, O'Reilly KM. Comparing new treatments for idiopathic pulmonary fibrosis—a network meta-analysis. *BMC Pulm Med.* 2015;15:37.

40. Raghu G, Rochwerg B, Zhang Y, et al. An official ATS/ERS/JRS/ALAT clinical practice guideline: treatment of idiopathic pulmonary fibrosis. An update of the 2011 clinical practice guideline. *Am J Respir Crit Care Med.* 2015;192(2):e3–e19.

41. Hoppo T, Komatsu Y, Jobe BA. Gastroesophageal reflux disease and patterns of reflux in patients with idiopathic pulmonary fibrosis using hypopharyngeal multichannel intraluminal impedance. *Dis Esophagus.* 2014;27(6):530–537.

42. Gavini S, Borges LF, Finn RT, et al. Lung disease severity in idiopathic pulmonary fibrosis is more strongly associated with impedance measures of bolus reflux than pH parameters of acid reflux alone. *Neurogastroenterol Motil.* 2017;29(5).

43. Lee JS, Collard HR, Anstrom KJ, et al. Anti-acid treatment and disease progression in idiopathic pulmonary fibrosis: an analysis of data from three randomised controlled trials. *Lancet Respir Med.* 2013;1(5):369–376.

44. Chen B, Jiang HD. Idiopathic pulmonary fibrosis and gastro-esophageal reflux. *Zhonghua Jie He He Hu Xi Za Zhi.* 2016;39(2):137–139.

45. Moran TJ. Experimental aspiration pneumonia. IV. Inflammatory and reparative changes produced by intratracheal injections of autologous gastric juice and hydrochloric acid. *AMA Arch Pathol.* 1955;60(2):122–129.

46. Savarino E, Carbone R, Marabotto E, et al. Gastro-oesophageal reflux and gastric aspiration in idiopathic pulmonary fibrosis patients. *Eur Respir J.* 2013;42(5):1322–1331.

47. Perng DW, Chang KT, Su KC, et al. Exposure of airway epithelium to bile acids associated with gastroesophageal reflux symptoms: a relation to transforming growth factor-beta1 production and fibroblast proliferation. *Chest.* 2007;132(5):1548–1556.

48. Lee JS, Ryu JH, Elicker BM, et al. Gastroesophageal reflux therapy is associated with longer survival in patients with idiopathic pulmonary fibrosis. *Am J Respir Crit Care Med.* 2011;184(12):1390–1394.

49. Ghebre YT, Raghu G. Idiopathic pulmonary fibrosis: novel concepts of proton pump inhibitors as antifibrotic drugs. *Am J Respir Crit Care Med.* 2016;193(12):1345–1352.

50. Linden PA, Gilbert RJ, Yeap BY, et al. Laparoscopic fundoplication in patients with end-stage lung disease awaiting transplantation. *J Thorac Cardiovasc Surg.* 2006;131(2):438–446.

51. Lee DH. Guidelines for the treatment of gastroesophageal reflux disease. *Korean J Gastroenterol.* 2011;57(3):203; author reply 203.

52. Allaix ME, Rebecchi F, Morino M, Schlottmann F, Patti MG. Gastroesophageal reflux and idiopathic pulmonary fibrosis. *World J Surg.* 2017;41(7):1691–1697.

53. Hamada K, Nagai S, Tanaka S, et al. Significance of pulmonary arterial pressure and diffusion capacity of the lung as prognosticator in patients with idiopathic pulmonary fibrosis. *Chest.* 2007;131(3):650–656.

54. Kimura M, Taniguchi H, Kondoh Y, et al. Pulmonary hypertension as a prognostic indicator at the initial evaluation in idiopathic pulmonary fibrosis. *Respir Int Rev Thorac Dis.* 2013;85(6):456–463.

55. Lettieri CJ, Nathan SD, Barnett SD, Ahmad S, Shorr AF. Prevalence and outcomes of pulmonary arterial hypertension in advanced idiopathic pulmonary fibrosis. *Chest.* 2006;129(3):746–752.

56. Minai OA, Santacruz JF, Alster JM, Budev MM, McCarthy K. Impact of pulmonary hemodynamics on 6-min walk test in idiopathic pulmonary fibrosis. *Respir Med.* 2012;106(11):1613–1621.

57. Shorr AF, Wainright JL, Cors CS, Lettieri CJ, Nathan SD. Pulmonary hypertension in patients with pulmonary fibrosis awaiting lung transplant. *Eur Respir J.* 2007; 30(4):715–721.

58. Corte TJ, Wort SJ, Gatzoulis MA, Macdonald P, Hansell DM, Wells AU. Pulmonary vascular resistance predicts early mortality in patients with diffuse fibrotic lung disease and suspected pulmonary hypertension. *Thorax.* 2009;64(10):883–888.

59. Glaser S, Noga O, Koch B, et al. Impact of pulmonary hypertension on gas exchange and exercise capacity in patients with pulmonary fibrosis. *Respir Med.* 2009; 103(2):317–324.

60. Armstrong HF, Schulze PC, Bacchetta M, Thirapatarapong W, Bartels MN. Impact of pulmonary hypertension on exercise performance in patients with interstitial lung disease undergoing evaluation for lung transplantation. *Respirology.* 2014;19(5):675–682.

61. Zisman DA, Karlamangla AS, Ross DJ, et al. High-resolution chest CT findings do not predict the presence of pulmonary hypertension in advanced idiopathic pulmonary fibrosis. *Chest.* 2007;132(3):773–779.

62. Nathan SD, Shlobin OA, Barnett SD, et al. Right ventricular systolic pressure by echocardiography as a predictor of pulmonary hypertension in idiopathic pulmonary fibrosis. *Respir Med.* 2008;102(9):1305–1310.

63. Arcasoy SM, Christie JD, Ferrari VA, et al. Echocardiographic assessment of pulmonary hypertension in patients with advanced lung disease. *Am J Respir Crit Care Med.* 2003;167(5):735–740.

64. Alkukhun L, Wang XF, Ahmed MK, et al. Non-invasive screening for pulmonary hypertension in idiopathic pulmonary fibrosis. *Respir Med.* 2016;117:65–72.

65. Alhamad EH, Al-Boukai AA, Al-Kassimi FA, et al. Prediction of pulmonary hypertension in patients with or without interstitial lung disease: reliability of CT findings. *Radiology.* 2011;260(3):875–883.

66. Galie N, Humbert M, Vachiery JL, et al. 2015 ESC/ERS guidelines for the diagnosis and treatment of pulmonary hypertension: the joint task force for the diagnosis and treatment of pulmonary hypertension of the European Society of Cardiology (ESC) and the European respiratory Society (ERS): Endorsed by: association for European Paediatric and Congenital Cardiology (AEPC), International Society for heart and lung transplantation (ISHLT). *Eur Heart J.* 2016;37(1):67–119.

67. Weitzenblum E, Chaouat A, Canuet M, Kessler R. Pulmonary hypertension in chronic obstructive pulmonary disease and interstitial lung diseases. *Sem Respir Crit Care Med.* 2009;30(4):458–470.

68. Bell EC, Cox NS, Goh N, et al. Oxygen therapy for interstitial lung disease: a systematic review. *Eur Respir Rev.* 2017; 26(143).

69. King Jr TE, Behr J, Brown KK, et al. BUILD-1: a randomized placebo-controlled trial of bosentan in idiopathic pulmonary fibrosis. *Am J Respir Crit Care Med.* 2008;177(1): 75–81.

70. King Jr TE, Brown KK, Raghu G, et al. BUILD-3: a randomized, controlled trial of bosentan in idiopathic pulmonary fibrosis. *Am J Respir Crit Care Med.* 2011;184(1): 92–99.

71. Raghu G, Million-Rousseau R, Morganti A, Perchenet L, Behr J, Group MS. Macitentan for the treatment of idiopathic pulmonary fibrosis: the randomised controlled MUSIC trial. *Eur Respir J.* 2013;42(6):1622–1632.

72. Raghu G, Behr J, Brown KK, et al. Treatment of idiopathic pulmonary fibrosis with ambrisentan: a parallel, randomized trial. *Ann Intern Med.* 2013;158(9):641–649.

73. Han MK, Bach DS, Hagan PG, et al. Sildenafil preserves exercise capacity in patients with idiopathic pulmonary fibrosis and right-sided ventricular dysfunction. *Chest.* 2013;143(6):1699–1708.

74. Zisman DA, Schwarz M, Anstrom KJ, Collard HR, Flaherty KR, Hunninghake GW. A controlled trial of sildenafil in advanced idiopathic pulmonary fibrosis. *N Engl J Med.* 2010;363(7):620–628.

75. Nathan S, Behr J, Collard HR, et al. RISE-IIP: riociguat for the treatment of pulmonary hypertension associated with idiopathic interstitial pneumonia. *Eur Respir J.* 2017; 50(suppl 61).

76. Seeger W, Adir Y, Barbera JA, et al. Pulmonary hypertension in chronic lung diseases. *J Am Coll Cardiol.* 2013; 62(suppl 25):D109–D116.

77. Brewis MJ, Church AC, Johnson MK, Peacock AJ. Severe pulmonary hypertension in lung disease: phenotypes and response to treatment. *Eur Respir J.* 2015;46(5): 1378–1389.

78. Prins KW, Duval S, Markowitz J, Pritzker M, Thenappan T. Chronic use of PAH-specific therapy in World Health Organization Group III pulmonary hypertension: a systematic review and meta-analysis. *Pulm Circ.* 2017;7(1): 145–155.

79. Saggar R, Khanna D, Vaidya A, et al. Changes in right heart haemodynamics and echocardiographic function in an advanced phenotype of pulmonary hypertension and right heart dysfunction associated with pulmonary fibrosis. *Thorax.* 2014;69(2):123–129.

80. Degani-Costa LH, Levarge B, Digumarthy SR, Eisman AS, Harris RS, Lewis GD. Pulmonary vascular response patterns during exercise in interstitial lung disease. *Eur Respir J.* 2015;46(3):738–749.

81. Weill D, Benden C, Corris PA, et al. A consensus document for the selection of lung transplant candidates: 2014—an update from the pulmonary transplantation Council of the International Society for Heart and Lung Transplantation. *J Heart Lung Transpl.* 2015;34(1):1–15.

82. Orens JB, Estenne M, Arcasoy S, et al. International guidelines for the selection of lung transplant candidates: 2006 update—a consensus report from the pulmonary scientific Council of the International Society for Heart and Lung Transplantation. *J Heart Lung Transpl.* 2006;25(7):745–755.

83. Chambers DC, Yusen RD, Cherikh WS, et al. The Registry of the International Society for heart and lung transplantation: thirty-fourth adult lung and heart-lung transplantation Report-2017; focus theme: Allograft ischemic time. *J Heart Lung Transpl.* 2017;36(10):1047–1059.

84. Valapour M, Lehr CJ, Skeans MA, et al. OPTN/SRTR 2016 Annual data report: lung. *Am J Transplant.* 2018;(18 suppl 1):363–433.

85. Brown AW, Kaya H, Nathan SD. Lung transplantation in IIP: a review. *Respirology.* 2016;21(7):1173–1184.

86. Kilic A, Merlo CA, Conte JV, Shah AS. Lung transplantation in patients 70 years old or older: have outcomes changed after implementation of the lung allocation score? *J Thorac Cardiovasc Surg.* 2012;144(5):1133–1138.

87. Merlo CA, Weiss ES, Orens JB, et al. Impact of U.S. Lung Allocation Score on survival after lung transplantation. *J Heart Lung Transpl.* 2009;28(8):769–775.

88. Crawford TC, Grimm JC, Magruder JT, et al. Lung transplant mortality is improving in recipients with a lung allocation score in the upper quartile. *Ann Thorac Surg.* 2017; 103(5):1607–1613.

Index

A

A-a oxygen. *See* Alveolar–arterial oxygen (A-a oxygen)
Acid instillation, 12
Acute exacerbation (AE), 43–44, 55, 56f, 89, 99
  biomarkers, 105–106
Acute exacerbation of idiopathic pulmonary fibrosis (AE-IPF), 102
Adenocarcinoma, 44
AE. *See* Acute exacerbation (AE)
AE-IPF. *See* Acute exacerbation of idiopathic pulmonary fibrosis (AE-IPF)
AECs. *See* Alveolar epithelial cells (AECs)
Aerobic training, 113–114
Aging lung, 23
AHRR genes, 99–100
Air trapping, 43
Alveolar epithelial cells (AECs), 13–14, 101
Alveolar macrophages, 19–20
Alveolar type II epithelial cells, 14
Alveolar–arterial oxygen (A-a oxygen), 92
Amiodarone, 84
ANA. *See* Antinuclear antigen (ANA)
Animal models, 117
  acid instillation, 12
  asbestosis, 13
  bleomycin model, 11
  FITC, 13
  Hermansky-Pudlak models, 13
  of pulmonary fibrosis, 9–13, 10f, 12t
  radiation-induced fibrosis, 13
  repetitive bleomycin model, 12
  silica, 13
  TGF-β overexpression, 12–13
Anterior upper lobe, 47
Anticoagulants, 21
Antifibrotic therapies, 116–117
Antinuclear antigen (ANA), 82
Apoptosis of AECs, 14
Architectural distortion, 55
ARTEMIS-IPF study, 92
Asbestos, 13
  asbestos-induced pulmonary fibrosis, 48
  asbestos-related pleural disease, 48
Asbestosis, 13, 48–49, 58–59, 84
Aspiration, 55, 117
Assessment of Pirfenidone to Confirm Efficacy and Safety in Idiopathic Pulmonary Fibrosis (ASCEND), 89–90
Asymmetric fibrosis, 43
Autoantibodies, 82
  in rheumatic conditions, 83t

B

B cells, 20
BAL fluid. *See* Bronchoalveolar lavage fluid (BAL fluid)
Bile acid, 117
Biomarkers
  diagnostic, 101–103
  of disease activity and AE, 105–106
  of disease susceptibility, 99–101
  prognostic, 103–105
Bleomycin, 84
  fibrosis model, 11, 16, 21
  murine model, 10–11
    pathologic findings in, 11f
Body mass index (BMI), 92
Bone marrow failure, 34
Bronchiolectasis, 39–40
Bronchoalveolar lavage fluid (BAL fluid), 17, 21, 46, 68, 73–76, 102, 117–118

C

C-X-C motif chemokine 13 (CXCL13), 20, 105
C57BL/6J mouse, 11
N-Cadherin, 14
Canada, trends in IPF incidence and prevalence, 5
Canonical signaling, 17–18
CAPACITY studies. *See* Clinical Studies Assessing Pirfenidone in Idiopathic Pulmonary Fibrosis: Research of Efficacy and Safety Outcomes (CAPACITY studies)
Cardiopulmonary exercise test (CPET), 114
$CD4^+CD28^{null}$ cells, 104
CF. *See* Cystic fibrosis (CF)
Chemokine (C-C motif) ligand 2 (CCL2), 19, 101
Chemokine (C-C motif) ligand 7 (CCL7), 19
Chemokine (C-C motif) ligand 18 (CCL18), 19, 104

Chemokines, 17–19
Chemotherapy, 11
Chest imaging, 118
Chlorambucil, 84
Chronic hypersensitivity pneumonitis (CHP), 46, 73–77
  approach to suspected HP, 78f
  BAL and histopathology, 75–76
  diagnosis, 73
  epidemiology, 73
  IA identification, 73–75
  imaging, 75
  serologic evaluation, 75
  SIC, 75
Chronic inflammation, 55–57
Chronic lung injury, 55
Chronic obstructive pulmonary disease (COPD), 99, 113, 122
Cigarette smoking, 6
Cilium genes, 36
Circulating fibrocytes, 105
Circulating mesenchymal progenitor cells, 105
Clinical Studies Assessing Pirfenidone in Idiopathic Pulmonary Fibrosis: Research of Efficacy and Safety Outcomes (CAPACITY studies), 89–90
Clinical–radiographic–physiologic score (CRP score), 93
Coagulation, 21
  clotting cascade, 22f
Collagen, 9
  cross-linking, 16–17
  deposition, 14–17
    MMPs, 16
  and extracellular matrix, 16–17
  turnover, 16
Collagenase-1. *See* Matrix metalloproteinases 1 (MMP1)
Combined pulmonary fibrosis and emphysema (CPFE), 45–46, 69
Composite physiologic index (CPI), 93
Computed tomography (CT), 1, 3–4, 35, 39, 118
  features of fibrotic lung disease, 39–40
  prognostic value of, 41
Connective tissue disease (CTD), 46–48, 69, 77
  clinical diagnostic criteria, 80t–81t

Note: Page numbers followed by "f" indicate figures, "t" indicate tables.

Connective tissue disease (CTD) *(Continued)*
   CTD–associated ILD, 77–84
      background, 77
      clinical presentation, 77–82
      histopathologic features, 82
      imaging differences, 82
      pulmonary function testing, 82
      role of autoantibodies, 82
      survival differences, 83
      treatment differences, 82–83
Connective tissue disease–related interstitial lung disease (CTD-ILD), 20
Connective tissue growth factor (CTGF), 18
   signaling, 18
COPD. *See* Chronic obstructive pulmonary disease (COPD)
Cough, 91–92
CPET. *See* Cardiopulmonary exercise test (CPET)
CPFE. *See* Combined pulmonary fibrosis and emphysema (CPFE)
CPI. *See* Composite physiologic index (CPI)
CRP score. *See* Clinical–radiographic–physiologic score (CRP score)
CT. *See* Computed tomography (CT)
CT-GAP, 93–94
CTD. *See* Connective tissue disease (CTD)
CTD-ILD. *See* Connective tissue disease–related interstitial lung disease (CTD-ILD)
CTGF. *See* Connective tissue growth factor (CTGF)
CXCL13. *See* C-X-C motif chemokine 13 (CXCL13)
Cyclophosphamide, 84
Cystic fibrosis (CF), 122
Cytokines, 17–19
   IFN-γ, 19
   IL-13, 18–19
   TNF-α, 19

D

DAD. *See* Diffuse alveolar damage (DAD)
DC. *See* Dyskeratosis congenita (DC)
Defensins, 105
Demethylation, 99–100
Dense fibrosis, 55–57, 56f–57f
Dermatomyositis (DM), 82
Diagnosis
   CHP, 73
   IPF, 67–68
      challenges, 68–69
      clinical evaluation, 66
      ILD categorization by etiology and pattern, 65–66
      pathologic evaluation, 67
      radiographic evaluation, 66–67
      special considerations, 68

Diagnostic biomarkers, 101–103
   KL-6, 101–102
   MMPs, 102–103
   osteopontin, 103
   surfactant proteins, 102
Diarrhea, 116–117
Diffuse alveolar damage (DAD), 55, 65
Diffuse capacity of lung for carbon monoxide (DLCO), 82, 92, 118
DILD. *See* Drug-induced lung disease (DILD)
Disease activity biomarkers, 105–106
Disease course, 89
Disease monitoring, 93–94
Disease susceptibility biomarkers, 99–101
   genetic risk in familial fibrosis, 100
   genetic risk in sporadic IPF, 100–101
DLCO. *See* Diffuse capacity of lung for carbon monoxide (DLCO)
DM. *See* Dermatomyositis (DM)
Double lung transplantation, 122–123
Drug-induced lung disease (DILD), 84
Drug-related pulmonary fibrosis, 48
Dyskeratosis congenita (DC), 34, 100
Dyskerin, 34

E

ECM. *See* Extracellular matrix (ECM)
Efferocytosis, 20
Elastin, 17
ELMOD2, 33–34
Emphysema, 46
EMT. *See* Epithelial-mesenchymal transition (EMT)
End-stage honeycomb lung, 62f, 63
Endoplasmic reticulum stress (ER stress), 13–14, 22, 33–34
Endothelin receptor antagonists (ERAs), 118–119
Endothelin-A receptor antagonist (ET-A receptor antagonist), 118–119
Environmental exposures, occupational and, 6–7
Epigenome-wide association studies, 99–100
Epithelial cells in fibrosis, 13–14
   developmental program reactivation, 14
   EMT, 14
   endoplasmic reticulum stress, 14
Epithelial-mesenchymal transition (EMT), 14
ER stress. *See* Endoplasmic reticulum stress (ER stress)
ERAs. *See* Endothelin receptor antagonists (ERAs)
ET-A receptor antagonist. *See* Endothelin-A receptor antagonist (ET-A receptor antagonist)
European Respiratory Society Guidelines (2015), 119

Exome sequencing, 34
Extracellular matrix (ECM), 9, 16–17, 102
   materials, 14–15
"Exuberant honeycomb", 47

F

F2RL3 genes, 99–100
Factor Xa, 21
Familial fibrosis, genetic risk in, 100
Familial pulmonary fibrosis (FPF), 6, 33, 43, 100
   to identifying rare variants, 33
FDA. *See* Food and Drug Administration (FDA)
FEV1 second. *See* Forced expiratory volume in 1 second (FEV1 second)
Fibroblast growth factor (FGF), 18
Fibroblastic activity, 55
Fibroblastic foci, 16–17, 55, 56f
Fibroblasts, 9, 14–17, 15f
   fibrocytes, 15–16
   myofibroblasts, 15
   pericytes, 16
Fibrocytes, 9, 15–16, 105
Fibroelastotic scarring, 62
Fibronectin, 17
Fibrosing interstitial lung disease (fILD), 1
Fibrosing interstitial processes, 63
Fibrosis, 41, 46, 55–57, 84
   aging lung, 23
   animal models of pulmonary fibrosis, 9–13, 10f, 12t
   coagulation, 21
   epithelial cells in, 13–14
   fibroblasts and collagen deposition, 14–17
   growth factors, cytokines, and chemokines, 17–19
   inflammation and immune cells, 19–21
   mucociliary dysfunction, 22
   therapeutic perspectives, 23
Fibrotic lung disease, CT features of
   ground glass, 40
   honeycombing, 39
   reticulation, 39
   traction bronchiectasis, 39–40
Fibrotic nonspecific interstitial pneumonia (fibrotic NSIP), 57
Fibrotic nonspecific interstitial pneumonia (fNSIP), 115
fILD. *See* Fibrosing interstitial lung disease (fILD)
FITC. *See* Fluorescein isothiocyanate (FITC)
Fleischner Society, 39, 67–68
Fleischner Society criteria, 43
Fluorescein isothiocyanate (FITC), 13
fNSIP. *See* Fibrotic nonspecific interstitial pneumonia (fNSIP)
Food and Drug Administration (FDA), 82–83, 113

Force vital capacity (FVC), 89, 92, 102, 116

Forced expiratory volume in 1 second (FEV1 second), 92

FPF. *See* Familial pulmonary fibrosis (FPF)

Frozen lung tissue, 68

FVC. *See* Force vital capacity (FVC)

G

GAP index. *See* Gender, age, and physiology index (GAP index)

Gastroesophageal reflux (GER), 43, 45, 117–118

Gastroesophageal reflux disease (GERD), 92–93, 113

Gaucher's disease, 36

Gender, age, and physiology index (GAP index), 93–94

Gene profiling, 104

Genetic risk
  in familial fibrosis, 100
    surfactant protein mutations, 100
    telomerase abnormalities, 100
  in sporadic IPF, 100–101
    MUC5B promoter variant as molecular biomarker, 100–101
    TOLLIP gene, 101

Genetic(s), 100
  polymorphisms, 100
  predisposition in IPF, 100
  syndromes, 36

Genome-wide association studies (GWAS), 33
  variant identification, 35–36

Genome-wide scan, 34

GER. *See* Gastroesophageal reflux (GER)

GERD. *See* Gastroesophageal reflux disease (GERD)

GPR15 genes, 99–100

Ground glass opacity, 40

Growth factors, 17–19
  CTGF, 18
  FGF, 18
  PDGF, 18
  in pulmonary fibrosis pathogenesis, 16t
  TGF-β, 17–18
  VEGF, 18

GWAS. *See* Genome-wide association studies (GWAS)

H

Haplotypes, 35

Hermansky-Pudlak syndrome (HPS), 13, 36, 85

Herpesvirus saimiri proteins, 21

γ-Herpesvirus, 21

HHV-7. *See* Human herpesvirus 7 (HHV-7)

High-resolution computed tomography (HRCT), 4, 39, 66, 73, 75, 92, 117–118
  diagnosis of UIP, 40

Honeycombing, 39, 41
  change, 55–57, 57f
  diagnostic dilemma, 41–43

HP. *See* Hypersensitivity pneumonia (HP)

HPS. *See* Hermansky-Pudlak syndrome (HPS)

HRCT. *See* High-resolution computed tomography (HRCT)

Human herpesvirus 7 (HHV-7), 21

Human herpesvirus 8 (HHV-8), 21

Hydrochloric acid instillation, 12

Hypersensitivity pneumonia (HP), 55–57

Hypersensitivity pneumonitis (HP), 43, 65, 73, 76t

I

IA. *See* Inciting antigen (IA)

ICD. *See* International Classification of Diseases (ICD)

iCPET. *See* Invasive cardiopulmonary exercise testing (iCPET)

Ideal biomarker, 99

Idiopathic interstitial pneumonias (IIPs), 44, 65

Idiopathic pulmonary fibrosis (IPF), 1, 3, 9, 15f, 22f, 33, 39, 58, 65, 68, 73, 89, 99, 113, 115, 122. *See also* Usual interstitial pneumonia (UIP)
  atypical appearance, 43
  biomarkers
    diagnostic, 101–103
    of disease activity and acute exacerbation, 105–106
    of disease susceptibility, 99–101
    prognostic, 103–105
  complications
    acute exacerbation, 44
    CPFE, 45–46
    GER, 45
    lung cancer, 44
    PH, 44–45
  CT features of fibrotic lung disease, 39–40
  differential diagnosis, 46–49
    asbestosis and occupational lung disease, 48–49
    chronic HP, 46
    CTD, 47–48
    drug-related pulmonary fibrosis, 48
    NSIP, 46
  epidemiology
    background, 3–7
    countries, 5
    mortality rates and trends over time, 5–6
    risk factors, 6–7
    trends in IPF incidence and prevalence, 3–5
  fibroblasts, 14–15
  management of PH in, 121t
  multidisciplinary evaluation, 43–44

Idiopathic pulmonary fibrosis (IPF) *(Continued)*
  natural history
    of treated, 89–91, 90f
    of untreated, 89
  prognostic indicators, 91–93
  prognostic value of computed tomography, 41
  recommendations for disease monitoring, 93–94
  therapeutic options for patients with
    antifibrotic therapies, 116–117
    exercise and pulmonary rehabilitation, 113–115
    gastroesophageal reflux, 117–118
    lung transplantation, 121–123
    PH, 118–121
    supplemental oxygen, 115–116

IFN-γ. *See* Interferon-γ (IFN-γ)

IIPs. *See* Idiopathic interstitial pneumonias (IIPs)

ILD. *See* Interstitial lung disease (ILD)

ILD unspecified (ILD-U), 5

Immune cells, 9, 17, 19–21
  infections, 21
  lymphocytes, 20
  macrophages, 19–20

Immunohistochemical staining, 35

Inciting antigen (IA), 73
  identifying, 73–75, 74t

Indeterminate UIP pattern, 41

Infections, 21, 55

Inflammation, 19–21
  infections, 21
  neutrophils, 20

Inflammatory cells, 19

Inhalational model, 13

Inhaled asbestos, 14
  fibers, 13

Interferon regulatory factors 3 (IRF3), 104

Interferon-γ (IFN-γ), 19

Interleukins (ILs)
  IL-8, 19
  IL-13, 18–19, 106

International Classification of Diseases (ICD), 3

Interstitial fibrosis, 55

Interstitial lung disease (ILD), 3, 33, 35, 43, 65, 73, 77, 100–101, 115
  categorization by etiology and pattern, 65–66
  clinical trials of vasodilator therapy in, 120t
  CTD–associated, 77–84

Interstitial pneumonia with autoimmune features (IPAF), 69, 77, 79t

Interstitial pneumonia-pattern lung injury, 84–85
  asbestosis, 84
  DILD, 84
  HPS, 85
  radiation-induced lung disease, 84

Intratracheal administration, 11

Invasive cardiopulmonary exercise testing (iCPET), 121
Ionizing radiation, 13
IPAF. *See* Interstitial pneumonia with autoimmune features (IPAF)
IPF. *See* Idiopathic pulmonary fibrosis (IPF)
IPF Network (IPFnet), 118
IPF-clinical syndrome (IPF-CS), 5
IPFnet. *See* IPF Network (IPFnet)
IRF3. *See* Interferon regulatory factors 3 (IRF3)

K

Krebs von den Lungen-6 (KL-6), 101–102
   KL-6/MUC1, 101

L

LAS. *See* Lung allocation score (LAS)
LES. *See* Lower esophageal sphincter (LES)
Linkage analysis, 34
Liver enzymes, 116–117
Lobular air trapping, 43, 46
Lower esophageal sphincter (LES), 117
Lung. *See also* Nonspecific interstitial pneumonia (NSIP); Usual interstitial pneumonia (UIP)
   cancer, 44
   disease, 48–49, 119
   fibrosis, 118
   function, 44
   histology, 36
   transplantation, 121–123
Lung allocation score (LAS), 122
Lymphocytes, 20

M

Macrophages, 19–20
Matricellular protein, 18
Matrilysin. *See* Matrix metalloproteinases (MMPs)—MMP7
Matrix metalloproteinases (MMPs), 16–17, 102–103
   degradation products, 103–104
   MMP1, 102
   MMP3, 103
   MMP7, 17, 35, 102–103
Mean pulmonary artery pressure (mPAP), 119
Methotrexate, 84
Methyl-CCNU, 84
Milk fat globule-epidermal growth factor 8 (Mfge8), 17
Misfolded proteins, 14
MMPs. *See* Matrix metalloproteinases (MMPs)
Modified Medical Research Council score (mMRC score), 91–92
Molecular biomarkers, 99
   MUC5B promoter variant as, 100–101

Monoclonal antibody, 16–17
Monocyte chemoattractant protein 1 (MCP-1). *See* Chemokine (C-C motif) ligand 2 (CCL2)
Mortality rates and trends over time, 5–6
   countries, 6
   United States, 5–6
Mosaic pattern, 43
mPAP. *See* Mean pulmonary artery pressure (mPAP)
Mucin 1 (MUC1), 101
Mucin 5B (MUC5B), 22, 33, 35, 101
   gene, 35
   polymorphism, 100–101
   promoter polymorphism, 35
   promoter SNP, 35
   promoter variant, 22
      as molecular biomarker, 100–101
   SNP, 35
Mucins, 22
Mucociliary dysfunction, 22
Multidisciplinary
   discussion, 67
   evaluation, 43–44
Murine model
   of asbestosis, 13
   of bleomycininduced fibrosis, 105–106
Mutant SFTPA2 protein, 34
6MW distance. *See* Six-minute walk distance (6MW distance)
6MWT. *See* 6-min walk test (6MWT)
Myofibroblasts, 9, 14–15
   development and activation of profibrotic, 99
   and fibroblasts, 16
   phenotype, 117

N

N-terminal prohormone of brain natriuretic peptide (NT-proBNP), 119
Nasal cannula, 115–116
Neurofibromatosis, 36
Neutrophils, 20
Niemann-Pick disease, 36
Nintedanib, 18, 23, 89, 116
Nitrofurantoin, 84
Non-IPF diagnosis, 41
Noncanonical signaling, 17–18
Nonspecific interstitial pneumonia (NSIP), 33, 39, 46–47, 65, 75, 102
   NSIP-like areas, 57, 58f
Notch pathways, 14
NSIP. *See* Nonspecific interstitial pneumonia (NSIP)
NT-proBNP. *See* N-terminal prohormone of brain natriuretic peptide (NT-proBNP)

O

Occupational and environmental exposures, 6–7
Organizing pneumonia (OP), 55, 65
Osteopontin, 102–103

P

PA. *See* Pulmonary artery (PA)
PAH. *See* Pulmonary arterial hypertension (PAH)
PAI-1. *See* Plasminogen activator inhibitors 1 (PAI-1)
PaO$_2$. *See* Partial pressure of arterial oxygen (PaO$_2$)
PAR-2 signaling, 21
Parenchymal cells, 17
Parenchymal injury, 65
Parenchymal lung disease, 119
PARN. *See* Poly(A)-specific ribonuclease deadenylation nuclease (PARN)
Partial pressure of arterial oxygen (PaO$_2$), 92
Pathogenesis, 113
   of IPF, 13
   of pulmonary fibrosis, 12–13
Pathologic evaluation, 67
PDGF. *See* Platelet-derived growth factor (PDGF)
Peribronchiolar metaplasia, 57, 58f
Pericytes, 16
Periostin, 105–106
Peripheral blood, 104–105
PF. *See* Pulmonary fibrosis (PF)
PH. *See* Pulmonary hypertension (PH)
Pindolol, 84
PIPF. *See* Postinflammatory pulmonary fibrosis (PIPF)
Pirfenidone, 23, 90–91, 116
Plasminogen activator inhibitors 1 (PAI-1), 21
Plasminogen activator inhibitors 2 (PAI-2), 21
Platelet-derived growth factor (PDGF), 18
PLCH. *See* Pulmonary Langerhans cell histiocytosis (PLCH)
Pleuroparenchymal fibroelastosis (PPFE), 59–62, 62f, 69
PM. *See* Polymyositis (PM)
Pneumoconiosis, 63
Poly(A)-specific ribonuclease deadenylation nuclease (PARN), 23, 33–34
Polymyositis (PM), 82
Positive predictive value (PPV), 4
Postinflammatory pulmonary fibrosis (PIPF), 4
PPFE. *See* Pleuroparenchymal fibroelastosis (PPFE)
PPV. *See* Positive predictive value (PPV)
Probable UIP pattern, 41, 67–68
Prognosis, 93, 94t, 99
Prognostic biomarkers, 103–105
   CCL18, 104
   CXCL13, 105
   gene profiling, 104
   MMPs degradation products, 103–104

Prognostic biomarkers *(Continued)*
T cells, 104—105
TLRs, 104
YKL40 protein, 104
Prognostic indicators, 91—93, 91t
Promoter polymorphism, 35
Protein tyrosine phosphatase-α
(PTP-α), 17—18
Proteins, 14
extracellular matrix, 15
herpesvirus saimiri, 21
mesenchymal, 14
misfolded, 14
Smad, 17—18
surfactant, 102
Pseudomonas aeruginosa, 21
PTP-α. *See* Protein tyrosine phosphatase-α (PTP-α)
Pulmonary arterial hypertension
(PAH), 122
phenotype, 119
therapy, 119—121
Pulmonary artery (PA), 44—45
Pulmonary fibrosis (PF), 4, 49, 73
animal models, 9—13, 10f, 12t
genetics
ELMOD2, 34
using FPF to identifying rare
variants, 33
genetic syndromes, 36
genome-wide association studies,
35—36
mucin 5B, 35
SFTPC mutations, 33—34
surfactant protein A mutations, 34
telomerase mutations, 34
transcriptional profiling, 36
models, 17
UIP differentiation from, 59—63
Pulmonary function testing, 82, 118
Pulmonary hypertension (PH),
44—45, 82, 92, 113, 118—121, 121t
Pulmonary Langerhans cell histiocytosis (PLCH), 59—63
Pulmonary physiologic dysfunction,
117
Pulmonary rehabilitation, 113—115
Pulmonary surfactant, 33
Pulmonary vascular disease, 118, 121

R

RA. *See* Rheumatoid arthritis (RA)
RA-ILD. *See* Rheumatoid arthritis
associated interstitial lung disease
(RA-ILD)
Radiation-induced fibrosis, 13
Radiation-induced lung disease, 84
Radiographic evaluation, 66—67
Reactivation, developmental program,
14
Regulator of telomere elongation
helicase 1 (RTEL1), 33—34
Regulatory T cells (Tregs), 20,
104—105

Repetitive acid instillation model, 12
Repetitive bleomycin model, 12
Repetitive microinjuries, 9
Reticulation, 39
RF. *See* Rheumatoid factor (RF)
Rheumatoid arthritis (RA), 65, 77
Rheumatoid arthritis associated interstitial lung disease (RA-ILD), 47, 77
Rheumatoid factor (RF), 82
Right ventricular systolic dysfunction
(RV systolic dysfunction), 119
Risk stratificatiOn ScorE index (ROSE
index), 93
Rodent models, 13
ROSE index. *See* Risk stratificatiOn
ScorE index (ROSE index)
RTEL genes, 23
RTEL1. *See* Regulator of telomere
elongation helicase 1 (RTEL1)
RV systolic dysfunction. *See* Right
ventricular systolic dysfunction (RV
systolic dysfunction)

S

Scleroderma, 47
Secreted phosphoprotein 1. *See*
Osteopontin
Semaphorin 7a (Sema7a), 104—105
Serologic evaluation, 75
Serum, 17
amyloid P, 23
of IPF patients, 20
SP-A, 102
SP-D, 102
SIC. *See* Specific inhalation challenge
(SIC)
Silica, 13
Single nucleotide polymorphism
(SNP), 100
6-min walk test (6MWT), 114
Six-minute walk distance (6MW
distance), 92
Sjögren syndrome, 47, 77—82
αSMA. *See* α-Smooth muscle actin
(αSMA)
Smoking-related interstitial fibrosis
(SRIF), 59—62, 62f
α-Smooth muscle actin (αSMA), 14
Smooth muscle hyperplasia, 57, 57f
SNP. *See* Single nucleotide polymorphism (SNP)
Sonic hedgehog pathways, 14
SP-A. *See* Surfactant protein A (SP-A)
SP-D. *See* Surfactant protein D (SP-D)
SPC. *See* Surfactant protein C (SPC)
Specific inhalation challenge (SIC), 75
Squamous cell carcinoma, 44
Squamous cell metaplasia, 57, 57f
SRIF. *See* Smoking-related interstitial
fibrosis (SRIF)
SSc. *See* Systemic sclerosis (SSc)
Stem cells in distal airway, 22
Stiff matrix, 17
Subpleural sparing, 46

Supplemental oxygen, 115—116
mutations, 100
surfactant proteins, 102
Surfactant protein A (SP-A), 101
mutations, 34
SP-A1, 100
SP-A2, 100
Surfactant protein C (SPC), 33—34,
100
Surfactant protein D (SP-D), 101
Systemic sclerosis (SSc), 77

T

T cells, 20, 104—105
Telomerase reverse transcriptase
(TERT), 23, 33, 100
Telomerase RNA component (TERC),
23, 33
Telomerase(s), 23
abnormalities, 100
complex, 34
mutations, 34
TERC. *See* Telomerase RNA component (TERC)
TERT. *See* Telomerase reverse transcriptase (TERT)
TGF-β. *See* Transforming growth factor-β (TGF-β)
TGV. *See* Thoracic gas volume (TGV)
Th17 cells, 20
Th2-type inflammatory responses,
18—19
Therapeutic perspectives, 23
Thoracic gas volume (TGV), 92
Thrombin, 21
Tissue inhibitors of metalloproteinases (TIMPs), 17
TLC. *See* Total lung capacity (TLC)
TLR3 gene L412F, 104
TLRs. *See* Toll-like receptors (TLRs)
TNF-α. *See* Tumor necrosis factor-α
(TNF-α)
Toll-interacting protein gene (TOLLIP
gene), 101
Toll-like receptors (TLRs), 101, 104
TOLLIP gene. *See* Toll-interacting
protein gene (TOLLIP gene)
Torque teno virus DNA, 21
Total lung capacity (TLC), 92
Traction bronchi-/bronchiolectasis, 57
Traction bronchiectasis, 39—40
Transbrachial biopsy, 68
Transbronchial biopsy, 76
Transbronchial cryobiopsy, 68
Transcriptional profiling, 36
Transforming growth factor-β (TGF-
β), 12—13, 17—18
Transthoracic echocardiography, 44—45
Transtracheal oxygen (TTO),
115—116
Tregs. *See* Regulatory T cells (Tregs)
TTO. *See* Transtracheal oxygen (TTO)
Tumor necrosis factor-α (TNF-α), 19
gene polymorphisms, 19

U

UCD. *See* Underlying cause of death (UCD)
UCTD-ILD. *See* Undifferentiated CTD–associated ILD (UCTD-ILD)
UIP. *See* Usual interstitial pneumonia (UIP)
Underlying cause of death (UCD), 5–6
Undifferentiated CTD–associated ILD (UCTD-ILD), 77
Unfolded protein response (UPR), 14, 33–34
United Kingdom, trends in IPF incidence and prevalence, 4–5
United States
    IPF incidence and prevalence, 3–4
    mortality rates and trends over time, 5–6
UPR. *See* Unfolded protein response (UPR)
Usual interstitial pneumonia (UIP), 1, 9, 33, 39, 46, 55, 56f, 73, 101.

See also Idiopathic pulmonary fibrosis (IPF); Lung
area with increased alveolar septal chronic inflammation, 58f
causes, 58–59
challenges in classification
    asymmetric fibrosis, 43
    atypical appearance of IPF, 43
    diagnostic dilemma of honey-combing, 41–43
    familial pulmonary fibrosis, 43
    mosaic pattern and air trapping, 43
classification, 40–41
computed tomography in, 41
differentiation, 59–63
geographic heterogeneity and fibroblastic activity, 55
histologic features, 55
histopathologic findings in interstitial fibrosing processes, 60t–61t
honeycomb change, 55–57, 57f
idiopathic, 59
and NSIP-like areas, 57

Usual interstitial pneumonia (UIP) *(Continued)*
    pattern, 4, 41, 65, 67, 92
    thickened pulmonary artery, 58f
    vascular changes, 57

V

Vanderbilt Familial Pulmonary Fibrosis Registry, 34
Vascular changes, 57
Vascular endothelial growth factor (VEGF), 18
Viral infection, 21
Viral proteins, 21

W

Wnt pathways, 14
Working diagnosis, 68
World Health Organization (WHO), 119

Y

YKL40 protein, 104

Printed in the United States
By Bookmasters